AF382851

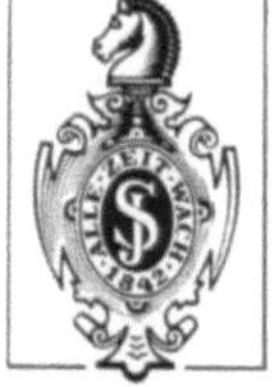

A. Berger A. Delbrück P. Brenner
R. Hinzmann (Eds.)

Dupuytren's Disease

Pathobiochemistry and Clinical Management

With 143 Figures and 45 Tables

Springer-Verlag
Berlin Heidelberg New York London Paris
Tokyo Hong Kong Barcelona Budapest

Prof. Dr. med. Alfred Berger
Dr. med. Peter Brenner
Klinik für Plastische, Hand- und
Wiederherstellungschirurgie

Prof. Dr. med. Axel Delbrück
Dr. rer. nat. Rolf Hinzmann
Institut für Klinische Chemie II

Krankenhaus Oststadt, Medizinische Hochschule Hannover
Podbielskistraße 380, 30659 Hannover, Germany

ISBN-13: 978-3-540-57239-8   e-ISBN-13: 978-3-642-78517-7
DOI: 10.1007/978-3-642-78517-7

Library of Congress Cataloging-in-Publication Data
Dupuytren's disease: pathobiochemistry and clinical management/
A. Berger . . . [et al.], (eds.). p. cm. Includes index.
1. Dupuytren's contracture. I. Berger, Alfred.
[DNLM: 1. Dupuytren's Contracture-physiopathology. 2. Dupuytren's
Contracture-therapy. WE 830 D9453 1994]
RD778.5.D88 1994 617.5'75-dc20 DNLM/DLC 93-34322

The use of general descriptive names, registered names, trademarks, etc.
in this publication does not imply, even in the absence of a specific statement, that such names are exempt from the relevant protective laws and
regulations and therefore free for general use.

Product Liability: The publishers cannot guarantee the accuracy of any
information about dosage and application contained in this book. In every
individual case the user must check such information by consulting the
relevant literature.

Typesetting: Best-set Typesetter Ltd., Hong Kong
24/3130-5 4 3 2 1 0 – Printed on acid-free paper

Preface

Dupuytren's disease has been known to physicians for centuries. Although much effort has been spent on clarifying its origin and pathogenesis, our knowledge of it is still limited. However, recent growth in our knowledge of the pathobiochemistry of connective tissue diseases in general has opened up new research and clinical perspectives regarding Dupuytren's contracture.

To encourage work in this field, it is necessary for the individual groups concerned with problems of the pathogenesis and therapy of the disease to discuss continuously the state of the art in Dupuytren's research and to exchange clinical experiences and results of biochemical research. Following the meetings in Vienna (1983) and London, Ontario (1985), the progress in this field over the last 6 years was presented at the Hannover Symposium on Pathobiochemistry and Clinical Management of Dupuytren's Disease in 1991. In particular, the impact of biochemical findings on the diagnosis and therapy of Dupuytren's disease was discussed. Therefore, this volume starts with the presentation of new morphological aspects of the pathogenesis of Dupuytren's disease (part I). In parts II to VI a comprehensive delineation of general connective tissue pathobiochemistry is followed by an extensive discussion of metabolic aberrations and abnormities of the macromolecular extracellular structure of the palmar fascia in Dupuytren's contracture. Finally, parts VII and VIII deal with the methods to detect these chrateristics and the progress in diagnosis and surgical treatment procedures.

Let us add one comment to the term "Dupuytren's disease". Although this disease has frequently been referred to as "Dupuytren's contracture" in past, we agree with numerous others that disease is the more appropriate word, reflecting the fact that this condition involves more than a medical shortening.

This report of the Hannover conference should aid those colleagues and research groups who could not attend the meeting and enourage and challenge them to actively participate in further enlightenment of the problems we are all faced with in our work on this disease.

December 1993   The Editors

Contents

List of Contributors

Babyof, I., M.D.
Connective Tissue Research Laboratory
Hebrew University of Jerusalem
P.O. Box 1172
Jerusalem, Israel

Bailey, A.J., M.D.
Muscle and Collagen Research Group
Department of Veterinary Medicine
Langford, Bristol BS18 7DY, Great Britain

Berger, A., Prof. Dr.
Klinik für Plastische, Hand- und Wiederherstellungschirurgie
Krankenhaus Oststadt, Medizinische Hochschule Hannover
Podielskistraße 380
30659 Hannover, Germany

Borchert, M., Dr.
Um Unter Dorf 30
38527 Meine, Germany

Borchert, W., Dr.
Medizinische Klinik I
Städtisches Klinikum Braunschweig
Salzdahlumer Straße 90
38126 Braunschweig, Germany

Botz, J.S., M.D.
Department of Pathology, Victoria Hospital
University of Western Ontario
375 South Street
London, Ontario N6A 4G5, Canada

Brandes, G., Dr.
Abteilung Zellbiologie und Elektronenmikroskopie
Medizinische Hochschule Hannover
Konstanty-Gutschow-Straße 8
30625 Hannover, Germany

Brenner, P., Dr.
Klinik für Plastische, Hand- und Wiederherstellungschirurgie
Krankenhaus Oststadt, Medizinische Hochschule Hannover
Podbielskistraße 380
30659 Hannover, Germany

Burge, P., F.R.C.S.
Consultant Hand Surgeon
Nuffield Orthopaedic Centre, University of Oxford
Windmill Road
Headington, Oxford OX3 7LD, Great Britain

Coleman, D.J., M.D.
The School of Pharmacy, University of Bradford
Richmond Road
Bradford West, Yorkshire BD7 1DP, Great Britain

Coleman, R.A., M.D.
The School of Pharmacy, University of Bradford
Richmond Road
Bradford West, Yorkshire BD7 1DP, Great Britain

Cross, S.E., M.D.
The School of Pharmacy, University of Bradford
Richmond Road
Bradford West, Yorkshire BD7 1DP, Great Britain

Delbrück, A., Prof. Dr.
Institut für Klinische Chemie II
Krankenhaus Oststadt, Medizinische Hochschule Hannover
Podbielskistraße 380
30659 Hannover, Germany

Euler, E., Dr.
Chirurgische Klinik und Poliklinik, Klinikum Innenstadt
Ludwig-Maximilians-Universität München
Nußbaumstraße 20
80336 München, Germany

Foo, I.T.H., M.D.
The School of Pharmacy, University of Bradford
Richmond Road
Bradford West, Yorkshire BD7 1DP, Great Britain

Francis, M.J.O., M.D.
The Nuffield Orthopaedic Centre, University of Oxford
Windmill Road
Headington, Oxford OX3 7LD, Great Britain

Funk, S., M.D.
Department of Biological Structure
University of Washington
Seattle, WA, USA

Gabbiani, G., Prof. Dr.
Department of Pathology, CMU, University of Geneva
1 rue Michel-Servet
1211 Geneva 4, Switzerland

Gässler, N., Dr.
Zentrallabor der Caritas Trägergesellschaft Trier e.V.
St. Elisabeth-Krankenhaus Wittlich
Postfach 1660
54506 Wittlich, Germany

Geldmacher, J., Prof. Dr.
Chirurgische Universitätsklinik
Krankenhausstraße 12
91054 Erlangen, Germany

Gressner, A.M., Prof. Dr.
Abteilung für Klinische Chemie und
Zentrallaboratorium, Klinikum der Philipps-Universität
Baldingerstraße
35033 Marburg, Germany

Grinnell, F., M.D.
Department of Anatomy and Neuroscience
University of Texas
Dallas, TX, USA

Gurr, E., Priv. Doz. Dr.
Zentrallaboratorium
Zentralkrankenhaus "Links der Weser"
Senator-Weßling-Straße 1
28277 Bremen, Germany

Hamilton, G., Dr.
Abteilung für Plastische und Rekonstruktive Chirurgie
I. Chirurgische Universitätsklinik
Alserstraße 4
1090 Wien, Austria

Hasegawa, B., M.D.
Department of Pathology, Victoria Hospital
University of Western Ontario
375 South Street
London, Ontario N6A 4G5, Canada

Hinzmann, R., Dr. rer. nat.
Institut für Klinische Chemie II
Krankenhaus Oststadt, Medizinische Hochschule Hannover
Podbielskistraße 380
30659 Hannover, Germany

Hoch, J., Dr.
Klinik für Plastische Chirurgie, Universität Lübeck
Ratzeburger Allee 160
23562 Lübeck, Germany

Howlett, C.R., M.D.
The Nuffield Orthopaedic Centre, University of Oxford
Windmill Road
Headington, Oxford OX3 7LD, Great Britain

Hueston, J.T., Dr.
B.P. 2
Sainte-Saturini d'Apt. 844 90, France

Körner, T., Dr.
Abteilung Zellbiologie und Elektronenmikroskopie
Medizinisiche Hochschule Hannover
Konstanty-Gutschow-Straße 8
30625 Hannover, Germany

Kreusser, T., Dr.
Chirurgische Klinik und Poliklinik, Klinikum Innenstadt
Ludwig-Maximilians-Universität München
Nußbaumstraße 20
80336 München, Germany

Leclercq, C., Dr.
Institut Francaise de la Main
15 rue Franklin
75116 Paris, France

Mailänder, P., Dr.
Klinik für Plastische, Hand-und Wiederherstellungschirurgie
Krankenhaus Oststadt, Medizinische Hochschule Hannover
Podbielskistraße 380
30659 Hannover, Germany

Mallinger, R., Dr.
Abteilung für Plastische und Rekonstruktive Chirurgie
I. Chirurgische Universitätsklinik
Alserstraße 4
1090 Wien, Austria

McFarlane, R.M., Prof., M.D.
Department of Pathology, Victoria Hospital
University of Western Ontario
375 South Street
London, Ontario N6A 4G5, USA

Meinel, A., Dr.
Abteilung für Chirurgie, Kreiskrankenhaus
Albert Schweitzer-Straße 37
97941 Tauberbischofsheim, Germany

Menzel, E.J., Prof. Dr.
Institut für Immunologie, Universität Wien
Borschkegasse 8a
1090 Wien, Austria

Messina, A., M.D.
Centro Chirurgia della Mano
CTO-Via Zannetti 29
10126 Torino, Italy

Millesi, H., Prof. Dr.
Abteilung für Plastische und Rekonstruktive Chirurgie
I. Chirurgische Universitätsklinik
Alserstraße 4
1090 Wien, Austria

Mohr, W., Prof. Dr.
Abteilung für Pathologie, Universität Ulm
Albert-Einstein-Allee 11
89081 Ulm, Germany

Mosler, S., Dipl. Biol.
Institut für Medizinische Molekularbiologie
Universität Lübeck
Ratzeburger Allee 160
23538 Lübeck, Germany

Murell, G.A.C., M.D.
The Nuffield Orthopaedic Centre, University of Oxford
Windmill Road
Headington, Oxford OX3 7LD, Great Britain

Naylor, I.J., Prof., M.D.
The School of Pharmacy, University of Bradford
Richmond Road
Bradford West, Yorkshire BD7 1DP, Great Britain

Neumüller, J., M.D.
Ludwig Boltzmann-Institut
für Rheumatologie und Balneologie
Kurbadstraße 10
1107 Wien-Oberlaa, Austria

Notbohm, H., Dr.
Institut für Medizinische Molekularbiologie
Universität Lübeck
Ratzeburger Allee 160
23538 Lübeck, Germany

Peleg, I., M.D.
Connective Tissue Research Laboratory
Hebrew University of Jerusalem
P.O. Box 1172
Jerusalem, Israel

Pringle, G., M.D.
Department of Pathology, Victoria Hospital
University of Western Ontario
375 South Street
London, Ontario N6A 4G5, Canada

Reale, E., Prof. Dr.
Abteilung Zellbiologie und Elektronenmikroskopie
Medizinische Hochschule Hannover
Konstanty-Gutschow-Straße 8
30625 Hannover, Germany

Reihsner, R., Dr.
Abteilung für Plastische und Rekonstruktive Chirurgie
I. Chirurgische Universitätsklinik
Alserstraße 4
1090 Wien, Austria

Rietsch, A., Dr.
Ludwig-Boltzmann-Institut
für Rheumatologie und Balneologie
Kurbadstraße 10
1107 Wien-Oberlaa, Austria

Ron, J., M.D.
Connective Tissue Research Laboratory
Hebrew University of Jerusalem
P.O. Box 1172
Jerusalem, Israel

Sachse, C., Dr.
Institut für Klinische Chemie II
Krankenhaus Oststadt, Medizinische Hochschule Hannover
Podbielskistraße 380
30659 Hannover, Germany

Sage, E.H., M.D.
Department of Biological Structure
University of Washington
Seattle, WA, USA

Schröder, H.
Institut für Klinische Chemie II
Krankenhaus Oststadt, Medizinische Hochschule Hannover
Podbielskistraße 380
30659 Hannover, Germany

Scott, J.E., Prof., M.D.
Institute of Chemical Morphology
University of Manchester
Oxford Road
Manchester M13, 9PL, Great Britain

Shoshan, S., Prof., Ph.D.
Connective Tissue Research Laboratory
Hebrew University of Jerusalem
P.O. Box 1172
Jerusalem 91010, Israel

Shum, D.T., M.D.
Department of Pathology, Victoria Hospital
University of Western Ontario
375 South Street
London, Ontario N6A 4G5, Canada

Tubiana, R., Prof. Dr.
Institut Francaise de la Main
15 rue Franklin
75116 Paris, France

Varian, J., M.D.
Consultant Hand Surgeon, Blackrock Clinic
Rock Road
Blackrock, Co. Dublin, Ireland

Wessinghage, D., Prof. Dr.
Abteilung für Pathologie, Universität Ulm
Oberer Eselsberg
89081 Ulm, Germany

Wilhelm, K., Dr.
Chirurgische Klinik und Poliklinik, Klinikum Innenstadt
Ludwig-Maximilians-Universität München
Nußbaumstraße 20
80336 München, Germany

Morphology

Morphology of Dupuytren's Disease

W. Mohr and D. Wessinghage

Dupuytren's disease has a prevalence of 1%–3% (Viljanto 1973) and usually occurs in middle aged or elderly men (>40 years). Females suffer much less frequently from this disorder (Fig. 1), as shown by Yost et al. (1955), who found a male:female ratio of 3:1. Although there is an often mentioned "causal" association with diabetes mellitus (Pal et al. 1987), this is not etiologically significant.

Histologically, the disease is characterized by cellular nodules inside the fibrous tissue of the palmar aponeurosis. These foci are irregularly demarcated with regard to the normal surrounding tendon tissue; no capsule is present between the hypercellular areas and the aponeurosis (Fig. 2). This situation is also reflected in the electron microscopic appearance of the disease. Ultrastructurally, there is no clear distinction between the accumulation of fibroblast-like cells and normal tissue, which is rich in collagenous fibrils (Fig. 3). The fibroblasts of the hypercellular foci seem to become intermingled with the

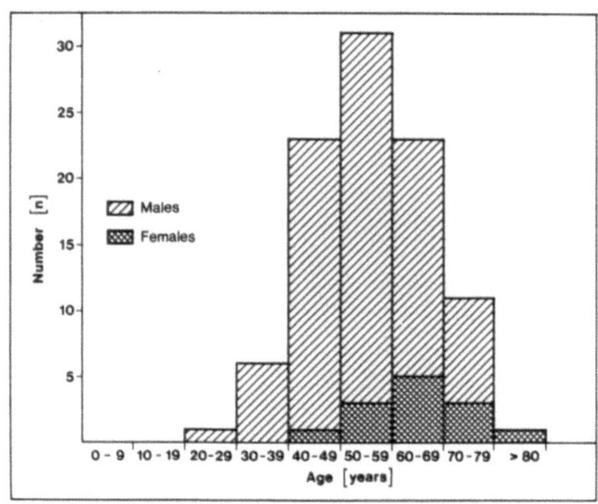

Fig. 1. Age and sex distribution of patients with histologically proven Dupuytren's disease (1980–6/1990; Orthop. Klinik Bad Abbach)

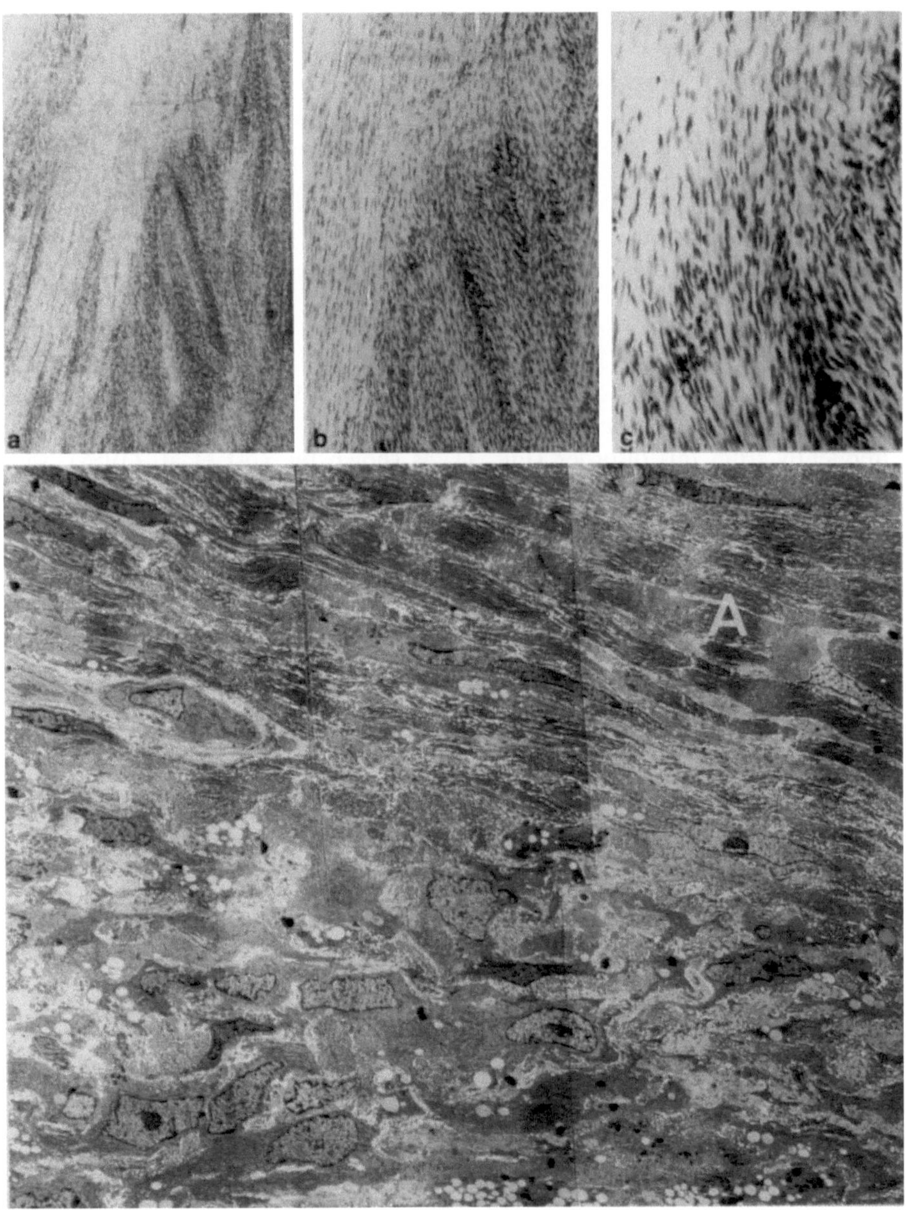

Fig. 2a–c *(above)*. Histological appearance of a fibromatous focus in the proliferative phase. H and E, ×35 (**a**), ×85 (**b**), ×220 (**c**)

Fig. 3 *(below)*. Ultrastructure of a cellular focus in the proliferative phase with irregular demarcation from the surrounding tendon tissue of the aponeurosis (*A*). ×3000

collagenous tissue of the preserved aponeurosis. In contrast to desmoid tumors, no invasion of voluntary muscles occurs (Allen 1977).

The clinical course and corresponding histological appearance of the disease are usually divided into three more or less distinct phases. According to Luck (1959), the initial proliferative phase is followed by an increase in collagen synthesis by the infiltrating cells, leading to the involution phase. The final residual phase is characterized by scar tissue with few fibroblasts and a dominant, extracellular, fibrillar matrix. Histologically, it is apparent that the aponeurotic tissue may contain disease foci that are in the various phases of development (Mohr 1987).

Ultrastructural investigations have shown that different cell populations predominate in each of the three phases (Vossbeck 1986). During the proliferative phase, there is an abundance of fibroblasts with prominent rough endoplasmatic reticulum (Fig. 4a), some myofibroblasts, and few collagenous fibrils. During the involution phase myofibroblasts with indented nuclei and intracellular microfilaments surrounded by collagenous fibrils predominate (Fig. 4b). These cells (specialized contractile fibroblasts: Tomasek et al. 1987) are surrounded by bundles of filamentous material, presumably fibronectin (Tomasek et al. 1987). In the residual phase the tissue consists of collagenous fibrils with few fibroblasts (Fig. 4c).

From these observations and from the results of Meister et al. (1979) it may be assumed that the appearance of myofibroblasts is not the initial step in the evolution of Dupuytren's disease. Furthermore, doubt as to the specifity of myofibroblasts has recently arisen. Comparing the ultrastructure of the fibrous tissue in carpal tunnel syndrome and Dupuytren's disease, Murrell et al. (1989) observed identical myofibroblastic cells in both conditions. It should also be mentioned that the occurrence of myofibroblasts is by no means restricted to Dupuytren's disease (Mohr 1983).

From immunohistological investigations it may be concluded that in the proliferative phase only some cells express vimentin, which is more prominent in scar tissue. Skalli et al. (1989) observed that vimentin is usually present in cells inside the foci of Dupuytren's disease and is often coexpressed with α smooth muscle actin. In most instances, there is also coexpression of vimentin, α smooth muscle actin, and desmin (Table 1). Recently it has been found that cells of aggressive fibromatoses express the Ki-1 antigen (CD30), which had been considered to be restricted to activated lymphocytes and related tumors (Mechtersheimer and Möller 1990).

Table 1. Distribution of cytoskeletal proteins in Dupuytren's disease, total of 25 cases

Protein	Cases detected	Percent of cells
Vimentin	25	not mentioned
Vimentin and α smooth muscle actin	25	70–90
Vimentin, α smooth muscle actin, and desmin	22	10–30

From Skalli et al. 1989.

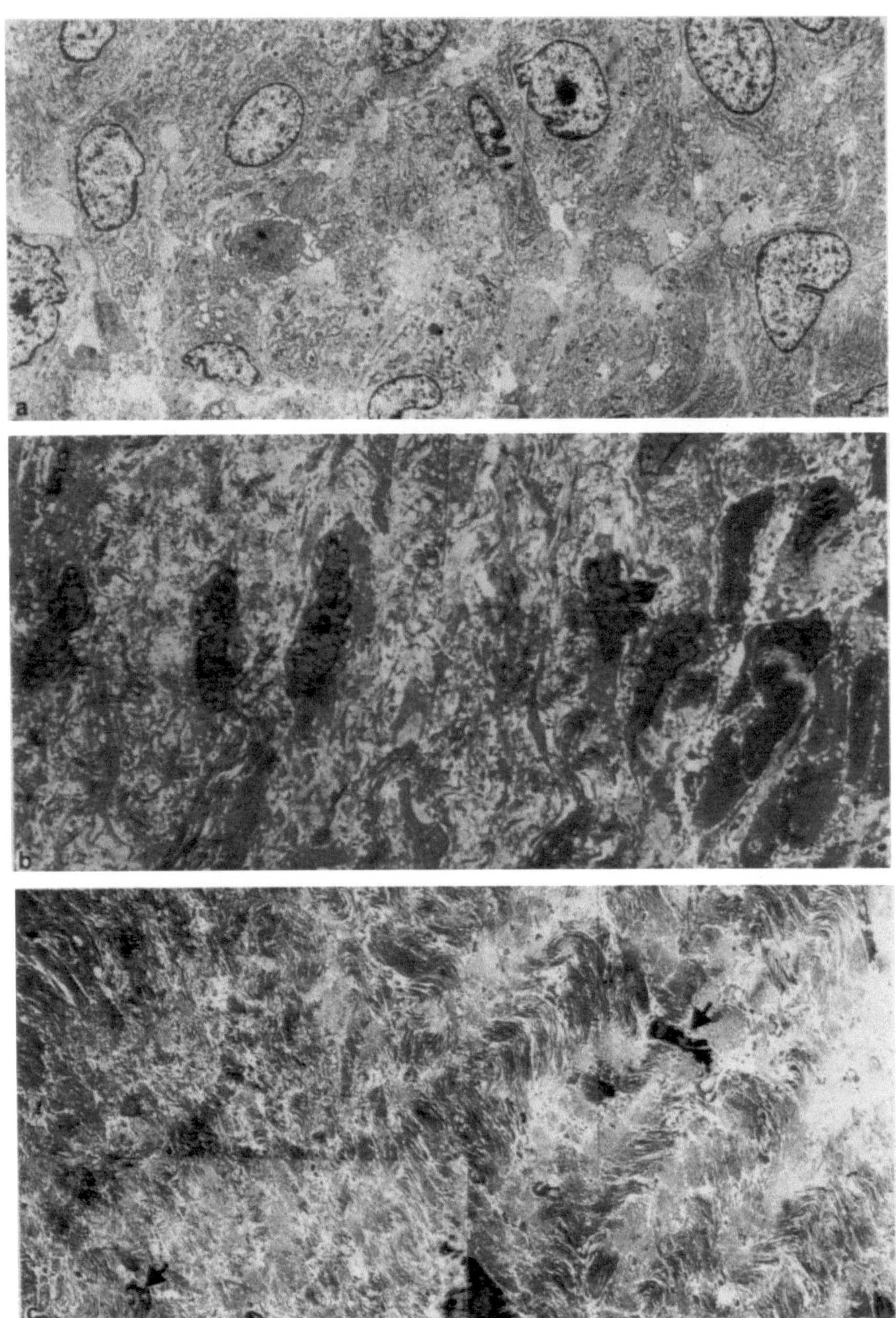

Fig. 4a–c. Electron micrographs of the different phases of Dupuytren's disease. **a** Proliferative phase with predominance of fibroblasts. **b** Involution phase with myofibroblasts surrounded by collagenous fibrils. **c** Residual phase with a predominance of collagenous fibrils and only some fibroblasts (*arrows*). ×2500

6   W. Mohr and D. Wessinghage

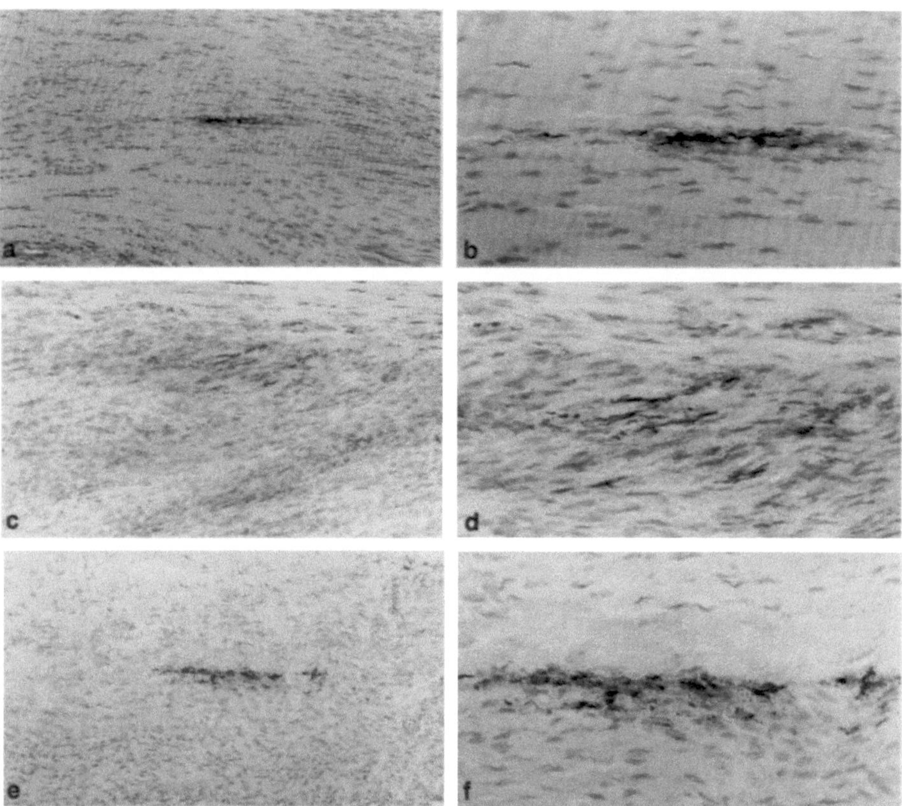

Fig. 5a–f. Iron deposits in Dupuytren's foci. a Small focus of iron deposits; ×85. b Spindle-shaped cells with siderin; ×220. c Irregular focus of siderin deposits; ×85. d Spindle-shaped cells with iron deposits; ×220. e Small focus with iron deposits; ×85. f Granular deposits of iron inside round and spindle-shaped cells; ×220. All sections stained with Prussian blue and nuclear fast red

Nodules of Dupuytren's disease may also contain other constituents. Not infrequently iron deposits are present in the cellular foci (Fig. 5). According to Viljanto (1973) siderin is present in about 20% of the cases; in our own sample, we found that in about 40% of 24 unselected cases some iron deposits could be observed. Ushijima et al. (1984) noted that iron is present especially in early stages of the disease.

Elastic fibers are rarely encountered; they may be observed either as small fibers running parallel to the woven collagenous fibrils or as irregular depositions of elastin (Fig. 6).

Alcian blue staining showed a slightly increased stainability for glycosaminoglycans inside the fibromatous foci in the proliferative phase compared to the normal fibrous aponeurotic tissue.

In recent years the relationship between mast cells and fibrotic diseases has been extensively studied, and it has been suggested that either mast cells or

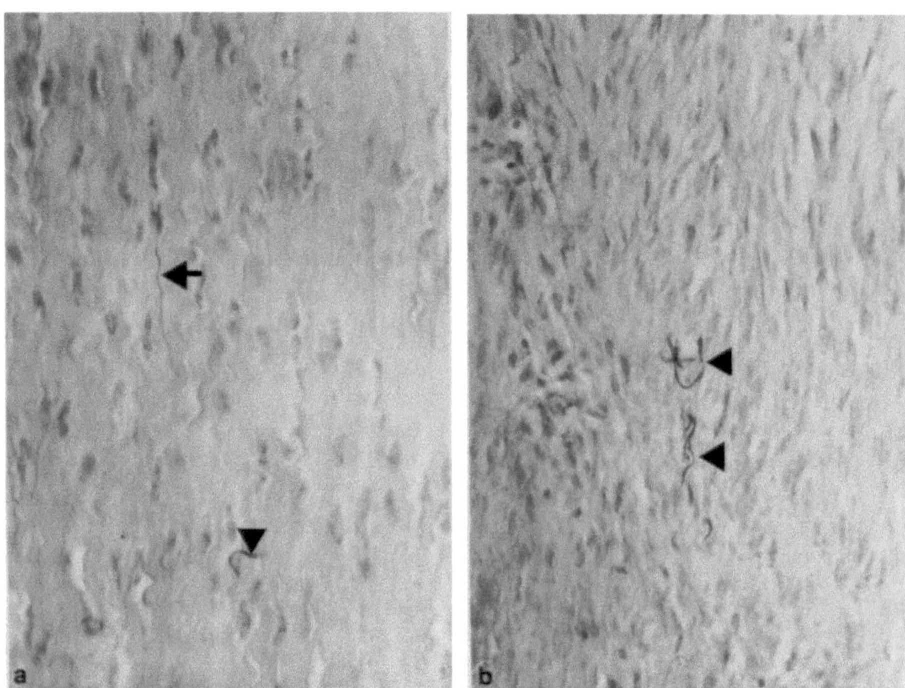

Fig. 6a,b. Elastic fibers in Dupuytren's focus either arranged in parallel with the woven collagenous fibers (*arrow*) or occurring as irregular deposits of elastin (*arrowheads*). Weigert's resorcin-fuchsin, nuclear fast red. **a** ×220, **b** ×350

Table 2. Role of mast cells in fibrotic diseases

Disease or condition	Findings	Reference
Systemic sclerosis	Elevated plasma histamine level; activated mast cells	Falanga et al. (1990) Claman (1989)
Tsk mouse with cutaneous fibrosis	Increased number and increased proportion of degranulated mast cells	Walker et al. (1985)
Tsk mouse with cutaneous fibrosis and blocking mast cell degranulation	Inhibition of fibrosis	Walker et al. (1987)
Collagen synthesis in polyvinyl sponges with compound 48/80	Increased collagen synthesis	Sandberg (1962)
Rat mesentery in vitro treated with compound 48/80	Increased proliferation of fibroblasts	Druvefors and Norrby (1988)
Cultured fibroblasts and histamine	Increased collagen synthesis	Hatamochi et al. (1985)
Cultured microvascular endothelial cells and histamine	Increased proliferation	Marks et al. (1986)
Cultured capillary endothelial cells and mast cells or lysate	Increased migration (no increased proliferation)	Azizkhan et al. (1980)

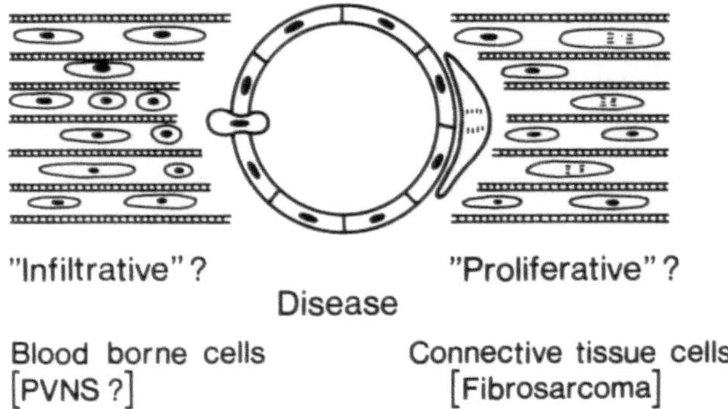

Fig. 7. Hypothetical mechanisms that may lead to Dupuytren's disease. *PVNS*, pigmented villonodular synovitis

histamine is responsible for the increased fibroblast proliferation and collagen synthesis (Table 2). Histological examination of Dupuytren's disease only rarely reveals mast cells, located either perivascularly or between connective tissue cells of the foci. This may indicate that neither mast cells nor their products are involved in the pathogenesis of the disease.

Except for the study by Andrew et al. (1990), there have been no reports on the presence of macrophages in Dupuytren's nodules.

With regard to the pathogenesis of the disease, two mechanisms may be discussed (Fig. 7). On the one hand, Dupuytren's disease may be regarded as an infiltrative disease caused by the differentiation of blood-borne cells. Such a mechanism has recently been assumed as the basic process in the development of nodules in pigmented villonodular synovitis (Ghadially 1983). No reports, however, are found in the literature that would support such an idea for Dupuytren's disease. On the other hand, Dupuytren's disease may be interpreted as a proliferative disease, resembling tumorous connective tissue proliferation such as occurs in fibrosarcoma.

To acquire more information about the proliferative aspect of the disease, we have performed autoradiographic investigations on specimens of Dupuytren's disease after [^{3}H]thymidine labeling in vitro (Mohr and Vossbeck 1985). For this purpose the tissues were divided into normal tendon, cords, nodules, and scars (Fig. 8). Labeled cells were rarely encountered in the normal tendon, while an increased number of labeled cells was present in the cords and nodules and especially in the perivascular region (Fig. 9). With regard to the distribution of the proliferating cell population, we did not observe areas in which labeling was more intense, either in the border or center zones of the fibromatous foci (Fig. 10). From the quantitative evaluation presented in Fig. 11 it may be concluded that proliferating cells are preferentially present in vascular or perivascular areas. This is in accordance with the findings of Murrell et al. (1989) who "suggest that the crucial phenomenon of fibroblast proliferation begins around narrowed microvessels."

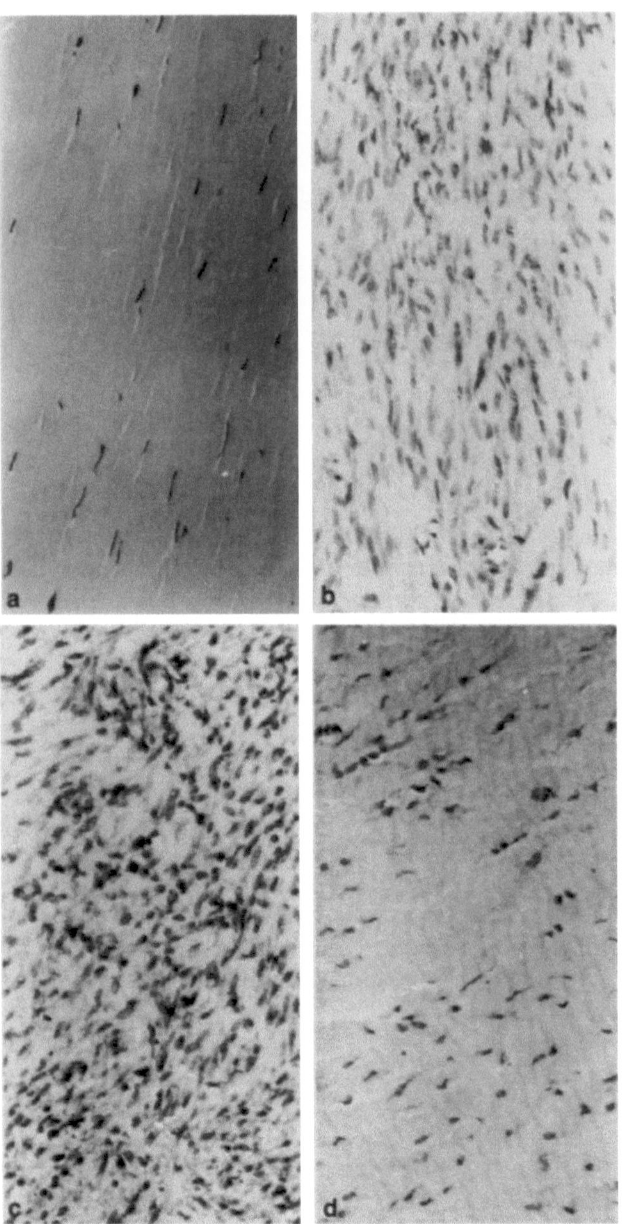

Fig. 8a–d. Structures evaluated for evidence of cell proliferation: **a** tendon; **b** cord; **c** nodule; **d** scar. H and E, ×220

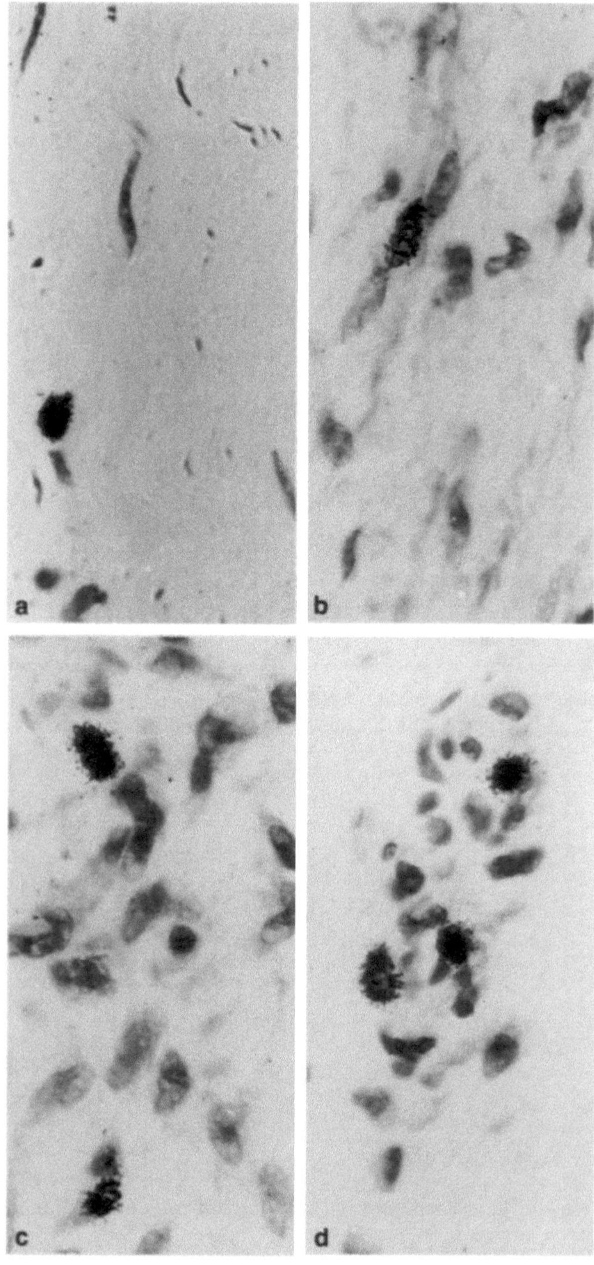

Fig. 9a–d. Autoradiography of [^{3}H]thymidine incorporation in: **a** normal tendon tissue of the aponeurosis; **b** Dupuytren's cord; **c** Dupuytren's nodule; **d** perivascular cells inside a fibromatous focus. Hematoxylin, ×875

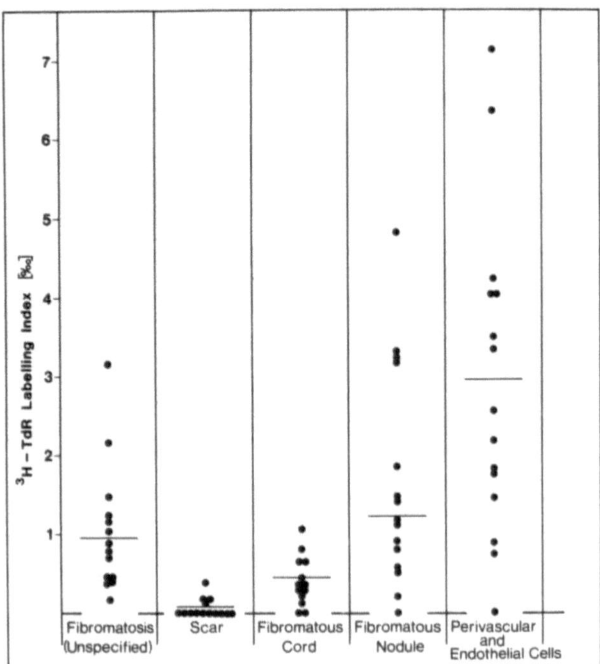

Fig. 10. [^{3}H]thymidine labeling index of cells in the different anatomical structures of Dupuytren's disease (*unspecified* refers to all cells of the fibromatosis)

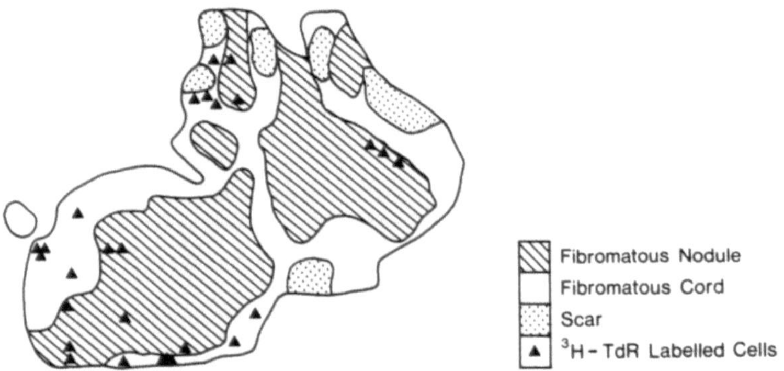

Fig. 11. Localization of proliferating cells in different areas of Dupuytren's disease

It is difficult, however, to histologically differentiate cells after ^{3}H-thymidine labeling. Therefore, it is not clear which cell population the proliferating cells belong to. Nevertheless, these investigations may lead to the hypothesis that precursor cells of the perivascular region are responsible for development of the hypercellular foci.

12   W. Mohr and D. Wessinghage

Table 3. Pericytes as a source of increased cellularity

Disease	Reference
Hemangiopericytoma	Stout and Murray (1942)
Intimal thickening (blood vessels)	Diaz-Flores and Dominguez (1985)
	Sarkisov et al. (1989)
	Beranek and Cavarocchi (1990)
Dupuytren's disease	Andrew et al. (1990)
Pigmented villonodular synovitis	Brax (1992)

Table 4. Immunohistological demonstration of smooth muscle actin and muscle actin in different tissue cells

Cell type	Smooth muscle actin		Muscle actin
	α	γ	
Smooth muscle cells	+	+	+
Myofibroblasts (Dupuytren's disease)	+	+	+
Pericytes	+	+	+
Fibroblasts	−	−	−

From Roholl et al. (1990).

Perivascular connective tissue may contain a peculiar type of cell that has been termed "pericyte" (Fig. 12; Zimmermann 1923). Different conditions are known in which pericytes are said to be responsible for a tumorous or nontumorous increase of cellularity in tissues (Table 3). The assumption that pericytes may also be involved in the pathogenesis of Dupuytren's disease is supported by the immunohistochemical investigations of Andrew et al. (1990), who found that pericyte proliferation was present around occluded capillaries in the fibromatous foci. The expression of smooth muscle actin α and γ and muscle actin in pericytes and myofibroblasts (Table 4) further supports this finding.

Brooks (1986) has developed a different hypothesis concerning the origin of connective tissue cells (Fig. 13). According to this author, there is an intermediate cell, the fibrohistiocyte, that is responsible for differentiation into various types of connective tissue cells. Thus, it may be that either an undifferentiated stem cell or an intermediate precursor cell is stimulated to proliferate and terminally differentiate into a fibroblast.

Since neither the etiology nor the pathogenesis of Dupuytren's disease has been clarified, the opinion of Viljanto (1973) remains valid: "The reader may feel frustrated by noticing that the puzzle of DC (Dupuytren's contracture) is still unsolved, even to so a great an extent, that the number of speculations can be compared with those concerning cancer or collagenoses."

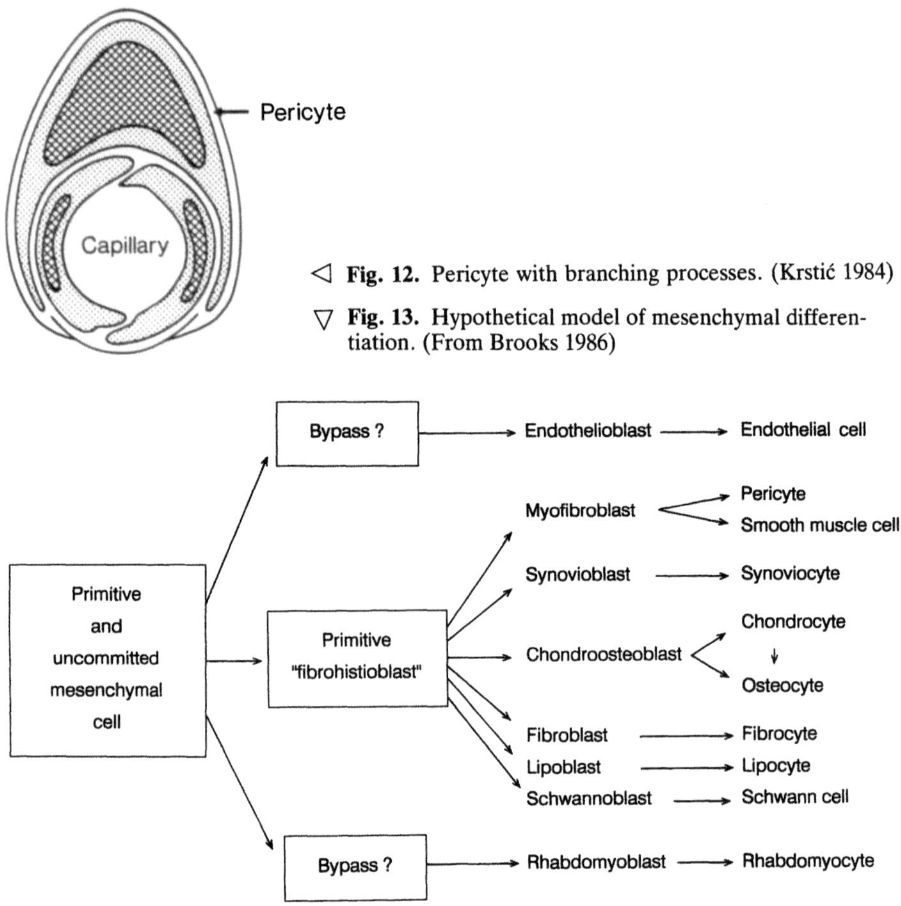

◁ **Fig. 12.** Pericyte with branching processes. (Krstić 1984)

▽ **Fig. 13.** Hypothetical model of mesenchymal differentiation. (From Brooks 1986)

References

Allen PW (1977) The fibromatoses: a clinicopathologic classification based on 140 cases. Am J Surg Pathol 1:255–270

Andrew JG, Ash A, Turner B, Andrew SM (1990) The role of inflammatory cells in Dupuytrens contracture: an immunohistochemical study (Abstr). J Bone Joint Surg [Br] 72:1110

Azizkhan RG, Clifford Azizkhan J, Zetter BR, Folkman J (1980) Mast cell heparin stimulates migration of capillary endothelial cells in vitro. J Exp Med 152:931–944

Beranek JT, Cavarocchi NC (1990) Histogenesis of the intimal thickening in atherosclerosis and of hyperplastic processes in connective tissue. Hum Pathol 21:1082–1083

Brax P (1992) Pathologisch-anatomische und pathogenetische Aspekte der pigmentierten villomodulären Synovialitis. Medical dissertation, University of Ulm

Brooks JJ (1986) The significance of double phenotypic patterns and markers in human sarcomas. A new model of mesenchymal differentiation. Am J Pathol 125:113–123

Claman HN (1989) Mast cell changes in a case of rapidly progressive scleroderma – ultrastructural analysis. J Invest Dermatol 92:290–295

Diaz-Flores L, Dominguez C (1985) Relation between arterial intimal thickening and the vasa-vasorum. Virchows Arch [A] 406:165–177

Druvefors P, Norrby K (1988) Molecular aspects of mast-cell-mediated mitogenesis in fibroblasts and mesothelial cells in situ. Virchows Arch [Cell Pathol] 55:187–192

Falanga V, Soter NA, Altman RD, Kerdel FA (1990) Elevated plasma histamine levels in systemic sclerosis (scleroderma). Arch Dermatol 126:336–338

Ghadially FN (1983) Fine structure of synovial joints. Butterworth, London

Hatamochi A, Fujiwara K, Ueki H (1985) Effects of histamine on collagen synthesis by cultured fibroblasts derived from guinea pig skin. Arch Dermatol Res 277:60–64

Krstić RV (1984) Illustrated encyclopedia of human histology. Springer, Berlin Heidelberg New York

Luck JV (1959) Dupuytren's contracture. J Bone Joint Surg [Am] 41:635–664

Marks RM, Roche WR, Czerniecki M, Penny R, Nelson DS (1986) Mast cell granules cause proliferation of human microvascular endothelial cells. Lab Invest 55:289–294

Mechtersheimer G, Möller P (1990) Expression of Ki-1 antigen (CD30) in mesenchymal tumors. Cancer 66:1732–1737

Meister P, Gokel JM, Remberger K (1979) Palmar fibromatosis – "Dupuytren's contracture". A comparison of light electron and immunofluorescent microscopic findings. Pathol Res Pract 16:402–412

Mohr W (1983) Pathologie der Dupuytren'schen Krankheit. Med Welt 34:397–404

Mohr W (1987) Pathologie des Bandapparates. Sehnen, Sehnenscheiden, Faszien, Schleimbeutel. In: Doerr W, Seifert G (eds) Spezielle pathologische Anatomie, vol 19. Springer, Berlin Heidelberg New York

Mohr W, Vossbeck G (1985) Untersuchungen zur Proliferation und ^{3}H-Prolin-Inkorporation von Zellen der Palmarfibromatose (Morbus Dupuytren). Z Rheumatol 44:226–230

Murrell GAC, Francis MJO, Howlett CR (1989) Dupuytren's contracture. Fine structure in relation to aetiology. J Bone Joint Surg [Br] 71:367–373

Pal B, Griffiths ID, Anderson J, Dick WC (1987) Association of limited joint mobility with Dupuytren's contracture in diabetes mellitus. J Rheumatol 14:582–585

Roholl PJM, Elbers HR, Prinsen I, Claessens JAJ, van Unnik JAM (1990) Distribution of actin isoforms in sarcomas: an immunohistochemical study. Hum Pathol 21:1269–1274

Sandberg N (1962) Accelerated collagen formation and histamine. Nature 194:183

Sarkisov DS, Kolocolchicova EG, Varava BN, Tjurmin AV, Peclo MM, Printseva OY (1989) Morphogenesis of intimal thickening in nonspecific aortoarteritis. Hum Pathol 20:1048–1056

Skalli O, Schürch W, Seemayer T, Lagacé R, Montandon D, Pittet B, Gabbiani G (1989) Myofibroblasts from diverse pathologic settings are heterogeneous in their content of actin isoforms and intermediate filament proteins. Lab Invest 60:275–285

Stout AP, Murray MR (1942) Hemangiopericytoma. A vascular tumor featering Zimmermanns' pericytes. Ann Surg 116:26–33

Tomasek JJ, Schultz RJ, Haaksma CJ (1987) Extracellular matrix-cytoskeletal connections at the surface of the specialized contractile fibroblast (myofibroblast) in Dupuytren disease. J Bone Joint Surg [Am] 69:1400–1407

Ushijima M, Tsuneyoshi M, Enjoji M (1984) Dupuytren type fibromatoses. A clinicopathologic study of 62 cases. Acta Pathol Jpn 34:991–1001

Viljanto JA (1973) Dupuytren's contracture: a review. Semin Arthritis Rheum 3:155–176

Vossbeck G (1986) Zur Pathogenese der Palmarfibromatose (Morbus Dupuytren) – autoradiographische und elektronenmikroskopische Untersuchung. Medical dissertation, University of Ulm

Walker MA, Harley RA, Maize J, DeLustro F, LeRoy EC (1985) Mast cells and their degranulation in the Tsk mouse model of scleroderma. Proc Soc Exp Biol Med 180:323–328

Walker MA, Harley RA, LeRoy EC (1987) Inhibition of fibrosis in Tsk mice by blocking mast cell degranulation. J Rheumatol 14:299–301

Yost J, Winter T, Fett HC (1955) Dupuytrens contracture. A statistical study. Am J Surg 90:568–571

Zimmermann KW (1923) Der feinere Bau der Blutcapillaren. Z Anat Entwicklungsgesch 68:29–109

Interactions Between Proteoglycans and Collagen Fibrils in the Palmar Fascia in Dupuytren's Disease

G. Brandes, E. Reale, P. Brenner, and T. Körner

Introduction

In Dupuytren's disease the morphology and function of palmar fascia change resulting in a progressive and irreversible flexion of the fingers. The pathogenesis is not known, although many efforts has been made to describe the histology and biochemistry of Dupuytren's tissue. In the nodules, the cells proliferate and differentiate to myofibroblasts (Gabbiani and Majno 1972, reviewed by Schürch et al. 1992) and the amount and types of collagen and glycosaminoglycans are altered (Bailey et al. 1977; Bazin et al. 1980; Brickley-Parsons et al. 1981; McFarlane et al. 1990; Gelbermann et al. 1980; Hanyu et al. 1984; Hunter et al. 1975; Meister et al. 1979; Menzel et al. 1979; Tunn et al. 1988). Later, tendon-like cords are formed; these contain only a few fibroblasts in an excessive collagenous matrix (Luck 1959; Chiu and McFarlane 1978).

In the present investigation the extracellular matrix of the normal and diseased palmar fascia were compared. The proteoglycans were stained by two different histochemical procedures: (1) acridine orange, according to the method of Shepard and Mitchell (1981) and (2) reduced osmium tetroxide, according to the method of Karnovsky (1971). The localization of the reaction products in the matrix and their interaction with the collagen fibrils were analyzed and compared. The alterations seen during the disease demonstrate the importance of these proteoglycans in the correct function of the palmar fascia. Preliminary results have been published (Brandes et al. 1991a).

Materials and Methods

Specimens from four individuals with normal palmar fascia and from 20 men (mean age 50 years) with Dupuytren's contracture were fixed in 3% glutaraldehyde in $0.1\,M$ sodium cacodylate buffer (pH 7.2) immediately after surgery. After rinsing in the same buffer the specimens were placed in 1% osmium tetroxide and 1.5% potassium ferrocyanide in water (Karnovsky 1971). Other specimens were fixed in aldehyde with addition of 0.01% acridine orange (Polysciences, Warrington, USA), their postfixation was performed in 2% osmium tetroxide in $0.1\,M$ cacodylate buffer. All the specimens were

"

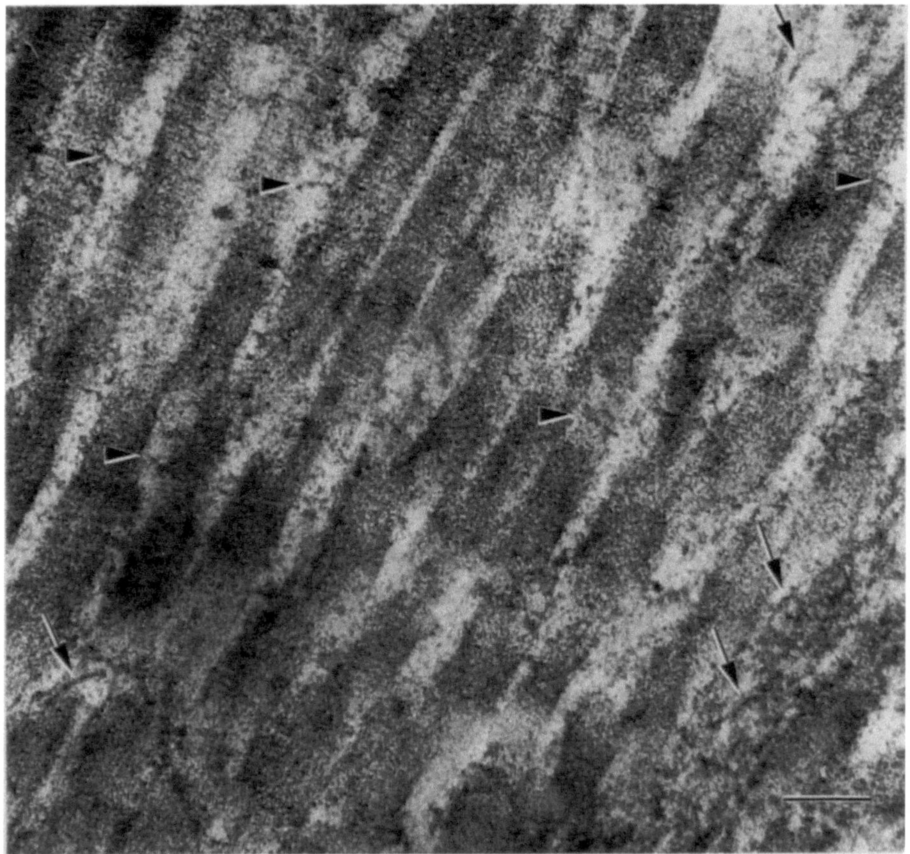

Fig. 1. Normal palmar fascia fixed in the presence of acridine orange. Parallel oriented collagen fibrils are surrounded by fine reaction products appearing as short (*arrowheads*) and long (*arrows*) filaments. The long filaments form a large interfibrillar assembly on the *right* side of the micrograph. *Bar* = 0.1 µm; ×120 000

dehydrated in graded alcohols and embedded in Epon. Thin sections, stained with uranyl acetate and lead citrate, were examined in a Siemens Elmiskop 101 electron microscope.

Results

In the normal palmar fascia, the fibroblasts were embedded in an extracellular matrix containing parallel bundles of collagen fibrils with a diameter of about 50–80 nm connected to each other by 3–4 nm thick, short, filamentous reaction products. These were orthogonally oriented along the fibrils at distances of 10–25 nm (Fig. 1, 3b). Long branched filaments with a similar thickness and a length of about 100 nm lay mainly parallel to the collagen fibrils and formed a network in the broader interfibrillar spaces (Fig. 1).

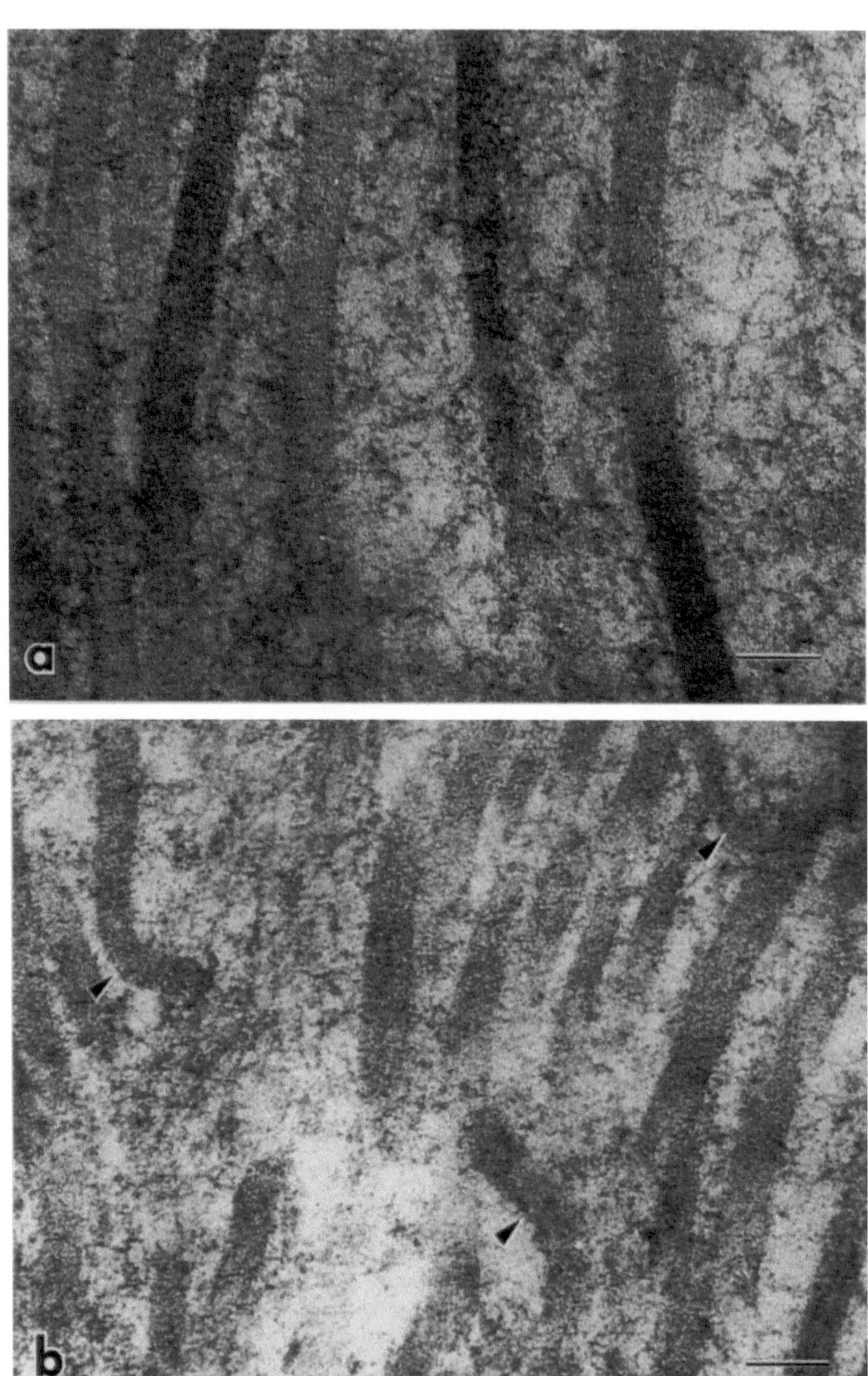

18   G. Brandes et al.

In the Dupuytren's disease fascia, the nodules were characterized by a predominance of myofibroblasts. These cells were surrounded by a tight network of 2–3 nm thick and about 100 nm long branched filaments. They bound at distances of 10–25 nm to collagen fibrils, about 40–60 nm thick, which were intermingled with the network (Fig. 2a). At greater distances from the cells, the collagen fibrils were very irregularly oriented, abruptly changing their course but packed closer together than in the pericellular matrix (Fig. 2b). They were surrounded by abundant, short fine filaments connected to the fibrils at distances of 10–25 nm (Fig. 2b).

The cords contained only a few fibroblasts, which were closely packed between large bundles of collagen fibrils. After fixation with glutaraldehyde and acridine orange, the fibrils disaggregated into helicoidal microfibrils (Fig. 3a). Therefore, the diameter of the fibrils measured from 350 nm to 850 nm. The interfibrillar spaces disappeared. A fine network stained by acridine orange could only be seen within the fibrils (Fig. 3a). After using reduced osmium tetroxide the swelling of the collagen fibrils was limited. Fine filaments extended from the narrow interfibrillar spaces into the outer zone of each collagen fibril (Fig. 4).

Discussion

The present study demonstrates that the extracellular matrix changes both qualitatively and quantitatively during the course of Dupuytren's disease. Whereas in the ultrastructural analysis the collagen fibrils could be seen with the usual preparation techniques, special methods were needed to visualize the proteoglycans. Acridine orange and reduced osmium tetroxide can be used to localize sulfated glycosaminoglycans as demonstrated in hyaline cartilage by digestion with specific enzymes (Brandes and Reale 1988, 1990). Therefore, the fine filamentous reaction products in the palmar fascia are presumably proteoglycans.

In the nodule the matrix around the myofibroblasts usually contains predominantly proteoglycans which connect the cells with the collagen fibrils and these to each other (Badalamente et al. 1983; Chiu and McFarlane 1978; Gabbiani and Majno 1972). Therefore, contraction of the myofibroblasts seems to cause the parallel orientation of the newly formed collagen fibrils (Badalamente et al. 1983; Brickley-Parsons et al. 1981; Chiu and McFarlane 1978). Additionally, the proteoglycans themselves have an important influence on the cells and matrix (reviewed by Ruggeri and Benazzo 1984): First, due to their high water-binding capacity, they fill the whole matrix regulating the

◁ **Fig. 2a,b.** Dupuytren's disease. In the nodule close to the myofibroblasts (**a**) a tight filamentous network can be seen in which the collagen fibrils are intermingled. Far away from the cells (**b**) prevailing short filaments connect the fibrils which are packed closer together and are more disorderly than in the pericellular matrix. *Arrowheads* indicate fibrils following an irregular pathway. *Bar* = 0.1 μm; ×120 000

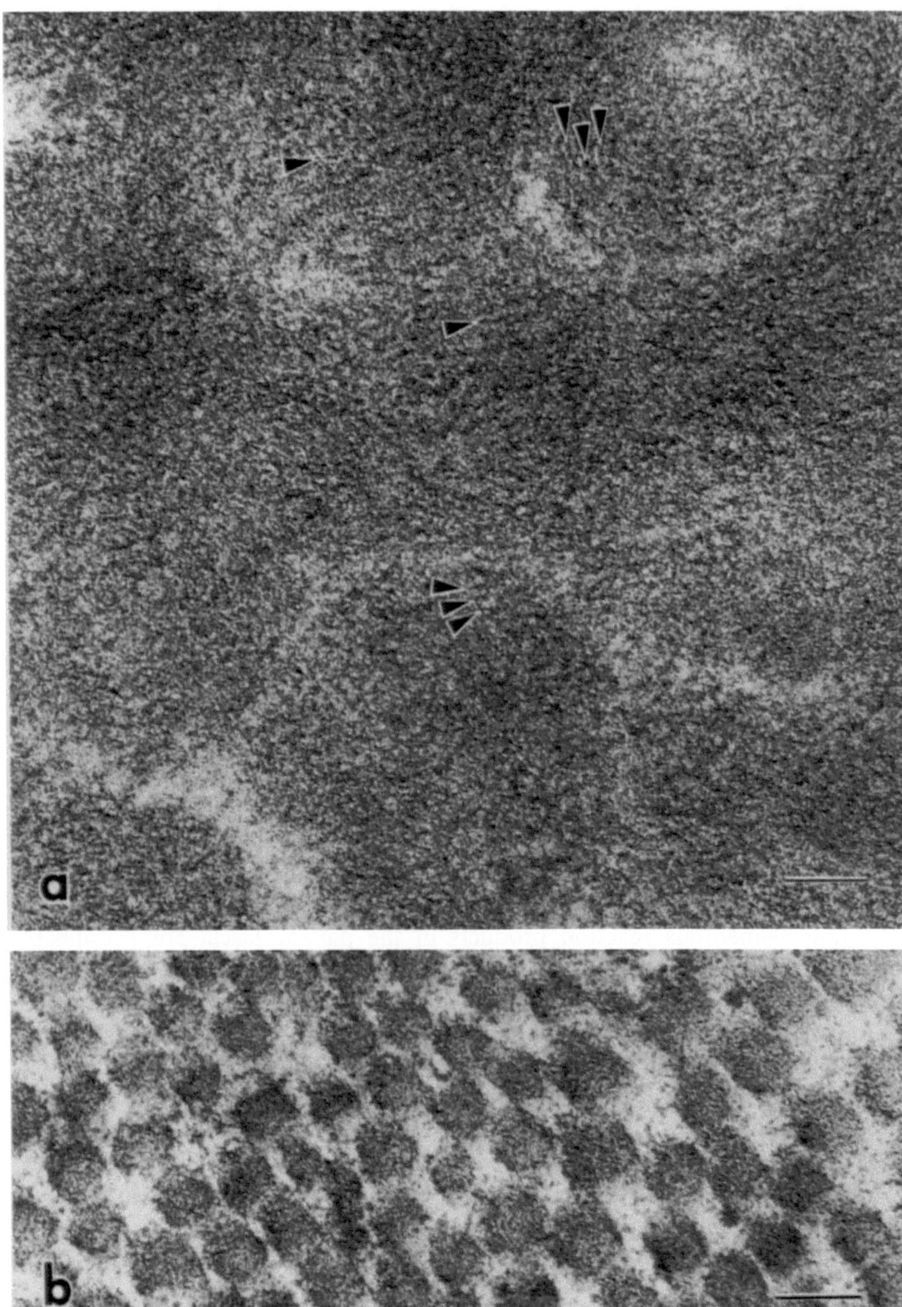

Fig. 3. a Dupuytren's disease, cord. After fixation in the presence of acridine orange the collagen fibrils are swollen. A finely stained network (*arrowheads*) lies between the helicoidal microfibrils. **b** Normal palmar fascia fixed in the same solution as in **a**. *Bar* = 0.1 μm; ×120 000

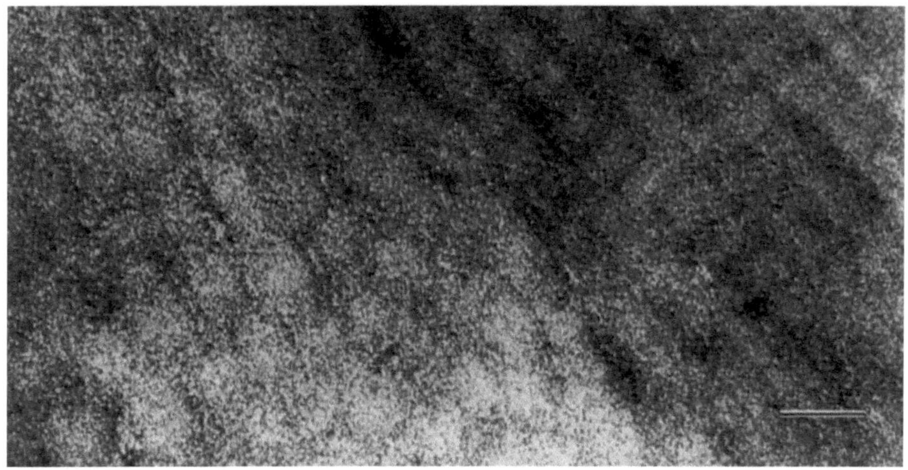

Fig. 4. Dupuytren's disease, cord. Reduced osmium tetroxide induces a limited swelling of the collagen fibrils. Staining is present between and within the outer zone of the collagen fibrils. *Bar* = 0.1 µm; ×120 000

transport of substances to the cells and of cell products to the surrounding matrix. Second, they influence fibrillogenesis, as shown by in vivo and in vitro experiments.

During the pathological process not only the amount but also the type of the proteoglycans changes. In the normal palmar fascia hyaluronan and dermatan sulfate predominate; in Dupuytren's tissue hyaluronan decreases, and chondroitin sulfate increases more than dermatan sulfate in the nodule but does not change quantitatively in the cords (Flint et al. 1982; Gurr et al. 1984; Tunn et al. 1988). Based on comparing the reaction products seen after staining with acridine orange or reduced osmium tetroxide, the shorter filaments connected to the collagen fibrils could be composed of dermatan sulfate proteoglycans, since they are present in the normal and diseased fascia. The tight network of long branched filaments predominantly seen in the nodule around the myofibroblasts could contain most of the chondroitin sulfate, which reacts with acridine orange and with reduced osmium tetroxide. Although this hypothesis has to be proven by digestion with specific glycosaminoglycan lyases, it is in agreement with the results on other connective tissues (reviewed by Ruggeri and Benazzo 1984).

The functional characteristics of the connective tissue are mainly affected by proteoglycans and collagen: The small dermatan sulfate proteoglycans seem to have an important role in the fibrillogenesis and alignment of the newly formed collagen fibrils, for example, in the tendon (Öbrink 1973; Ruggeri and Benazzo 1984; Scott 1980) and probably in the normal palmar fascia as well. In comparison, the large chondroitin sulfate proteoglycans of the hyaline cartilage and also of Dupuytren's nodule fill the broad interfibrillar spaces and are typically found with small, randomly oriented collagen fibrills. These macromolecules are responsible for the resilience of the tissue: acting pressure forces the water between the glycosaminoglycan chains to be squeezed out and the fibrillar constituents to be stretched. Since after unloading the proteoglycans can again bind water, the tissue recovers to its previous state. Therefore, the functional characteristics of the nodule of Dupuytren's disease can be explained by its cartilage-like appearance, which is caused by a specific and mutual interaction between proteoglycans and collagen fibrils.

In the cords, where only a few proteoglycans can be recognized in the interfibrillar spaces, the collagen fibrils are swollen, probably through the prevailing intrafibrillar proteoglycans (Brandes et al. 1991a). Conceivably, the balance between interfibrillar and intrafibrillar proteoglycans is important for the buildup and maintenance of the collagen fibrils in the extracellular matrix of the palmar fascia.

In summary, the present study demonstrates that interaction of the different proteoglycans with collagen fibrils can explain the morphological and functional changes of the palmar fascia during Dupuytren's disease. Conclusions regarding the pathogenesis remain difficult, since this tissue retains its ability to adapting to acting forces (Brandes et al. 1991b).

References

Badalamente MA, Stern L, Hurst LC (1983) The pathogenesis of Dupuytren's contracture: contractile mechanisms of the myofibroblasts. J Hand Surg 8:235–243

Bailey A, Sims T, Gabbiani G, Bazin S, Le Lous M (1977) Collagen of Dupuytren's disease. Clin Sci 53:499–502

Bazin S, Le Lous M, Duance VC, Sims TJ, Bailey AJ, Gabbiani G, D'Andiran G, Pizzolato G, Browski A, Nicoletis C, Delaunay A (1980) Biochemistry and histology of the connective tissue of Dupuytren's disease lesions. Eur J Clin Invest 10:9–16

Brandes G, Reale E (1988) Proteoglycans of the articular cartilage stainable with ferrocyanide-reduced osmium tetroxide. 11th Meeting of the Federation of European Connective Tissue Societies, Amsterdam

Brandes G, Reale E (1990) The reaction of acridine orange with proteoglycans in the articular cartilage of the rat. Histochem. J 22:106–112

Brandes G, Körner T, Brenner P, Reale E (1991a) Histochemical localization of glycoconjugates in the palmar aponeurosis of Dupuytren's patients. J Submicrosc Cytol Pathol 23:551–558

Brandes G, Messina A, Reale E (1991b) Extracellular matrix of the palmar fascia. Its aspects after continuous elongation by TEC device. International Meeting on the Biology and Pathology of the Extracellular Matrix, Lorne

Brickley-Parsons D, Glimcher MJ, Smith RJ, Albin R, Adams JP (1981) Biochemical changes in the collagen of the palmar fascia in patients with Dupuytren's disease. J Bone Joint Surg [Am] 63A:787–797

Chiu HF, McFarlane RM (1978) Pathogenesis of Dupuytren's contracture: a correlative clinical-pathological study. J Hand Surg 3A:1–10

Flint MH, Gillard GC, Reilly HC (1982) The glycosaminoglycans of Dupuytren's disease. Connect Tissue Res 9:173–179

Gabbiani G, Majno G (1972) Dupuytren's contracture: fibroblast contraction? An ultrastructural study. Am J Pathol 66:131–146

Gelbermann RH, Amiel D, Rudolph RM, Vance RM (1980) Dupuytren's contracture: an electron microscopic, biochemical and clinic correlative study. J Bone Joint Surg [Am] 62A:425–432

Gurr E, Tizian C, Delbrück A, Berger A (1984) Glykosaminoglykane in der Dupuytren'schen Kontraktur. Handchirurgie 16:161–164

Hanyu T, Tajima T, Takagi T, Sasaki S, Fujimoto D, Isemura M, Yosizawa Z (1984) Biochemical studies on the collagen of the palmar aponeurosis affected with Dupuytren's disease. Tohoku J Exp Med 142:437–443

Hunter JAA, Ogdon C, Norris MG (1975) Dupuytren's contracture. I. Chemical pathology. Br J Plast Surg 28:10–18

Karnovsky MJ (1971) Use of ferrocyanide-reduced osmium tetroxide in electron microscopy. 11th Meeting of the American Society of Cell Biology, New York

Luck JV (1959) Dupuytren's contracture. A new concept of the pathogenesis correlated with surgical management. J Bone Joint Surg [Am] 41A:635–664

McFarlane RM, McGrouther DA, Flint MH (1990) Dupuytren's disease, biology and treatment. Churchill Livingstone, Edinburgh

Meister P, Gokel JM, Remberger K (1979) Palmar fibrosis – "Dupuytren's contracture". A comparison of light, electron and immunofluorescence microscopic findings. Pathol Res Pract 164:402–412

Menzel EJ, Piza H, Zielinski C, Endler AT, Steffen C, Millesi H (1979) Collagen types and anticollagen-antibodies in Dupuytren's disease. Hand 11:243–248

Neumüller J, Tohidast-Akrad AM, Ammer K, Hakimzadeh A, Stransky G, Weis S, Partsch G, Eberl R (1988) Ultrastructural and autoradiographic investigations of cell cultures derived from tendons or ligamentous material from patients with fibromatous disorders. Exp Cell Biol 56:113–130

Öbrink B (1973) A study of the interactions between monomeric topocollagen and glycosaminoglycans. Eur J Biochem 33:387–400

Ruggeri A, Benazzo F (1984) Collagen-proteoglycan interaction: In: Ruggeri A, Motta PM (eds) Ultrastructure of the connective tissue matrix. Nijhoff, Boston, pp 113–125

Schürch W, Seemayer TA, Gabbiani G (1992) Myofibroblast. In: Sternberg SS (ed) Histology for pathologists. Raven, New York, pp 109–144

Scott JE (1980) Collagen-proteoglycans interactions – localization of proteoglycans in tendon by electron microscopy. Biochem J 187:887–891

Shepard N, Mitchell N (1981) Acridine orange stabilization of glycosaminoglycans in beginning endochondral ossification. A comparative light and electron microscopic study. Histochemistry 70:107–114

Tunn S, Gurr E, Delbrück A, Buhr T, Flory J (1988) The distribution of unsulphated and sulphated glycosaminoglycans in palmar fascia from patients with Dupuytren's disease and healthy subjects. J Clin Chem Clin Biochem 26:7–14

Myofibroblasts Are Not Specific to Dupuytren's Disease

G.A.C. Murrell, M.J.O. Francis, and C.R. Howlett

Introduction

The etiology of Dupuytren's contracture has confounded clinicians and scientists since Dupuytren's first description in 1834. While the light and electron microscopic appearance of Dupuytren's contracture has been frequently described (MacCallum and Hueston 1962; Bazin et al. 1980; Millesi 1985; Nézelof 1985; Gabbiani and Majno 1972; Gokel and Hübner 1977; Iwasaki et al. 1984; Kischer and Speer 1984; Tomasek et al. 1987), little attention has been paid to palmar fascia sampled from patients without Dupuytren's contracture (Legge et al. 1981; Gabbiani and Montandon 1985).

We have compared the fine structure of palmar fascia from patients with Dupuytren's contracture and carpal tunnel syndrome and have been able to highlight significant morphological changes. These findings contradict previously held assumptions regarding the uniqueness of Dupuytren's contracture fibroblasts.

Methods

Patients

Palmar fascia was obtained from patients undergoing either fasciectomy for Dupuytren's contracture or carpal tunnel release for carpal tunnel syndrome. Skin for culture was obtained from a forearm biopsy. Informed consent was obtained from all patients prior to operation.

For the light microscopic studies, tissues were taken from nine patients with Dupuytren's contracture (seven men, two women; age range 45–73) and five with carpal tunnel syndrome (all women; age range 50–63); for electron microscopy, from eight patients with Dupuytren's contracture (six men, two women; age range 52–73) and six with carpal tunnel syndrome (all women; age range 50–65); and for tissue culture from six patients with Dupuytren's contracture (three men, three women; age range 53–70) and six with carpal tunnel syndrome (three men, three women; age range 53–90).

Light Microscopy

Samples were fixed in buffered formalin saline (pH 7.4) for 24 h, dehydrated and embedded in paraffin wax. Sections were cut at 5 µm and stained with hematoxylin and eosin. Fibroblasts and blood vessels were counted using a 21 mm eyepiece graticule (Graticules Ltd, Kent, UK) and a Cooke 100 1 mm graduated slide. Mann-Whitney U nonparametric statistical tests were used for all data.

Electron Microscopy

Tissue Samples. Tissue was immediately dissected into 1 mm cubes and placed in 3% glutaraldehyde, buffered in 0.1 M sodium cacodylate (pH 7.3), postfixed in 2% osmium tetroxide in the same buffer, dehydrated in ethanol, and embedded in Epikote 812 (Emscope Ltd, UK). Ultrathin sections, stained on formvar coated copper grids with 2% uranyl acetate and Reynold's lead citrate, were examined in a JEOL T8 electron microscope (Japan Electron Optics Laboratory, Tokyo, Japan). Analysis of the diameter of collagen fibrils was performed by tracing the outlines of 288 collagen fibrils with a Zeiss modulator system for quantitative digital image analysis (MOP AM02) (Oberkochen, West Germany).

In Vitro Culture. Tissue was immediately placed in 100% Dulbecco's modified Eagle's medium, pH 7.35 (Flow Laboratories Ltd, UK), with 10% foetal calf serum (Flow) and dissected into 1 mm cubes. Two cubes of tissue were placed into 25 cm^2 tissue culture flasks (Nunclan Ltd, Denmark) and cultured at 37°C. Media were changed every 3 days throughout the culture period. At confluence cells were harvested and frozen in 9:1 (v/v) foetal calf serum:dimethyl sulfoxide in a Kryo 10 series cell freezer (Planer Products Ltd, Sunbury-on-Thames, UK). Two weeks prior to electron microscopic examination appropriate cell lines were thawed and cultured, thus each cell line was passaged three times prior to electron microscopy. Flasks (25 cm^2) seeded with 25×10^4 cells were incubated for 4 days until cells were near confluence. Media were discarded, cell layers washed with phosphate buffered saline (pH 7.4) and fixed in 3% glutaraldehyde, buffered with 0.1 M sodium cacodylate (pH 7.3), postfixed with 2% osmium tetroxide in the same buffer and dehydrated in an ascending series of ethanol. The specimens were preliminarily infiltrated in 1:1 hydroxypropyl methacrylate:Epikote, then 100% Epikote before baking in a 60°C oven. Embedded cell layers were separated from flasks after immersion in liquid nitrogen. Appropriate zones were trimmed, reembedded and sectioned parallel to the culture surface. The staining and subsequent characterization was as for tissue samples.

Results

Carpal Tunnel Syndrome

Palmar fascia from patients with carpal tunnel syndrome consisted of a tough, thin (<1 mm thick), pale, shining, translucent membranous structure that arose from beneath the flexor retinaculum and extended as a sheet across the palm.

The microscopic appearance was one of infrequent, well-spaced, elongated and spindle-shaped fibroblasts lying parallel to the encompassing matrix of well-organized collagenous fibers (Fig. 1). Microvessels were occasionally observed, usually at the periphery of bundles of collagenous fibers. These vessels had patent lumina of greater diameter than vessel wall thickness. Hyalinization of vessel walls was rarely encountered as was any perivascular cellular accumulation.

Electron microscopic examination revealed collagen fibrils to be grouped into well-organized fibers (2–20 µm in diameter) and arranged in a regular lattice, the majority having a diameter of either 60 nm or 110 nm (ratio 1:3) with an overall density of 100 fibrils per µm^2.

Fibroblasts contained numerous microfilaments (6–8 nm) that coursed in bundles from the perinuclear region to or close to the plasmalemma and were

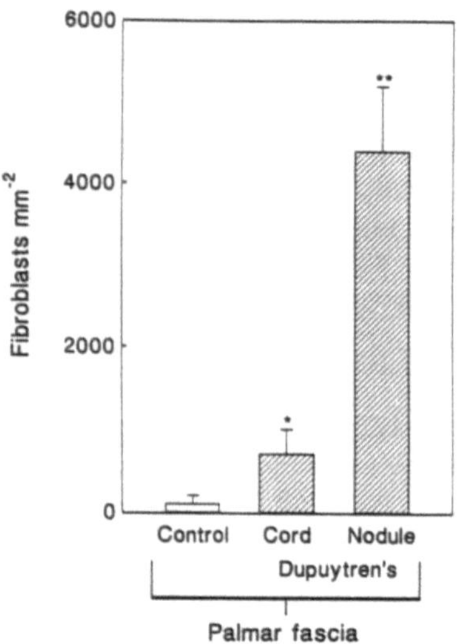

Fig. 1. Distribution of fibroblasts in Dupuytren's contracture and control palmar fascia. Expressed as mean (SEM) cells mm^{-2}; control ($n = 5$), cord ($n = 9$), nodule ($n = 8$). *$p <$ 0.05; **$p <$ 0.01; compared with control

Fig. 2a,b. Intracellular ultrastructure. Regular arrays of perinuclear, 6–8 nm microfilaments ▷ (*MF, mf*) and multiple 50–70 nm micropinocytotic vesicles (*arrows*) are prominent in fibroblasts from patients with carpal tunnel syndrome (**a**) and Dupuytren's contracture (**b**). *N*, nucleus, *CV*, coated vesicle; *CP*, coated pit; *F*, fibrils. (From Murrell et al. 1989) ×33 000

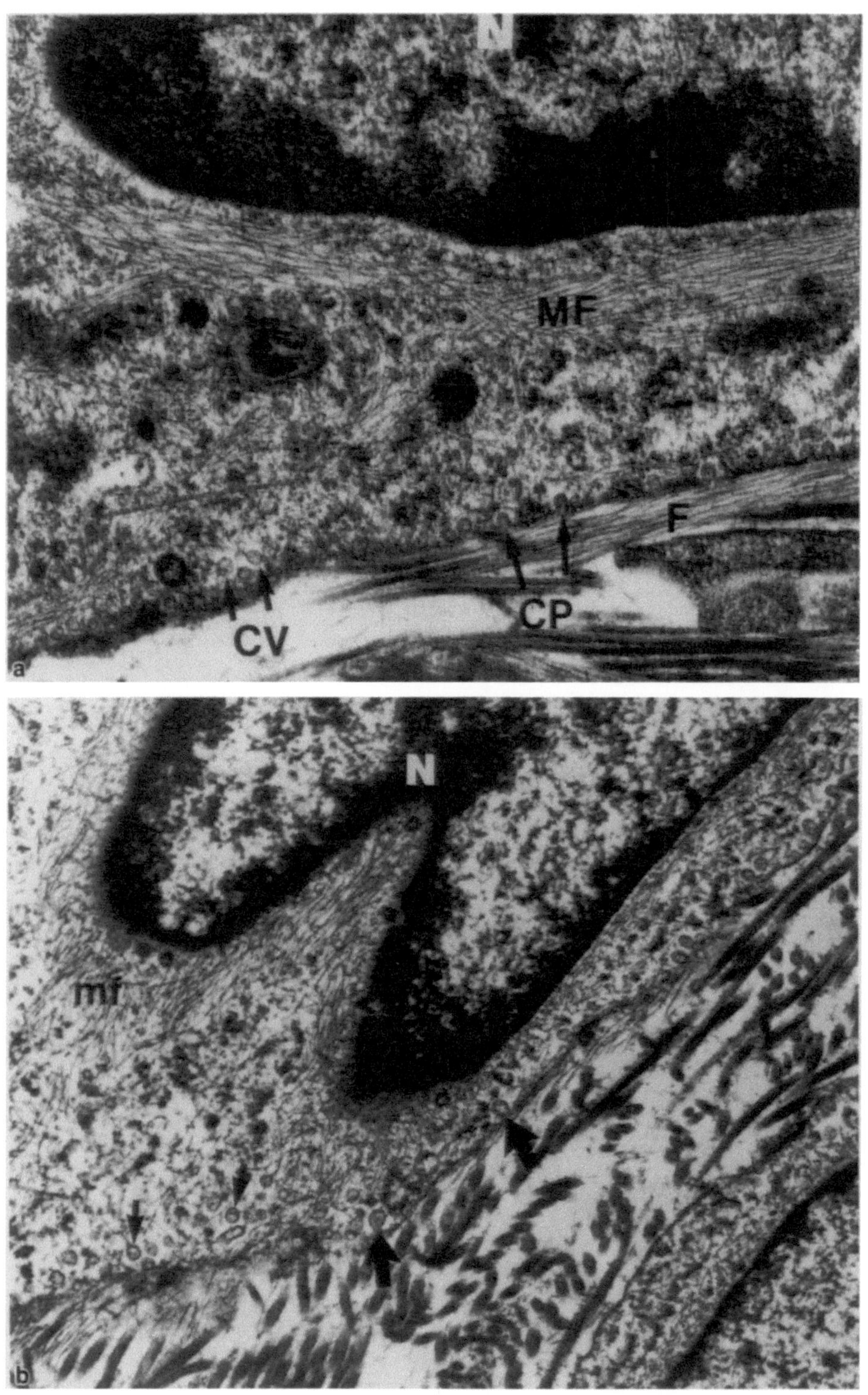

N
MF
F
CP
CV
N
mf

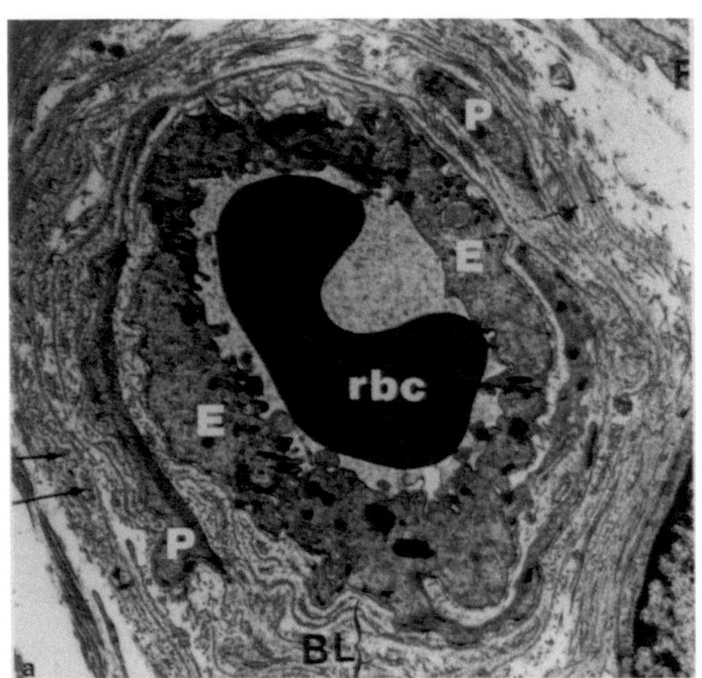

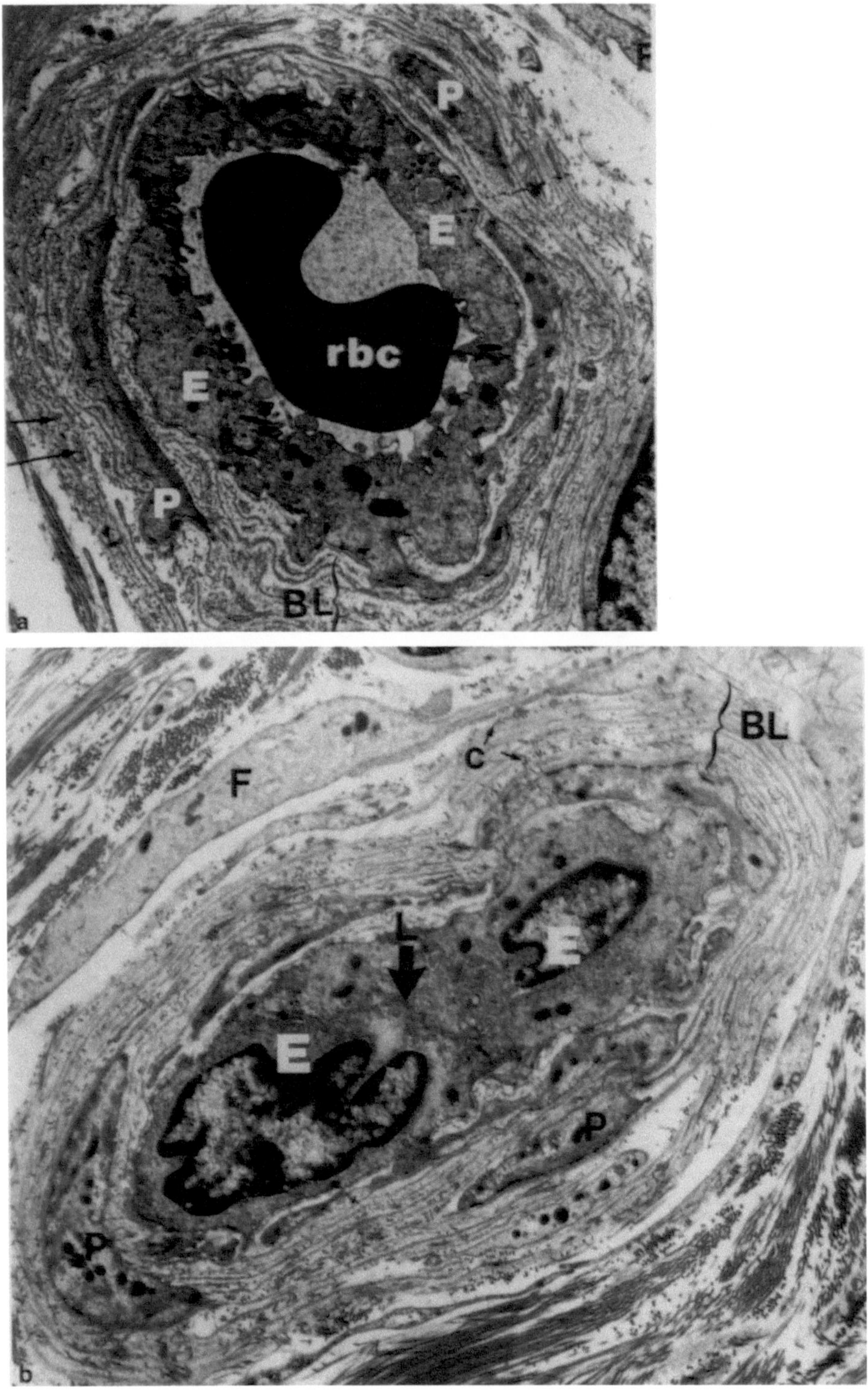

P
F
E
rbc
E
P
BL
a
BL
C
F
E
E
P
P
b

generally aligned in the long axis of the cell (Fig. 2a). Micropinocytic vesicles (50–70 nm in diameter) were abundant, particularly associated with the cell membrane. The nuclear membrane contained several large smooth indentations. No intercellular junctional complexes were observed.

Capillaries with luminal diameters of 4–6 μm were lined by a single continuous layer of endothelial cells and enveloped with one to six (mean three) circumferential layers of basal lamina. Pericytes and collagen fibrils lay circumferentially between layers of basal laminae (Fig. 3a).

Dupuytren's Contracture

Palmar fascia from patients with Dupuytren's contracture consisted of a variety of longitudinally arranged, glistening, opaque, yellow-white, firm fibrous cords (2–5 mm in diameter) often extending from nodules (5–10 mm in diameter).

The microscopic appearance was heterogeneous, with cord, nodular and intermediate forms observed in all sections (as described by Nézelof 1985). Scattered within and immediately peripheral to the nodular areas were a number of small vessels. The majority of these vessels coursed parallel to the long axis of collagen fibers and were surrounded by an irregular swirling proliferation of fibroblasts. Many vessels were markedly narrowed and their walls grossly thickened and hyalinized. Leukocytes and pigmentary deposits were not encountered.

Electron microscopic examination showed the fibrillary matrix to be markedly disorganized, being composed of haphazardly arranged fibrils with varying diameters between 60 and 100 nm. Clustered around these fibrils were smaller swirls of 8–10 nm filaments.

Within the fibroblast cytoplasm were numerous perinuclear and longitudinally arranged microfilaments (6–8 nm diameter) extending to the cell surface. Abundant swollen rough endoplasmic reticula were frequently filled with moderately electron dense material. Micropinocytic vesicles (40–80 nm) were also numerous. Nuclei were invariably indented (Fig. 3b).

Completely or partially occluded capillaries (lumina 0–4 μm in diameter) were consistently observed, particularly in the nodular areas. These vessels were lined by continuous, bulging endothelial cells and five to ten (mean seven) layers of basement membrane, interspersed by collagen fibrils and hypertrophied pericytes. The outermost layers of basal lamina were loosely textured, folded and frequently disrupted (Fig. 3b). Peripheral to these vascular walls were fibroblasts and associated fibrillary bundles of collagen.

◁ **Fig. 3a,b.** Capillaries from the palmar fascia of patients with carpal tunnel syndrome (**a**) and Dupuytren's contracture (**b**). Note the narrowing of the lumen (*L*) and lamination of the basal lamina (*BL*), collagen fibrils (*C*) and thickened pericytes (*P*) envelope the endothelial cells in (**b**). *rbc*, red blood cell; *E*, endothelial cells; *P*, pericytes; *small arrows*, collagen fibrils; *F*, fibrob-last. (From Murrell et al. 1989) ×8500

Cultured Fibroblasts

Cells cultured from each set of skin and of palmar fascia from patients with carpal tunnel syndrome or Dupuytren's contracture had a similar fine structure. The prominent subcellular feature was longitudinally arranged microfilaments (6–8 nm), coursing parallel to the long axis of the cell. Similar cytoskeletal components arose from within the cytoplasm and tapered outward to the surface of the flask forming apparent focal contacts (Fig. 4). In essence, all the cells in culture had features of myofibroblasts and their origin could not be distinguished by ultrastructural criteria.

Discussion

Although the fine structure of palmar fascia from patients with Dupuytren's contracture has been reported on extensively, palmar fascia from patients without Dupuytren's contracture (e.g., carpal tunnel syndrome) has rarely been examined. In this study the major difference between palmar fascia from patients with Dupuytren's contracture and carpal tunnel syndrome was *not* a difference in the ultrastructural characteristics of the fibroblasts, as previously suggested (Gabbiani and Majno 1972; Gokel and Hübner 1977; Iwasaki et al. 1984; Gabbiani and Montandon 1985). *All* fibroblasts examined had ultrastructural features of myofibroblasts. In addition *all* cultured cells derived from skin and palmar fascia from both groups of patients had prominent myofibroblastic characteristics including anchoring strands, features previously reported in other fibroblast cell lines (Abercrombie and Heaysman 1966; Goldman et al. 1976).

Fibroblast density was sixfold and 40-fold greater in cords and nodules from Dupuytren's contracture than in carpal tunnel syndrome. These observations and an increase in proliferation of perivascular fibroblasts (Mohr and Vossbeck 1985) suggest that the crucial phenomenon of fibroblast proliferation begins around narrowed microvessels.

Narrowing of capillary lumina and thickening and lamination of basal laminae were particularly pronounced in palmar fascia from patients with Dupuytren's contracture, changes consistent with those found by Kischer and Speer (1984). One of the striking features in Dupuytren's contracture capillaries was the hypertrophied and swollen, electron lucent endothelial cells; the latter appearance may represent damage to the integrity of the endothelial membrane. Swollen endothelial cells and occluded lumina have also been noted in hypertrophic scars and keloids (Kischer et al. 1982). Vracko (1974) proposed that noxious conditions cause pericytic necrosis in the microvasculature with subsequent regeneration within the old basal lamina tube. Repetition of this cycle adds further layers, progressively narrowing the lumen and trapping collagen fibers in a thickening wall. As the basal lamina widens, older outer layers become looser in texture, increase in width and electron lucency. Our observations are in keeping with such a hypothesis. We

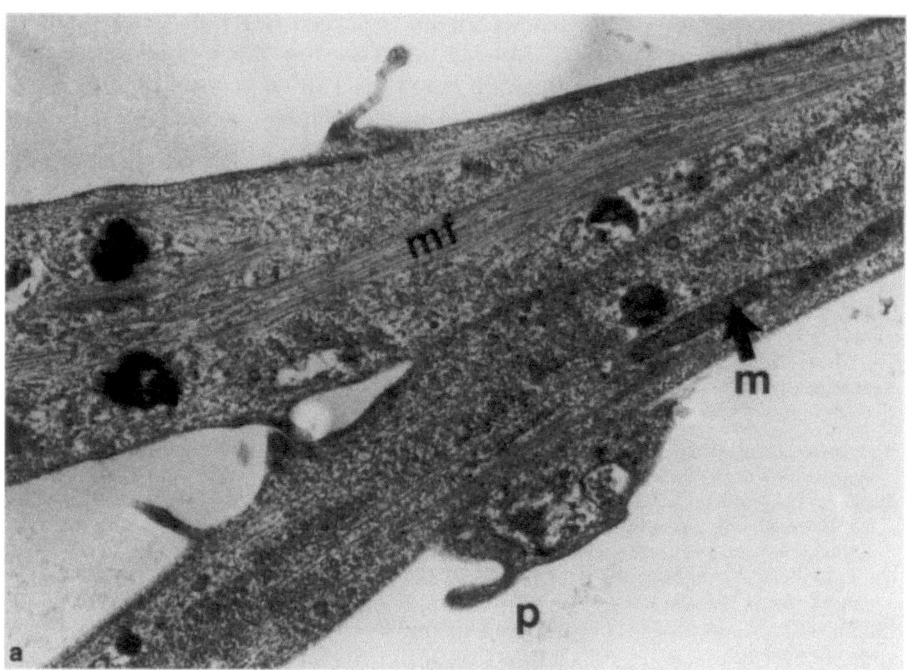
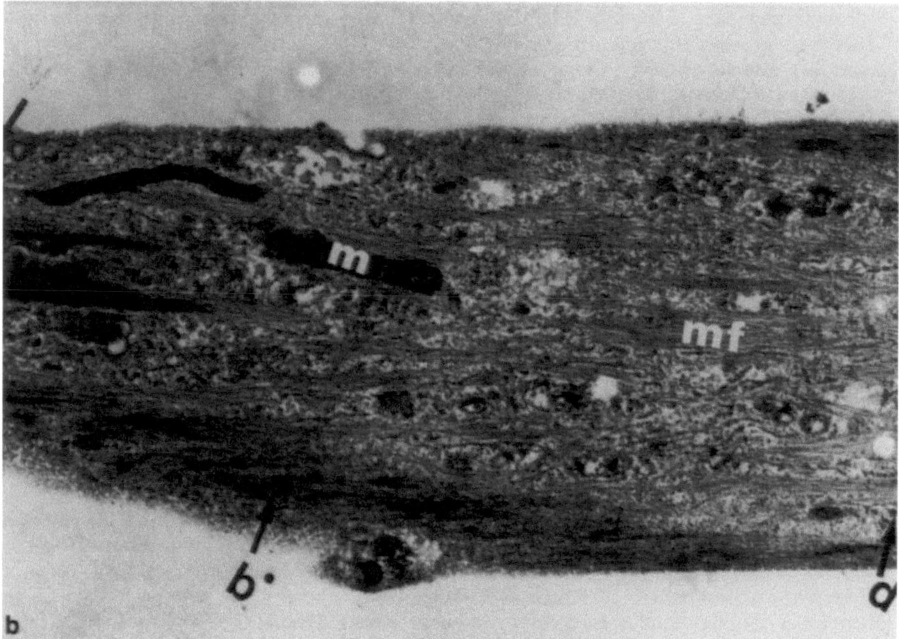

Fig. 4a,b. Cultured fibroblasts from palmar fascia of a patient with carpal tunnel syndrome (a) and from a patient with Dupuytren's contracture (b). Bundles of 6–8 nm microfilaments (*mf*) extend through the cytoplasm. *M*, mitochondria. (From Murrell et al. 1989) ×14 500 (a), ×5700 (b)

propose that one source of noxious stimuli is oxygen free radicals (Murrell et al. 1987a,b, 1988, 1989, 1990; Murrell and Hueston 1990). The source and effects of these species are outlined in our chapter titled Oxygen Free Radicals and Dupuytren's Disease. Vascular narrowing may occur both prior to the onset and during the progression of Dupuytren's contracture.

Acknowledgments. We thank Mrs. Joan Farmer for her excellent electron microscopic preparations, and the patients and surgeons of the Nuffield Orthopaedic Centre for tissue samples. GACM was supported by the Rhodes Trust.

References

Abercrombie M, Heaysman JEM (1966) The directional movement of fibroblasts emigrating from cultured explants. Ann Med Exp Fenn 44:161–165

Bazin S, LeLous M, Duance VC, Sims TJ, Bailey AJ, Gabbiani G, D'Andiran G, Pizzolato G, Browski A, Nicoletis C, Delaunay A (1980) Biochemistry and histology of the connective tissue of Dupuytren's disease lesions. Eur J Clin Invest 10:9–16

Dupuytren G (1834) Permanent retraction of the fingers produced by an affection of the palmar fascia: clinical lectures on surgery. Lancet 2:222–225

Gabbiani G, Majno G (1972) Dupuytren's contracture: fibroblast contraction? Am J Pathol 66:131–146

Gabbiani G, Montandon D (1985) The myofibroblasts in Dupuytren's disease and other fibromatoses. In: Hueston JT, Tubiana R (eds) Dupuytren's disease. Churchill Livingstone, Edinburgh, pp 86–93

Gokel JM, Hübner G (1977) Occurrence of myofibroblasts in the different phases of morbus Dupuytren (Dupuytren's contracture). Beitr Pathol 161:166–175

Goldman RD, Schloss JA, Stangen JM (1976) Organizational changes of actin-like microfilaments during animal cell movement. Cold Spring Harbour Conf Cell Prolif 3: 217

Iwasaki H, Müller H, Stutte HJ, Brennscheidt U (1984) Palmar fibromatosis (Dupuytren's contracture). Ultrastructural and enzyme histochemical studies of 43 cases. Virchows Arch [A] 405:41–53

Kilo C, Vogler N, Williamson JR (1972) Muscle capillary basement membrane changes related to ageing and to diabetes mellitus. Diabetes 21:881–905

Kischer CW, Speer DP (1984) Microvascular changes in Dupuytren's contracture. J Hand Surg 9:58–62

Kischer CW, Theis C, Chvapil M (1982) Perivascular myofibroblasts and microvascular occlusion in hypertrophic scars and keloids. Hum Pathol 13:819–824

Legge JWH, McFarlane RM (1981) Prediction of results of Dupuytren's disease. J Hand Surg 5:608–616

MacCallum P, Hueston JT (1962) The pathology of Dupuytren's contracture. Aust N Z J Surg 31:241–253

Millesi H (1985) The clinical and morphological course of Dupuytren's disease. In: Hueston JT, Tubiana R (eds) Dupuytren's disease. Churchill Livingstone, Edinburgh, pp 49–59

Mohr W, Vossbeck G (1985) Proliferation and ^{3}H-proline incorporation of cells of Dupuytren's fibromatosis. Z Rheumatol 44:226–230

Murrell GAC (1988) Studies on Dupuytren's contracture. Thesis, Oxford University

Murrell GAC, Hueston JT (1990) The aetiology of Dupuytren's contracture. Aust N Z J Surg 60:22–26

Murrell GAC, Francis MJO, Bromley L (1987a) Free radicals and Dupuytren's contracture. Br Med J 295:1373–1375

Murrell GAC, Pilowsky E, Murrell TGC (1987b) A hypothesis on the resolution of Dupuytren's contracture with allopurinol. Specul Sci Technol 10:107–112

Murrell GAC, Francis MJO, Howlett CR (1989) Dupuytren's contracture: fine structure in relation to etiology. J Bone Joint Surg [Br] 71:367–373

Murrell GAC, Francis MJO, Bromley L (1990) Modulation of fibroblast proliferation by oxygen free radicals. Biochem J 265:659–665

Nézelof C (1985) Histological aspects of Dupuytren's contracture. In: Hueston JT, Tubiana R (eds) Dupuytren's disease. Churchill Livingstone, Edinburgh, pp 22–27

Tomasek JJ, Schultz RJ, Episalla CW, Newman SA (1986) The cytoskeleton and extracellular matrix of the Dupuytren's disease "myofibroblast": an immunofluorescence study of a nonmuscle cell type. J Hand Surg 11:365–371

Tomasek JJ, Schultz RJ, Haaksma CJ (1987) Extracellular matrix-cytoskeletal connections at the surface of the specialized contractile fibroblast (myofibroblast) in Dupuytren's disease. J Bone Joint Surg [Am] 69:1400–1407

Vracko R (1970a) Skeletal muscle capillaries in diabetics: a quantitative analysis. Circulation 41:271–284

Vracko R (1970b) Skeletal muscle capillaries in nondiabetics: a quantitative analysis. Circulation 41:285–297

Vracko R (1974) Basal lamina layering in diabetes mellitus: evidence for accelerated rate of cell death and cell regeneration. Diabetes 23:94–104

Werner C, Elmqvist D, Ohlin P (1983) Pressure and nerve lesion in the carpal tunnel. Acta Orthop Scand 54:312–316

The Significance of Skin Anchoring Fibres in Palmar Fibrosis: Brief Comment

A. Meinel

In a postmortem study I examined the texture and dynamics of the fiber system in the distal palm. Using microdissection and, for the first time, sections from adult plastinated hands the following observations were made.

In contrast to the static fixed state of the skin in the central palm, in the distal palm an extremely mobile or dynamic skin anchoring system allows the enclosed tissue to fold during finger flexion and to extend during finger stretching. All fibers in this "crumble zone" anchor the dermis, more or less mobilely to the base of the first phalanx. Neither on the volar nor on the lateral apsects of the tendon sheaths could fascial structures or longitudinal bands be shown.

The cutis in the predigital region is fixed by shorter, delimitated osteocutaneous fibers. This is in contrast to the interdigital region, where the web cutis is anchored by cutaneous-cutaneous vertical fibers enclosing fatty tissue.

In the distal third of the crumble zone the so-called natatory ligament is present. In the intact dermis-covered tissue these fibers represent a special part of the osteocutaneous fiber network and not a transverse ligament between index and small fingers. This impression of a ligament, according to my findings, is nothing else but an artifact after classical preparation with skin removal. The cutanous ligaments described by Grayson and Cleland are actually the lateral part of the skin anchoring system in the digital zone.

In the crumble zone, the skin anchoring fibers are exposed to extensive movement – during finger stretching the fibers distend, while during finger flexion they are compressed. Dupuytren's disease starts with the well known nodule, which is established in the fibrofatty tissue, as described by Hueston, with limitation of fiber movement. As the ulnar fingers are mainly held in a flexed position and the radial fingers in a stretched position, the diseased and arrested fiber texture corresponds to these finger positions. The so interposed nodule is exposed to stress, with cord transformation as a result of stress adaptation, such as occurs in scars. If the Dupuytren tissue comes in contact with the palamar aponeurosis, its longitudinal bands are stretched and become hypertrophic. In this respect the Dupuytren tissue is a new tissue, with nodule or cord formation according to stress adaptation. Thus, there is no finger contraction, but rather retraction, as Dupuytren called it, in the predominant finger position. The anatomical structure of all other fibromatoses in positions arising from the palm can also be explained in this manner.

Pathobiochemistry of Fibrillar Component

Collagen Changes in Dupuytren's Disease

A.J. Bailey

Introduction

The major biochemical characteristic of Dupuytren's disease (DD) is the progressive and irreversible deposition of excess fibrous collagen. This proliferation of collagen certainly impairs normal function, but in some as yet unknown way it also provides the disease with its characteristic clinical feature, flexure of the fingers.

The major questions in DD are: (1) What are the stimuli that actuate the process of collagen proliferation? (2) Can one inhibit or reverse this excess deposition of collagen? (3) What is the mechanism by which the tissue contracts?

A prerequisite of any hypothesis to account for the characteristic features of DD is knowledge of the changes taking place in the collagenous structure of the aponeurosis. It cannot be assumed that all fibrotic situations are similar nor that any particular stimulating factor produces identical effects. For example, changes of collagen type follow different paths during fibrosis of the skin and kidney in scleroderma (Black et al. 1985) and during normal and hypertrophic scarring in the dermis (Bailey et al. 1975b). Any proposed stimulating factor must produce all the changes observed to occur in the collagen in DD. In contrast to most fibrotic situations, in DD one can distinguish the early and late stages of the disease. It is therefore possible to follow, at least in part, the course of the disease, and from the early stages it should be possible to distinguish between a variety of suggested stimulating factors.

The lesion primarily involves the palmar aponeurosis, i.e., the collagenous fascia or fibrous sheet separating the flexor tendon from the overlying fibrofatty layer. In the early stages discrete highly cellular nodules form, but in the later stages few nodules are present and the characteristic feature is dense fibrotic bands or cords along the aponeurosis. These changes result in flexural contraction of one or more fingers towards the palm. Studies on the collagenous tissue have therefore concentrated on comparing the nodules and the contracture bands.

Alterations in the Collagenous Tissue

Changes in: (a) physical appearance of the fibres and their composition in terms of genetic type of collagen; (b) posttranslational modification and extracellular cross-linking and (c) the organisation of the tissues have been reported (for recent review see McFarlane et al. 1990).

Biochemical Changes

Studies on DD have attempted to identify and analyse at least three regions of the aponeurosis: (1) the highly cellular nodules, (2) the fibrous bands and (3) the apparently unaffected regions.

Composition. There is a progressive increase in the proportion of collagen in the aponeurosis from the control, at about 60%, to the bands, at about 90% and even higher in the nodules (Bazin et al. 1980; Brinkley-Parsons et al. 1981; Hamamoto et al. 1982). The amount of neutral-salt soluble and acid soluble collagen was very small, about 0.2%, from the diseased tissue compared to virtually nothing from the control. Similarly, the amount of collagen digestible by pepsin treatment increased from 80% in the controls to almost complete solubilisation for the diseased tissue, as would be expected for immature collagen.

Compositional analysis of the collagen extracted revealed a higher level of hydroxylation, increasing from five to 13 residues of hydroxylysine per 1000 residues (Brinkley-Parsons et al. 1981). This increase was accompanied by a parallel increase in the number of glycosylated hydroxylysines so that the

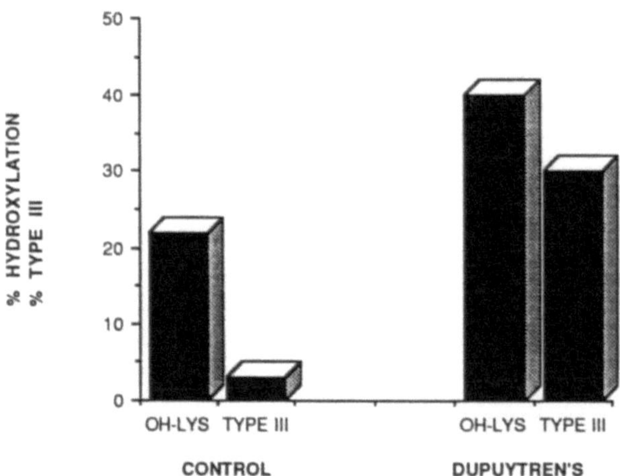

Fig. 1. Changes in the levels of hydroxylysine and type III collagen in Dupuytren's disease compared to control tissue

relative proportion of glycosylated hydroxylysines remained constant. Increased glycosylation occurred in both type I and type III collagens. The overall increase in the hydroxylation of the bands is illustrated in Fig. 1.

Collagen Types. Chemical determination of the ratio of type I to type III collagen has been carried out using either pepsin digestion, which solubilised over 90% of the collagen and therefore gave a representative sample (Bailey et al. 1977; Bazin et al. 1980; Gelberman et al. 1980), or complete dissolution of the sample by cyanogen bromide in formic acid (Brinkley-Parsons et al. 1981). Similar results were obtained for ratios of types I to III. Basically there was an increase from 1%–2% type III in the normal aponeurosis to 10%–15% in the apparently uninvolved, 10%–20% in the nodules, and 30%–40% in the fibrous bands (Fig. 1).
Murrell et al. (1989) have suggested that the change in the type I to III ratio is due to a decrease in the synthesis of type I collagen. However, this proposal is based on decreased synthesis of type I collagen from fibroblasts in high density culture and may not relate to in vivo conditions. The decrease in type I necessary to account for the apparent increase in type III from 3% to 30% would be dramatic and unlikely in a fibrotic condition.
These changes in collagen types determined by analysis of the tissue are analogous to those occurring in granulation tissue of dermal wounds (Bailey et al. 1975a) and in hypertrophic scars (Bailey et al. 1975b). One would expect the greatest amount of type III in the nodules, where there is a rapid proliferation of collagen, and decreasing amounts in the bands as they mature, if Dupuytren's contracture follows the pattern of normal wounds and fibrotic lesions. However, a large amount of type III would be retained over a long time period if the bands follow a similar course to those of the hypertrophic scar. Cross-link studies show that the DD bands do not mature, indicating more rapid turnover of collagen in the band. In addition, analysis of collagen from patients with long-standing Dupuytren's revealed biochemical changes similar to those in short-term disease (Brinkley-Parsons et al. 1981), indicating a failure to mature analogous to what occurs in the hypertrophic scar.
Other collagen types have been detected, as in granulation tissue, but in much smaller amounts. The relative proportions of type V and type I trimer were found to double from 5% to 9% and 2% to 5%, respectively. These increases are similar to those found in hypertrophic scars (Ehrlich et al. 1982). Type VI collagen (Timpl and Engel 1987) is not detectable in normal tendon, but examination of the aponeurosis of Dupuytren's revealed the presence of type VI in the fascicular sheath. Electron microscopic examination of the nodules and bands showed typical 100 nm banded fibrils, but supporting evidence that the fibrils were type VI has not yet been provided by immunofluorescent staining.

Cross-Linking. Distinct differences in the cross-link patterns were reported by Bailey and coworkers (Bailey et al. 1977; Bazin et al. 1980) and have been confirmed by others (Brinkley-Parsons et al. 1981; Gelberman et al. 1980;

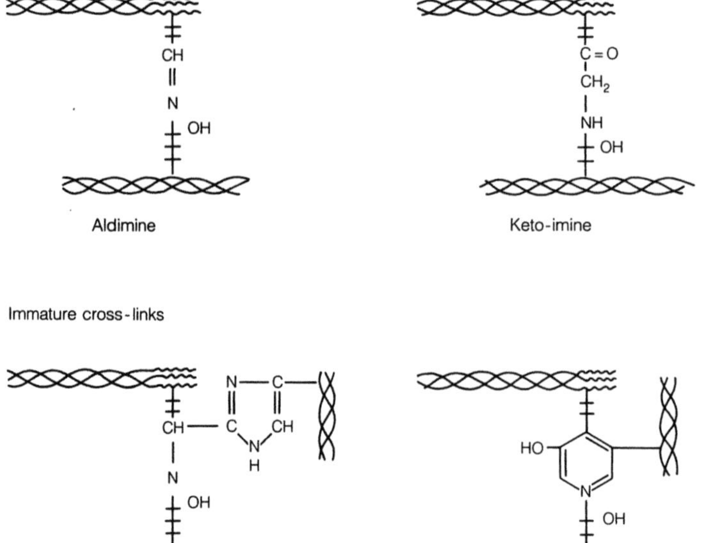

Fig. 2. *Top,* formation of the divalent reducible cross-links in developing collagen fibres. *Bottom,* further reaction of these cross-links to form the trivalent nonreducible cross-links found in mature tissues

Hanyu et al. 1984). As anticipated for mature collagen the control tissue revealed hexosyl lysines as the major reducible components, the divalent reducible cross-links being barely detectable. In contrast, the major reducible components of the nodules and the bands were the two reducible cross-links, the aldimine dehydro-hydroxylysinonorleucine and the keto-imine, hydroxylysino-keto-norleucine (Fig. 2). The reported increased levels of lysyl oxidase (Hamamoto et al. 1982) are consistent with the higher levels of these reducible cross-links. Surprisingly the apparently unaffected parts of the aponeurosis also showed increased amounts of the reducible cross-links, although a significant level of hexosyl lysines is still present. It should be remembered that the hexosyl lysines are not cross-links but can be considered good indicators of maturity (Bailey et al. 1974). Reducible cross-links are only present in immature tissues, and hexosyl lysine in mature tissue. Hanyu et al. (1984) reported equal amounts of pyridinoline in the normal and affected aponeurosis and concluded that the cross-link was not involved in the pathogenesis of the disease. Recently we have reanalysed the tissues for the non-reducible cross-links, histidino-hydroxylysinonorleucine (HHL) and pyridinoline (Fig. 2). The levels of HHL decreased by about 50% in the bands compared to the controls, as expected for an immature tissue. In contrast, a

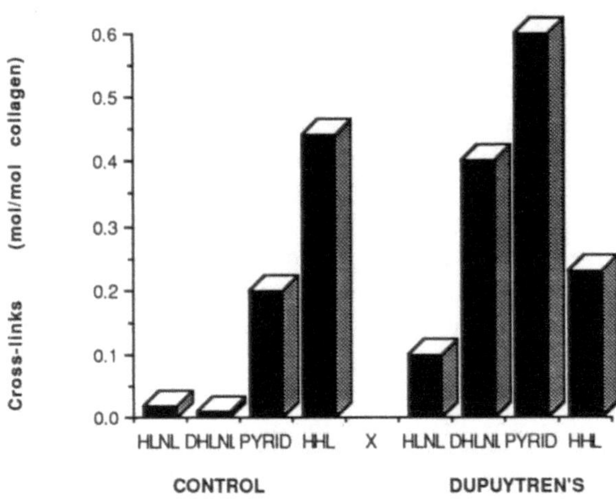

Fig. 3. Changes in the cross-linking levels in Dupuytren's disease compared to controls. *HLNL*, hydroxylysinonorleucine *DHLNL*, dihydroxylysinonorleucine; *Pyrid*, hydroxylysino-pyridinoline; *HHL*, histidino-hydroxylysinonorleucine the reduced forms of the aldimine and keto-imine respectively

significant increase of about threefold in the pyridinoline levels occurred in the DD bands compared to the controls (Fig. 3). This finding is consistent with the overall increase in hydroxylation and DHLNL, rather than indicating maturity of the tissue.

The apparently unaffected aponeurosis shows clear signs of some newly synthesised collagen, whilst the highly active nodules contain completely new collagen. The bands are mainly newly synthesised collagen but contain some mature features similar to the control, i.e., increased hexosyl lysines, clearly indicating that some maturation of the tissue has occurred.

Elastic Fibres. These fibres are a two component system consisting mainly of elastin but with a small proportion of microfibrils. Analysis of the amount of elastin was determined by the cross-links desmosine and iso-desmosine and found to be decreased by about 70% in the DD bands from a level of about 1% in the controls, consistant with increased amounts of newly synthesised collagen.

Structural Changes

Briefly, histological changes in DD (Hueston 1963; Larson et al. 1960; Millesi 1965; Millesi et al. 1983; Tubiana 1967) revealed two components, a highly cellular nodule and a virtually acellular scar tissue. The nodules are characterised by a network of thin collagen fibres and proteoglycans metachromatic to toluidine blue. In contrast, the fibres of the bands are more tightly packed and more orientated in a preferred direction than those of the normal aponeurosis.

Scanning electron microscopy has revealed similar changes (Hunter and Ogdon 1975; Legge et al. 1981). Using transmission electron microscopy it is seen that the individual collagen fibers possess the normal structure and typical axial banding pattern of 67 nm. Similarly, analysis of the fibres by both wide and low angle X-ray diffraction showed no detectable difference between normal tissue and that from DD patients (Brinkley-Parsons et al. 1981).

It would appear from these results that the structure of the individual collagen fibres in DD is indistinguishable from that of normal collagen fibres. However, using indirect immunofluorescence (von der Mark 1982) it is possible to determine the distribution of the various collagen types in tissues and a different picture emerges. When the normal aponeurosis was stained with antibodies to type I collagen uniform staining occurred as expected. With types III and V the staining was limited to the periphery of the regularly arranged bundles or fascicules (Bazin et al. 1980). This can be compared to the staining of Achilles tendon, where the fibre bundles of type I were surrounded mainly by fibres of type III with some IV and V collagen (Duance et al. 1977). A similar analysis of the diseased aponeurosis failed to reveal bundles with a surrounding sheath. The nodules were intensely stained with antibodies to type III and type V fibres, which were both distributed randomly amongst the major type I fibres, and the bundles were clearly grossly disorganised. The fibrous bands revealed aligned fibres which stained for both type I and type III, but the type III fibres were randomly distributed rather than confined to the bundle sheaths as observed in the normal aponeurosis (Fig. 4). Staining of the apparently unaffected areas revealed much the same picture as for the normal aponeurosis, except that in some areas the staining of the bundle sheath was more intense.

The immunohistochemical evidence clearly suggests that it is at the higher level of order of the fibre bundles or fascicules that the structure has broken down rather than at the level of the individual fibres themselves.

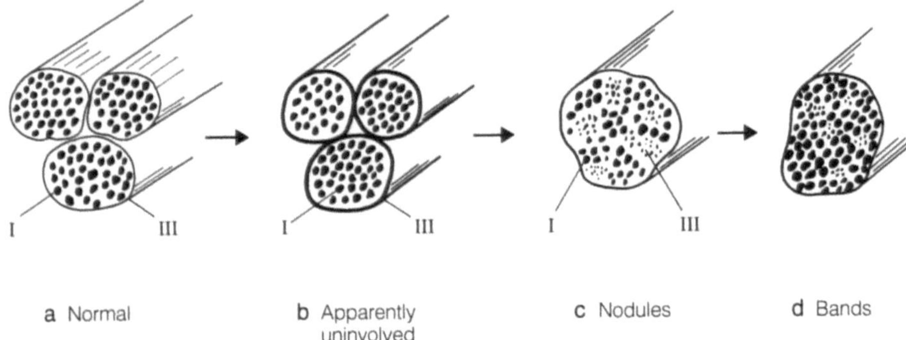

Fig. 4a–d. Development of Dupuytren's disease. **a** Normal aponeurosis: fascicular structure with type I fibres sheathed in type III collagen. **b** Apparently uninvolved: thickening of the fascicular sheath. **c** Nodules: loss of the fascicular structure and the formation of new fine fibres. **d** Bands or cords, tightly packed fibrils of type I and type III collagen but no fascicular structure

Discussion of the Biochemical and Structural Changes

The significance of the changes in collagen types in relation to DD is unknown. Excessive hydroxylation and the presence of type III collagen are typical of rapidly growing tissues with high plasticity, such as granulation tissue and embryonic tissue, rather than contracted tissues in particular. It is unlikely these changes are products solely of the myofibroblast since they are consistent in all cases compared to the sporadic appearance of the myofibroblasts themselves.

The major biochemical features of DD are similar to those of hypertrophic scar tissue in that the tissue fails to mature as in normal scars but, instead, maintains a high turnover rate.

We also observed that the disease is not strictly focal and limited to the nodules but is clearly evident in apparently unaffected parts of the aponeurosis (Bailey et al. 1979; Brinkley-Parsons et al. 1981). This is consistent with the well accepted clinical observation that DD can recur within the same aponeurosis, presumably due to failure to eliminate the disease by excision only of the grossly affected tissue. We have suggested (Bazin et al. 1980) that the disease could be initiated and/or propagated by cells migrating along the collagen bundle sheaths, that is, the equivalent in the aponeurosis of the endotendinium. The presence of myofibroblasts in the apparently unaffected aponeurosis (Bazin et al. 1980) supports this proposal, but this latter finding was not suported by Brinkley-Parsons (1981). However, Gelberman et al. (1980) have correlated recurrence of DD with those patients in whom myofibroblasts were detected.

As McGrouther (1982) and McFarlane (1974) have pointed out, the pattern of DD is not random but the nodules and tendonous bands follow anatomical pathways, that is, primarily the longitudinal fibres of the palmar fascia. This is precisely where there are lines of force passing from the palm to the fingers. Fibroblasts have long been known to be stimulated to lay down collagen along lines of force. This progression along the aponeurosis rather than specific localisation is consistent with the important finding that the apparently uninvolved part of the aponeurosis shows biochemical changes.

The aponeurosis has been shown to have a fascicular structure, the major type I fibre bundles being surrounded by a sheath of type III fibres. This structure is grossly disorganised in the highly cellular nodules and, although the fibres realign in the bands, the destroyed fascicular structure is not reformed, the type III being distributed at random. The ultrastructure studies have certainly demonstrated that the collagen fibres themselves are normal, but it is at the higher level of the fibre bundle structure of the aponeurosis that irreversible damage is seen.

Mechanism of Contraction

Several theories of contracture have been proposed, unfortunately none of which can be considered satisfactory. The early proposal, that contraction was due to the ability of collagen to shrink in vivo (Paylingwright 1954, cited in Ryan et al. 1974), can be discounted. Such shrinkage only occurs at 65°C or in strong denaturing agents and therefore cannot occur in vivo. Furthermore, it would be easy to demonstrate the presence of the denatured form of collagen, i.e., gelatin, by histological and physical techniques. However, the work did focus attention on the extracellular matrix. A further proposal suggested the fibres were shorter due to structural disorganisation (Hueston 1974) but there is little supporting evidence. In fact the fibres in the bands tend to be highly organized. More recently Legge et al. (1981) have proposed that the shorter wave form and helical twist of the fibres might account for the shortening.

In 1972 Gabbiani and Majno described the presence of the myofibroblast in DD tissue, and the emphasis switched to the cellular components. They proposed that as an active contractile cell the myofibroblast was involved in the contraction process. Since that time many investigators have confirmed the presence of these cells in the palmar fascia of DD patients. The role of these cells must involve physical connections between the cells and the collagen fibres. Although it is an attractive hypothesis which can account for contraction in all types of wounds, confirmation of their role and precise mechanism of action is still awaited.

The proliferation of collagen disrupts the normal smooth working surface of the aponeurosis and could lead to attachment to adjoining palmar fascia ligaments and possibly to the dermis. This would certainly prevent smooth movements of these ligaments in normal use of the hand, and the force exerted on flexing the fingers could lead to further proliferation of collagen at these points. Indeed, the fibrotic lesion can be seen to follow the lines of tension and look like a thickened tendon. This type of organisation would reduce extensibility of the tissue but quite why this leads to flexural contraction of the fingers rather than fibrotic swelling in the palmar fascia is ot clear. It is therefore worth considering a number of concepts and possible mechanisms of contraction.

First, a rather naive concept would be that, since the fingers' normal resting position is the relaxed 'fist' position, microadhesions could build up, slowly restricting the ability to flex the fingers; indeed, flexing would aggravate the fibrosis at just these attachment points. This hypothesis would not involve any 'contraction' of the collagenous tissue, only an inability to stretch.

Second, Glimcher and colleagues (Brinkley-Parsons et al. 1981) consider the fibres of the palmar fascia of DD to be structurally normal and that there is no folding or bunching of the fibres. They view the process of contraction as progressive replacement of the tissue fabric by a perfectly normal new piece of fabric but considerably shorter in length. However, this does not answer the question why part of the fascia is replaced by a shorter piece. The authors suggest that this can be achieved by myofibroblasts pulling the edges of the

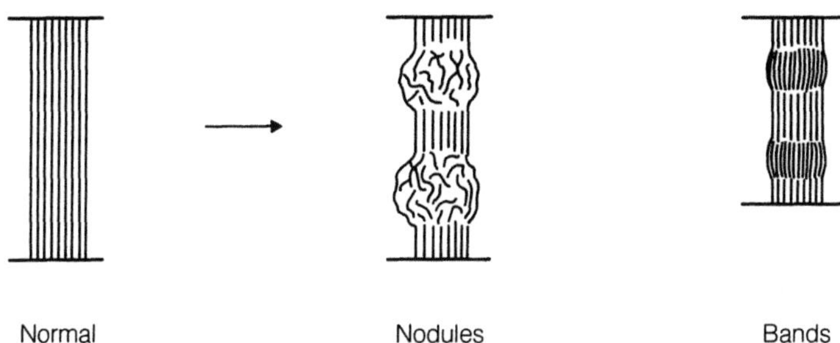

Fig. 5. Contracture of the aponeurosis. The multiple, highly cellular and grossly disorganized fibrous nodules formed in the aponeurosis contract like scar tissue to form the shorter organized fibrous bands, thus reducing the overall length of the aponeurosis. The actual mechanism of contraction is presumably through the same mechanism as scar tissue, possibly involving fibroblasts or myofibroblasts

affected tissue closer together. We are therefore back to the hypothesis that the basic mechanism is contraction of the tissue by myofibroblasts.

It is highly unlikely that contraction involves a smooth progressive renewal of the palmar fascia fibres with a structure similar to the original but considerably shorter, as proposed by Glimcher and coworkers. There is considerable disorganisation in the initial stages within the nodules and the final clinical manifestations are of thickened protruberances in the palm clearly demonstrating excessive collagenous tissue. This cannot all be laid down in the same manner as the original aponeurosis. The formation of a 'normal' aponeurosis would entail the orderly development of the fascicules bound together by type III collagenous sheaths as in normal aponeurosis. The high proportion of type III collagen suggested that this was unlikely and recent immunohistochemical studies of the bands clearly demonstrate the absence of a fasicular structure.

Third, an alternative simple theory involving contraction would then be as follows: The nodules formed along the aponeurosis contract like any wound as they progress to fibrous bands. The aponeurosis has a fixed length from the palm to the digits hence the additive effect of the contraction of multiple nodules by myofibroblasts would effectively shorten the aponeurosis which, having fixed anchorage points, would result in flexure of the fingers (Fig. 5). Further, the fibres in the bands are orientated to a greater degree than the normal aponeurosis and do not therefore possess the flexibility of the original fasicular organization.

The precise contractile mechanism is not yet clear but must involve fibroblasts or myofibroblasts contracting the nodular space (Gabbiani and Majno 1972). Fibroblasts certainly have the ability to contract fibrous collagen 'gels' and these cells are seen to possess bundles of intracellular actin filaments. It has been proposed that these filaments attach to the cell membrane through the integrins and that fibronectin acts as the extracellular adhesive between the integrins and the collagen fibres (Singer et al. 1984; Hynes 1987). The contractile ability of the cytoskeletal actin filaments remains to be elucidated.

Concluding Remarks

In our own studies we have shown that the first signs of change in DD are observed in the interfasicular connective tissue of the aponeurosis suggesting the disease is initiated in this region. Following progression from the nodules to the bands we have shown that, although the fibres are well orientated in the bands, there is no fascicular structure corresponding to the unaffected aponeurosis. Further, we have demonstrated that these changes are not unique but follow the same pattern as those occurring in wound granulation tissue and more particularly the hypertrophic scar. The inability of the collagen to mature suggests that the stimulating factor may be endogenous. Unfortunately, the reports of changes occurring when fibroblasts are grown in vitro are conflicting. Some workers report changes analogous to the in vivo observations whilst others report no differences from the controls. These differences may be due to the use of primary cultures as opposed to cells obtained after several passages.

It is of course possible that the collagen of DD patients is genetically defective and therefore responds in an abnornal way to stimuli that would not affect normal individuals. The genetic background to DD has been investigated. Welsh and Spencer (1990) concluded that it is not an HLA-linked disease but, based on the typing of patients using specific collagen type antibodies, suggested that a form of DD may indeed be an inherited disorder. If the collagen is abnormal then the change must be subtle since no biochemical difference has been reported to date.

The ultimate solution to the disease must be to identify the stimulating factor, an exogenous mediator or transformed cell which, based on the recurrence of the disease, albeit slow, appears to be retained in the tissue. A currently fashionable stimulating factor is the superoxide free radical (Halliwell and Gutteridge 1989), production of which has been invoked in the case of DD to account for the proliferation of fibroblasts (Murrell et al. 1990). However, it is not clear whether the earliest recognizable event, i.e., damage to the endothelium, is caused by free radicals or whether the damage results in ischaemia with consequent production of free radicals.

Unfortunately, in DD, fibrosis is already excessive before clinical presentation and knowledge of the stimulating factor is unlikely to help clinically at this stage. However, based on our understanding of the fundamentals of the synthesis and degradation of collagen, there are several approaches that might result in regression of the fibrosis: (1) control of the production of mRNA at the transcriptional level; (2) control of the posttranslational modification by specific inhibitors of, for example, prolyl hydroxylase, which are known to be effective in reducing synthesis; (3) controlled degradation of the collagen by selective use of collagenases and neutral proteinases. Unfortunately, at the present time inhibiting synthesis and the removal of excess collagen present formidable difficulties.

Although much has been learned about the changes of the collagen in DD, this knowledge has not yet helped our understanding of the nature of the stimulating factor nor the fundamental mechanism of contraction. However, the recent increased understanding of the nature of collagen, its complex biosynthetic and degradative pathways, together with a more detailed biochemical analysis of the progression of the disease will surely provide answers in the very near future to these two major questions in DD.

References

Bailey AJ, Robins SP, Balian G (1974) Biological significance of the intermolecular crosslinks of collagen. Nature 251:105

Bailey AJ, Sims TJ, Le Lous M, Bazin S (1975a) Collagen polymorphism in experimental granulation tissue. Biochem Biophys Res Commun 66:1160

Bailey AJ, Bazin S, Sims TJ, Le Lous M, Nicoletis C, Delaunay A (1975b) Characterisation of the collagen of human hypertrophic and normal scars. Biochim Biophys Acta 405:412

Bailey AJ, Sims TJ, Gabbiani G, Bazin S, Le Lous M (1977) Collagen of Dupuytren's disease. Clin Sci Mol Med 53:499

Bailey AJ, Shellswell GB, Duance VC (1979) Identification and change of collagen types indifferentiating myoblasts and developing chicken muscle. Nature 278:67–69

Bazin S, Le Lous M, Duance VC, Sims TJ, Bailey AJ, Gabbiani G, D'Andiran G, Pizzolato G, Browski A, Nicoletis C, Delaunay A (1980) Biochemistry and histology of the connective tissue of Dupuytren's disease lesions. Eur J Clin Invest 10:9–16

Black CM, Duance VC, Light ND, Bailey AJ (1985) Immunology and biochemical investigations into the collagen changes. In: Black CM, Jayson MIV (eds) Systemic sclerosis. Gower, New York, pp 192–197

Brinkley-Parsons D, Glimcher MJ, Smith RJ, Albin R, Adams IP (1981) Biochemical changes in the collagen of the palmar fascia in patients with Dupuytren's disease. J Bone Joint Surg [Am] 63:787

Duance VC, Restall DJ, Beard H, Bourne FJ, Bailey AJ (1977) The location of three collagen types in skeletal muscle. FEBS Lett 79:248–252

Ehrlich HP, Brown H, White BS (1982) Evidence for type V and I trimer collagens in Dupuytren's contracture palmar fascia. Biochem Med 28:273–284

Gabbiani G, Majno G (1972) Dupuytren's contracture: fibroblast contraction? An ultrastructural study. Am J Pathol 66:131

Gelberman RH, Amiel D, Rudolph RM, Vance RM (1980) Dupuytren's contracture. J Bone Joint Surg [Am] 62:425

Gokel JM, Hubner G (1977) Intracellular 'fibrous long spacing' collagen in morbus Dupuytren's. Beitr Pathol 161:176

Halliwell B, Gutteridge JMC (1989) Free radicals in biology and medicine. Clarendon, Oxford

Hamamoto M, Ueba Y, Sudo Y, Sanada M, Yamamuro Y, Takeda T (1982) Dupuytrens contracture: morphological and biochemical changes in the palmar aponeurosis. Hand 14:237

Hanyu T, Tajima T, Sasiki S, Fujimoto D, Isemura M, Yosizawa Z (1984) Biochemical studies on the collagen of the palmar aponeurosis affected with Dupuytren's disease. Tohoku J Exp Med 142:437

Hueston JT (1963) Dupuytrens contracture. Livingstone, Edinburgh

Hueston JT (1974) Aetiological questions in Dupuytren's contracture. In: Hueston JT, Tubiana R (eds) Dupuytren's disease. Churchill Livingstone, Edinburgh, p 29

Hunter JAA, Ogdon C (1975) Dupuytren's contracture. II. Scanning electron-microscopic observations. Br J Plast Surg 28:19

Hynes RO (1987) Integrins, a family of cell surface receptors. Cell 48:549

Larson RD, Takagishi N, Posch JL (1960) The pathogenesis of Dupuytren's contracture. J Bone Joint Surg 421:993

Legge JW, Finlay JB, McFarlane RM (1981) A study of Dupuytren's tissue with the scanning electron microscope. J Hand Surg 6:482

McFarlane RM (1974) Patterns of the diseased fascia in the fingers in Dupuytren's contracture. Plast Reconstr Surg 54:31

McFarlane RM, McGrouther DA, Flint MH (1990) Dupuytren's disease. Churchill Livingstone, Edinburgh

McGrouther DA (1982) The microanatomy of Dupuytren's contracture. Hand 14:215

Millesi H (1965) Zur Pathogenese und Therapie der Dupuytrenschen Kontraktur. Ergeb Chir Orthop 47:51–101

Millesi H, Menzel J, Kovac W, Walzer LR, Mallinger R (1983) Morphologic studies to the pathology of Dupuytren's contracture. In: Williams HB, Canadian Society of Plastic Surgeons (eds) Montreal. The congress 1983. Transactions of the 8th International Congress of Mastic and Reconstructive Surgery, June 26–July 1, 1983, pp 641–643

Murrell GAC, Francis MJO, Howlett CR (1989) Dupuytren's contracture. J Bone Joint Surg [Br] 71:367–373

Murrell GAC, Francis MJO, Bromley L (1990) Modulation of fibroblast proliferation by oxygen free radicals. Biochem J 265:659–665

Ryan GB, Cliff WJ, Gabbiani G et al. (1974) Myofibroblasts in human granulation tissue. Human Pathol 5:55–67

Singer II, Kawka DW, Kazazis DM, Clark RAF (1984) In vivo co-distribution of fibronectin and actin fibres in granulation tissue. J Cell Biol 98:2091–2106

Timpl R, Engel J (1987) Type VI collagen. In: Mayne R, Burgeson RE (eds) Structure and function of collagen types. Academic, Orlando, pp 105–143

Tubiana R (1967) Les conceptions actuelles du traitement chirurgical de la maladie de Dupuytren. In: Orthopédie et traumatologie. Conférences d'enseignement. Expansion Scientifique, Paris, p 7

Von der Mark K (1982) Localisation of collagen types in tissue. Int Rev Connect Tissue Res 9:265

Welsh KI, Spencer JD (1990) In: McFarlane RM, McGrouther DA, Flint MH (eds) Dupuytren's disease. Churchill Livingstone, Edinburgh, pp 99–104

Connective Tissue Autoantibodies in Dupuytren's Disease: Associations with HLA DR3

E.J. Menzel, J. Neumüller, A. Rietsch, and H. Millesi

Introduction

The hypothesis that autoimmune phenomena might be associated with the pathogenesis of Dupuytren's contracture (DC) was advanced by Gay and Gay in 1972 [1]. This hypothesis was bolstered by Menzel et al. [2], who demonstrated the presence of circulating antibodies to collagen (ACA) in DC patients. These results were confirmed by Pereira et al. [3], showing a whole spectrum of autoantibodies to different collagen types in these patients. The mere demonstration of autoantibodies to connective tissue components, however, does not imply that these antibodies are instrumental in the pathogenesis of a disease. It only proves that autoimmune processes accompany the development of the disease, if only as innocent bystanders. The suggestion that autoantibodies to collagen might contribute to the perpetuation of DC is problematic, since the inflammatory component of this disease is not very pronounced. This is in contrast to the situation in rheumatoid arthritis (RA), which is characterized by circulating immune complexes, complement activation and ACA.

The basis of collagen autoimmunity seems to be an immunogenetic disposition. Thus, as shown by Klimiuk et al. [4], RA patients presenting with autoantibodies to native type II collagen (cartilage collagen) represent a distinct genetic subset characterized by an association with HLA DR3. In contrast, antibodies to denatured type II collagen are associated with HLA DR4, the class II histocompatibility antigen to which susceptibility for RA has been strongly linked [5]. Interestingly, an analogous association was demonstrated by Pereira et al. [3] in patients with DC. The condition itself may be familial. Two early studies [6,7] showing no association with the HLA system were followed by two investigations including the HLA DR locus [8,9]. According to these more recent publications there is a suggestion of an association with HLA DR4 and HLA B12, with a raised overall prevalence of the HLA-A1-B8-DR3 haplotype, although these associations did not reach statistical significance. A synopsis of HLA associations with collagen or elastin autoimmunity is presented in Table 1.

The immediate cause for the formation of autoantibodies to the various collagen types is unknown. Pereira et al. [3] suggested that the raised incidence

Table 1. Autoimmunity to collagen and the HLA system

Disease	Anti-collagen antibodies (type)	HLA association	Reference
Thromboangiitis obliterans	I	A1/B8	Smolen et al. [13]
RA	II den	DR 4	Rowley et al. [5]
RA	II	DR3/7	Sanders et al. [22]
RA	None	DR 4	Sanders et al. [22]
DC	II den	DR 4	Pereira et al. [3]
DC	I	DR 3	Menzel et al.
	Elastin	DR 3	(this chapter)

den, denaturated collagen.

of antibodies to native type III collagen may result from the considerable increase in the production of this collagen type at the site of the fibrotic lesion [10]. In contrast to collagen from the aponeurosis of normal adult subjects, the nodules, contracted bands and even the apparently uninvolved palmar fascia of DC patients contain substantial amounts of type III (fetal) collagen. These results were obtained by qualitative examination of SDS-polyacrylamide gels performed with pepsin digests of tissue samples. No information was given regarding how much total collagen was solubilized. The incidence of antibodies to type II collagen in DC patients [3] is intriguing, since this collagen type is rarely found even in the diseased palmar fascia [11]. The only possible interpretation of such a finding would be cross reactivity of ACA with different collagen types.

Here, we have attempted to correlate HLA typing results with ACA to collagens type I–IV and antielastin antibodies (ELAB) in DC patients and controls. Antibodies to kappa-elastin of bovine origin were first described in sera of severely atheromatous patients by Stein et al. [12]. ELAB are also found together with ACA in patients with thrombangiitis obliterans [13], another disease showing significant associations with the HLA system. In addition, we describe a sensitive enzyme immunoassay (EIA) for collagen type III and its utilization for determining the ratio of collagen type I: collagen type III in normal palmar aponeurosis and Dupuytren's lesions.

Materials and Methods

Enzyme Immunoassay for Antielastin Antibodies

Solubilized forms of elastin retain their immunological reactivity and can therefore be used for the detection of ELAB in solid phase assays. Among the several published methods to solubilize elastin we chose the procedure described by Robert and Poullain [14]. Starting material was a commercial preparation of insoluble elastin from bovine ligamentum nuchae (Sigma E

1625). What follows is a description of the preparation of soluble kappa 2 elastin: elastin powder (10 g) is suspended in 250 ml of 1 N KOH/ethanol (80:20, v/v) and stirred at 37°C for 60 min. After centrifugation at 16 000 g for 15 min the pellet is resuspended in KOH/ethanol and again heated for 60 min. The neutralized supernatant is lyophilized and redissolved in 0.02 M acetic acid. The soluble elastin is chromatographed on a Sephacryl S 200 column (Pharmacia) of the dimensions 1.8 × 26.0 cm (Fig. 1). Calibration was performed with human IgG and bovine serum albumin as molecular weight markers. For the assay of ELAB the molecular weight fraction between 40 000 and 65 000 (corresponding to the maximal molecular weight eluted) was used as soluble elastin antigen in the EIA procedure. To this end, the wells of NUNC microtiter plates were coated with 0.2 ml of the kappa 2 elastin solution of defined molecular weight range (0.1 mg/ml in a pH 7.5 phosphate or Tris buffer, 0.02 M, containing 0.45 M NaCl and 0.02% sodium azide). Incubation was for 3 days at 4°C. The coated plates were washed and incubated for 2 h at room temperature with phosphate buffered saline (PBS), containing 0.4% bovine serum albumin (BSA), to reduce nonspecific binding effects. After washing, 0.2 ml of a 1:20 dilution with PBS-0.1% Tween of each sample to be tested was added to each well (triplicate assays). Incubation was for 30 min at 37°C and 60 min at 4°C. After a threefold washing procedure, the second antibody, a 1:1000 dilution of anti-human IgG coupled to horseradish-peroxidase, in PBS-BSA (1%) without azide was added. Incubation and washing cycles were as above. Finally, the substrate ABTS was added and extinction measured in an ELISA reader at 405 nm after 10–30 min, depending on the intensity of color developed.

Each result is reported as the mean of triplicate assays, converted to the number of standard deviations of the normal control population above the normal mean value, as described by Wener et al. [15].

Enzyme Immunoassay for Anticollagen Antibodies

Antibodies to collagen types I–IV were determined by an analogous procedure as for ELAB. Coating was done at a much lower antigen concentration (5 µg/ml). Collagen type I was prepared from human infant dura mater, type II from human cartilage, type III from human skin and type IV from a commercial preparation of human placenta (Sigma C 7521). All collagens were extracted by peptic digestion and purified by salt fractionation [16]. They were used only in native form as EIA antigens. Evaluation of results was as described above for ELAB. Only duplicate assays were performed.

Quantitation of Collagen Type III in Tissue Samples

Samples were obtained immediately postoperatively and deep frozen or immediately processed. After complete removal of blood by thorough washing with PBS, the soaked samples were dried with paper towels and wet weight was determined. After mincing with scissors the tissue fragments were frozen in liquid nitrogen and homogenized in a Braun Dismembrator II (Teflon chambers, 3.0 ml, 9 mm balls from a ball bearing). All samples were completely transformed into powder. Digestion with pepsin of high purity (Sigma P 6887) was performed at an enzyme to substrate ratio of 1:10 in 0.5 M acetic acid for three days at 4°C. After ultracentrifugation the supernatants were assayed for type III collagen and total collagen. The collagen type III fraction was quantitated by a sandwich EIA method: briefly, anti-type III antibody from goat (Southern Biotechnology) was coated to NUNC microtiter wells at a dilution of 1:100. The antigen extract was then incubated with the solid phase and – after thorough washing – the bound type III collagen detected by second antibody (monoclonal anti-type III collagen from mouse, Heyl) at a dilution of 1:200, followed by an incubation step with sheep anti-mouse Ig in peroxidase-linked form (Amersham) at a dilution 1:2000–1:4000. Color was developed after adding ABTS. Different concentrations of pure type III collagen were analyzed in the same way to obtain a standard curve in the range 0.1–100 µg/ml type III collagen. Total collagen in the pepsin extract was assayed via Stegemann's method [17]. A direct quantitation of type I collagen by an analogous EIA method proved not feasible since the anti-type I antibodies available were of low quality. As control, immunofluorescence staining of formalin-fixed or frozen tissue sections was performed using anti-type III antibodies and anti-Ig antibodies in FITC-linked form (second antibodies). As an alternative, peroxidase-labeled second antibodies were used.

HLA Typing

The determination of HLA antigens of class I (HLA A, B, C locus) was performed using the microlymphocytotoxicity test (MLCT), NIH standard technique [18], while testing of the class II HLA antigens (only HLA DR subregion) was performed by the double fluorescence MLCT [19]. Every specificity was tested with three antisera of a different serum charge.

Statistics

As usual in HLA investigations, the chi^2 test obtained from 2 × 2 contingency tables was carried out. If one or more fields of the contingency tables were occupied by numbers <10, the Yate correction was performed. From the 2 × 2 contingency table relative risk was calculated as follows [20]:

$$RR = \frac{\text{Concordance} \times \text{absence of antigen and disease}}{\text{Discordance} \times \text{presence of antigen in absence of disease}}$$

Patients

There were 45 patients who suffered from DC and underwent surgical therapy; 59 healthy controls were selected for this study. HLA typing was performed in 42 DC patients and 47 controls; ELAB were determined in 38 patients and 50 controls; ACA in 22 DC patients and 50 controls.

Results

Autoantibodies to Collagen in DC Patients

The highest incidence of ACA in DC patients was observed for antibodies to type III collagen, closely followed by those to type I collagen. Autoantibodies to type IV collagen (basement membrane collagen) and type II collagen (cartilage collagen) were present in a minority of DC patients (Table 2). It is interesting to note that ACA-positive patients became negative upon reinspection 6 months after the first venipuncture (with the exception of one of seven patients assayed at two different postsurgical time intervals). This is

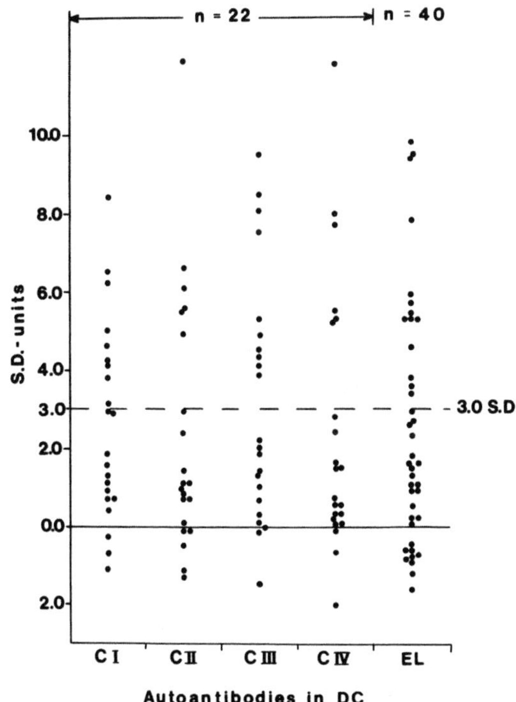

Fig. 1. Enzyme immunoassay results obtained by analysing Dupuytren's contracture (*DC*) sera for anti-collagen antibodies to collagen types I–IV and to elastin. *SD*, standard deviation

Table 2. Percentage of anti-collagen and anti-elastin antibodies in Dupuytren's contracture patients

Tissue antigen	Dupuytrens contracture ($n = 22/40$)	Controls[a] ($n = 50$)	Significance[b]
Collagen I	40.9	4.0	$p < 0.01$
Collagen II	27.3	8.0	$p < 0.01$
Collagen III	45.5	4.0	$p < 0.01$
Collagen IV	31.8	0	$p < 0.01$
Elastin kappa	40.0	15.1	$p < 0.05$

[a] For ELAB $n = 53$ controls.
[b] Dupuytren's contracture patients vs controls.

Table 3. Anticollagen antibody titer changes in 6 months[a]

Patient	I	II	III	IV
1	−/+	−/−	−/−	−/−
2	−/−	−/−	+/−	−/−
3	−/−	−/−	+/−	+/−
4	−/−	−/−	−/−	−/−
5	−/−	−/−	−/−	−/−
6	−/−	−/−	+/−	−/−
7	−/−	+/−	+/−	+/−

[a] Most antibodies disappear after 6 months.

shown in Tables 3 and 4. A graphical representation is given in Fig. 1, comparing high level ACA with low level ELAB. Individual results are shown in Table 5.

Autoantibodies to Elastin in DC Patients

Frequency and titer of ELAB are shown in Table 2 and Fig. 2. Individual results can be derived from Table 4. Interestingly, there was also a relatively high percentage of ELAB-positive control subjects (15% as opposed to 40% in the DC group).

Correlation with HLA Typing Results

HLA typing for class I antigens showed no remarkable difference between DC patients and controls or in ELAB-positive as compared to ELAB-negative individuals. Significant differences were found, however, for HLA class II antigen HLA-DR3, the only DR antigen with a statistically significant difference: 22 of 42 DC patients (52.4%) and 15 of 47 controls (31.9%) were

Table 4. Transitory nature of anti-collagen antibodies in a Dupuytren's contracture patient[a]

Collagen type	Anti-collagen antibody results (in SD units)	
	June 5, 1986	November 24, 1986
I	Negative	Negative
II	9.8	1.5
III	8.0	−1.1
IV	8.5	−2.0

[a] Patient number 7 (see Table 3); operated on Jan. 23, 1986.

Table 5. Autoantibodies to collagen and elastin in Dupuytren's contracture patients

Patient	Collagen type				Elastin (kappa)
	I	II	III	IV	
1	−	−	−	−	−
2	−	−	−	−	−
3	−	+	+	+	−
4	+	−	−	−	+
5	+	−	−	−	+
6	+	−	−	−	+
7	−	+	+	−	−
8	−	−	+	−	+
9	+	+	+	+	−
10	−	−	+	−	−
11	−	−	+	+	−
12	+	−	−	−	−
13	+	−	−	−	+
14	−	−	−	−	+
15	−	−	−	−	−
16	−	+	+	+	−
17	+	−	+	−	−
18	+	+	+	+	−
19	+	−	+	−	−
20	−	−	−	−	−
21	−	+	+	+	−
22	−	−	−	−	−

positive for HLA-DR3 (chi^2 = 3.82, of borderline significance; chi^2 value for p < 0.05 = 3.84; RR = 2.34). In addition, there was a significant correlation between presence of HLA-DR3 and increased concentration of ACA to type I collagen in DC patients (Table 6). Although no correlation of statistical significance was seen between ELAB positivity and HLA-DR3 in controls, the association of these autoantibodies with HLA-DR3 in the controls plus DC patients was statistically highly significant (Table 6).

Table 6. Association between Dupuytren's contracture (DC) and autoantibodies to connective tissue antigens and HLA DR3

Antibody	Dupuytren's contracture patients or controls	Significance
Collagen I	DC	$p < 0.05$
Collagen II	DC	n.s.
Collagen III	DC	n.s.
Collagen IV	DC	n.s.
Elastin	DC	n.s.
Elāstin	DC and controls	$p < 0.001$
ELAB and ACA	DC	n.s.
ELAB	DC: controls	$p < 0.05$
ACA	DC: controls	$p < 0.01$
Dupuytren	DC: controls	$p = 0.05$

ELAB, anti-elastin antibodies; ACA, anti-collagen antibodies.

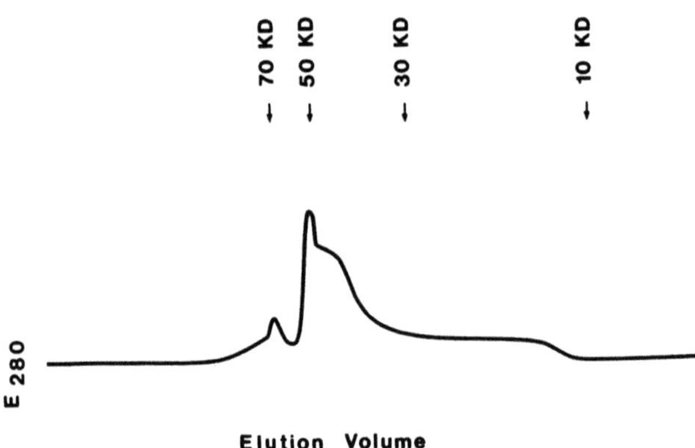

Fig. 2. Elution pattern of kappa-elastin chromatographed on Sephacryl S 200. *KD*, kilodaltons

Collagen Type III in DC Tissue

The type III sandwich EIA proved highly specific for this collagen type. Even a hundredfold excess of type I collagen did not significantly interfere with the quantitation of type III collagen (Figs. 3, 4). A much greater problem is the fact that collagen can be only partially solubilized by pepsin, even at the extreme enzyme to substrate ratio of 1:10 used in our study (Table 7). Therefore, only the percentage of type III collagen in the soluble fraction of total tissue collagen can be determined correctly, while the extrapolation to percentage of total collagen remains speculative. A significantly more efficient collagen solubilization may be achieved by peptic digestion at 14°C instead 4°C and/or by reducing pH to 2.5 or even 2.0 by addition of dilute hydrochloric acid.

Table 7. Type III collagen in Dupuytren's contracture tissue and control tissue as verified by sandwich ELISA technique

Sample	Localization	Collagen solubility by pepsin (%)	Type III in pepsin extract (%)[a]	Immuno-fluorescence
Carpal tunnel syndrome tendon	Long palmar muscle	5–38	0.3–4.2 (0.1–0.9)	Traces III
DC patient (apparently normal)	Third finger	11	3.3 (0.3)	III < I
Thickening of fibers, bands	Fourth finger	25–45	43–79 (10–35)	III > I
Contracture and nodules	Fifth finger	25	30 (7.5)	III > I
Rat tail tendons		95		
Human skin	Mammary	25	7	III < I

DC, Dupuytren's contracture.
[a] In estimated amount type as III percent of total collagen.

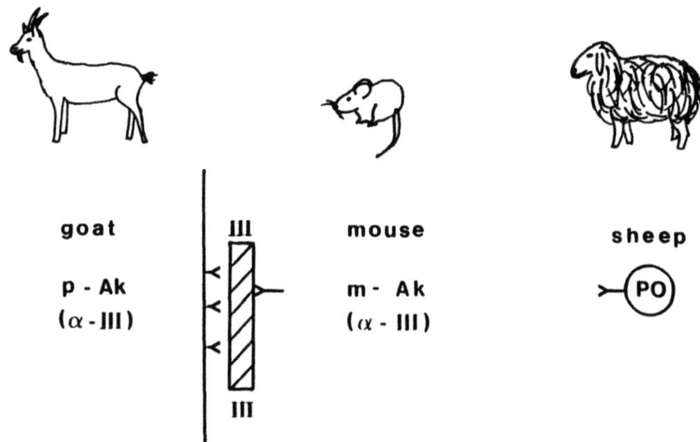

Fig. 3. Principle of type III collagen enzyme immunoassay quantitation

Discussion

In contrast to Pereira et al. [3], in DC we detected ACA to types III and I collagen at much higher frequency than ACA to type II collagen. This seems logical, since both these interstitial collagens are subject to an intense remodeling process in the course of DC, including neosynthesis and degradation by collagenase and other tissue proteases. Type II collagen, by contrast, is lacking in the normal palmar fascia and its appearance in involved aponeurosis is a rare finding (four out of 32 tissue samples contained type II collagen according to immunofluorescence studies by Meister et al. [11]). Why then should there be a significant titer of autoantibodies to this collagen type,

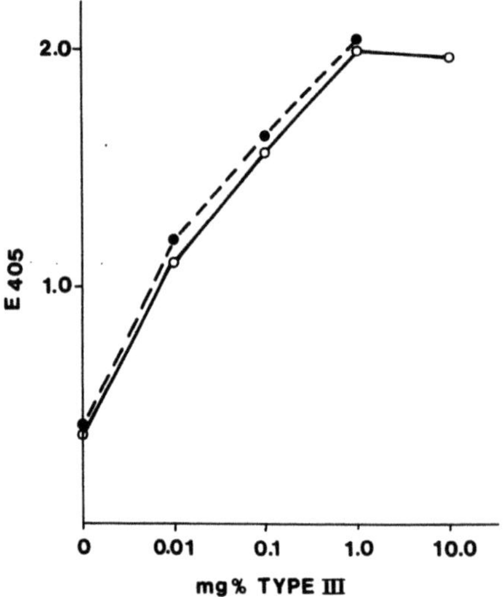

Fig. 4. Influence of type I collagen on type III sandwich enzyme immunoassay

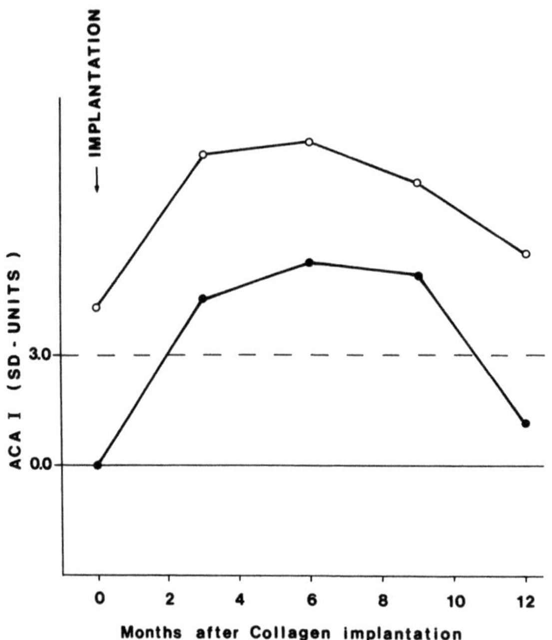

Fig. 5. Transitory nature of anti-collagen antibodies (*ACA*) in patients undergoing collagen implantation for diverse reasons. *Upper curve*, already existing autoantibody titer before collagen implantation; *lower curve*, autoimmunization to collagen as a consequence of collagen implantation

58   E.J. Menzel et al.

Table 8. Importance of anti-collagen antibodies Dupuytrens contracture (DC) and rheumatoid orthritis (RA)

Immune involvement	DC	RA
Local complement activation	−	+
Systemic compklement activation	−	+
Local immune Complexes	−	+
Systemic immune complexes	−	+
Systemic manifestation of disease	−	+ (EAM)
Other than connective tissue antibodies	−	+ (Rf)
HLA association	+	+
Anticollagen antibodies	I,III	II
Antibody class	?	IgG 2,3

as DC is a local and not a systemic disease like RA? The only explanation for ACA to type II collagen would be cross-reacting ACA, which should be more stringent for denatured collagens than native collagens. Another possibility is a genetic predisposition; HLA DR4 seems to be associated with ACA to denatured collagen type II and HLA DR3 with ACA to native type II collagen in RA patients [5,21,22].

ELAB were seen in a considerable percentage of DC patients. Here, however, the control population of healthy persons also displayed an astonishingly high percentage of ELAB-positive individuals (15%), in confirmation of the results of Stein et al. [12]. ELAB and ACA positivity was not correlated in DC patients. However, autoantibodies were significantly correlated with HLA DR3 in DC patients (this is valid only for ACA to type I collagen). The association between the presence of HLA DR3 and DC was only of borderline significance, meaning that there is a suggestion of an association. Accordingly, relative risk is low.

In seven patients ACA were assayed at two time intervals postoperatively (time increment approximately 6 months). We noted a disappearance of ACA positivity in six out of seven cases, suggesting that ACA were triggered by surgical therapy, much as ACA can be induced in HLA DR3- or DR4-positive individuals by implants of bovine collagen implanted for cosmetic or reconstructive reasons (Fig. 5).

Several facts point to a marginal importance of ACA and ELAB in the development of DC. First, in contrast to RA, inflammatory mechanisms are involved only to a minor degree in DC. As shown in Table 8 immune reactions such as complement activation or immune complex formation are not seen in this fibromatous process. Second, ACA appear after surgical intervention and disappear again (Tables 3, 4), indicating their transitory nature. Lastly, ELAB are also found in healthy controls of the right genetic background, although a strict association with HLA DR3 was not observed.

The increased presence of type III collagen in involved or even uninvolved regions of the DC aponeurosis is evident from our results and those of others [23,24]. The major problem in an assay for type III collagen that depends on the native collagen molecule is the restricted degree of collagen solubility, even in pepsin solutions of high enzyme activity, low pH and reaction temperatures above the normally used 4°C (e.g., 14°C). Most authors are rather reticent about the efficiency of collagen extraction procedures. The type III collagen EIA presented here proved, however, to be of high sensibitivity and good overall reproducibility and may be recommended for type III collagen quantitation, especially in the presence of the large excesses of type I collagen one usually has to cope with when analyzing connective tissue extracts of skin, tendon or dura mater.

References

1. Gay S, Gay B (1974) Ist die Dupuytren'sche Kontraktur eine Autoimmunerkrankung? Zentralbl Chir 97:728–733
2. Menzel EJ, Piza H, Zielinski C, Endler AT, Steffen C, Millesi H (1979) Collagen-types and anti-collagen antibodies in Dupuytren's contracture. Hand 11:243–248
3. Pereira RS, Black CM, Turner SM, Spencer JD (1986) Antibodies to collagen types I–VI in Dupuytren's contracture. J Hand Surg 11:58–60
4. Klimiuk PS, Clague RB, Grennan DM, Dyer PA, Smeaton I, Harris R (1985) Autoimmunity to native type II collagen- and distinct genetic subset of rheumatoid arthritis. J Rheumatol 12:865–870
5. Rowley M, Tait B, Mackay IR, Cunningham T, Phillips B (1986) Collagen antibodies in rheumatoid arthritis. Arthritis Rheum 29:174–184
6. Aron E (1977) Maladie de Dupuytren et alcoholism chronique: recherche d'un lien pathogénique groupes HL-A. Semin Hop Paris 53:139
7. Hunter T, Shanahan WR, Robertson GA, Strand MF, Schroeder ML (1981) The distribution of histocompatibility antigens in patients with Dupuytren's contracture. Arthritis Rheum 9:1218–1219
8. Tait BD, Mackay IR (1982) HLA-phenotypes in Dupuytren's contracture. Tissue Antigens 11:240–241
9. Spencer JD, Welsh KI (1984) Histocompatibility antigens in Dupuytren's contracture. J Hand Surg 9:276–278
10. Bailey AJ, Sims TJ, Gabbiani G, Bazin S, LeLous M (1977) Collagen of Dupuytren's disease. Clin Sci Mol Med 53:499–502
11. Meister P, Gokel JM, Remberger K (1979) Palmar fibromatosis-Dupuytren's contracture. A comparison of light, electron and immunofluorescence microscopic findings. Pathol Res Pract 164:402–412
12. Stein F, Pezess MP, Robert L, Poullain N (1965) Anti-elastin antibodies in normal and pathological human sera. Nature 207:312–313
13. Smolen JS, Youngchaiyud U, Weidinger P, Kojer M, Endler AT, Mayr WR, Menzel EJ (1978) Autoimmunological aspects of thrombangiitis obliterans (Buerger's disease). Clin Immunol Immunopathol 11:168–177
14. Robert L, Poullain N (1963) The preparation of soluble kappa-elastin. Bull Soc Chim Biol 45:1317–1321
15. Wener MH, Uwatoko S, Mannik M (1989) Antibodies to the collagen-like region of C1q in sera of patients with autoimmune rheumatic diseases. Arthritis Rheum 32: 544–551
16. Trelstad RL, Catanese VM, Rubin DF (1976) Collagen fractionation. Anal Biochem 71:114–118
17. Stegemann H, Stalder KH (1967) Determination of hydroxyproline. Clin Chim Acta 18:267–273
18. Terasaki PI, McClelland JD (1964) Microdroplet assay of human serum cytotoxins. Nature 206:998–1001

19. Van Rood JJ, van Leeuwen A, Ploem JS (1976) Simultaneous detection of two cell populations by two-colour fluorescence and application to the recognition of B-cell determinants. Nature 262:795–797
20. Festenstein H, Démant P (1978) Basic immunogenetics, biology and clinical relevance. Arnold, London, p 162
21. Terato K, Shimozuru Y, Katayama K, Nagai Y (1990) Specificity of antibodies to type II collagen in rheumatoid arthritis. Arthritis Rheum 33:1493–1500
22. Sanders PA, Grennan DM, Klimiuk PS, Clague RB, de Lange GG, Collins I, Dyer PA (1987) Gm allotypes and HLA in RA patients with circulating antibodies to native type II collagen. Ann Rheum Dis 46:391–394
23. Bazin S, LeLous M, Duance VL, Sims TJ, Bailey AJ, Gabbiani G, d'Andiran G, Pizzolato C, Browsk A, Nicoletis C, Delaunay A (1980) Biochemistry and histology of the connective tissue of Dupuytren's disease lesions. Eur J Clin Invest 10:9–16
24. Brickley-Parsons D, Glimcher MS, Smith RJ, Albin R, Astains JP (1981) Biochemical changes in the collagen of palmar fascia in patients with Dupuytren's disease. J Bone Joint Surg [Am] 63:787–797

Collagen Production by Cultured Dupuytren's Fibroblasts

G.A.C. Murrell and M.J.O. Francis

Introduction

Collagen is a major structural component of connective tissues and perhaps the most abundant protein in the animal world. More than ten types of collagen have been described, but the major fibrillar collagens are types I, II and III. Each consists of three triple helical polypeptide α-chains: type I collagen consists of $\alpha1(I)$, $\alpha1(I)$, $\alpha2$ and type III collagen consists of $\alpha1(III)$, $\alpha1(III)$, $\alpha1(III)$.

A major biochemical abnormality found in Dupuytren's tissue is an increase in total collagen associated with an increase in the ratio of type III to type I collagen (Bazin, 1980; Brickley-Parsons, 1981). The change in the ratio of type III/I collagen becomes more apparent as one progresses from control palmar fascia through uninvolved, mildly involved, cords and finally nodules of Dupuytren's contracture (Brickley-Parsons et al. 1981). Some authors have speculated that these changes may be a manifestation of a genetically inherited abnormality in collagen biosynthesis (Bazin et al. 1980; Gabbiani and Montandon 1985; Guber and Rudolph 1978).

Morphologically, the major difference between control and Dupuytren's contracture palmar fascia is a four- to 20-fold increase in fibroblast density in Dupuytren's palmar fascia (Murrell et al. 1989).

The aim of this study was to determine whether the collagen changes in Dupuytren's contracture are due to a genetic predisposition of fibroblasts to produce more type III collagen or to a response of the fibroblasts to an increase in cell density.

Current methods of measuring the amounts and proportions of the major fibrillar collagen types synthesized by cultured fibroblasts are tedious, expensive and only suitable for one or two cell lines at any given time (Bateman et al. 1984; Clore et al. 1979; Epstein 1974; Epstein and Munderloh 1975; Herrmann et al. 1980). For these reasons we developed a rapid reproducible micromethod. The method is similar to that employed by Bateman (1980), but adapted for multiple analysis of small samples of α-chains of type I and III collagen in the media and cell layers of fibroblasts cultured in conditions optimal for collagen synthesis (Uitto et al. 1980).

Materials and Methods

Sample Collection and Fibroblast Culture

Palmar fascia was obtained from patients during fasciectomy for Dupuytren's contracture and from patients undergoing carpal tunnel release operations. Skin was obtained from the forearm. All patients gave informed consent to sample collection. Each sterile tissue sample was immediately placed in cold (4°C) tissue culture medium (Dulbecco's modification of Eagle's medium; Flow Laboratories Ltd, UK) with a final concentration of 20 mM Hepes, 6 mM glutamine, 10 mM NaHCO$_3$, 27.5 U/ml benzyl penicillin, 13.75 µg/ml streptomycin base with 10% v/v fetal calf serum (Flow), pH 7.35 at 37°C. Tissue samples were dissected into 1 mm cubes and two cubes placed into 25 cm^2 tissue culture flasks (Nunclan Ltd, Denmark) and cultured at 37°C. Media were changed every 3 days throughout the culture period. Assays were performed immediately after the third passage. The morphology at both light and electron microscopy was checked in all cell lines (Murrell et al. 1989).

Collagen Type Micromethod

Each well of a 24 × 1.6 cm multiwell culture plate (Flow) was seeded with 8–20 × 10^4 cells in 1.0 ml of tissue culture medium and cultured at 37°C for 16 h. Six replicates were used for each cell line or culture condition. The medium was then replaced by 1.0 ml of preincubation medium (Bateman et al. 1984) and cultured for 4 h, before being replaced with 1.0 ml of incubation medium (identical to preincubation medium, but with 12.5 µCi [^{3}H]proline/ml; Amersham International Plc., UK) and incubated for a further 20 h at 37°C. Incubation medium was then removed from each well, the cell layer washed with 0.5 ml medium harvest solution (Bateman et al. 1984). The incubation medium and medium harvest solution from each well were combined. The cell layer was then trypsinized (with 1.0 ml of 0.25% trypsin with 0.025% w/v EDTA in phosphate-buffered saline, pH 7.35 at 37°C), removed and the well washed with 0.5 ml cell harvest solution (Bateman et al. 1984). The trypsinized cell solution and the cell harvest solution were added to a 4.5 ml polypropyline tube.

Carrier collagen of 20 µl of 5 mg/ml type III collagen (Sigma Ltd., UK) in 0.5 M acetic acid and 1.52 ml of 50% w/v (NH$_4$)$_2$SO$_4$ was added to each tube and the collagen allowed to precipitate at 4°C overnight and the following collagen extraction performed at 4°C: Tubes were spun at 1700 × g for 15 min, the supernatant discarded and the collagen pepsinized in 0.5 ml of pepsin solution (100 µg/ml pepsin; activity 1:60 000 (Sigma), 0.5 M acetic acid, 0.5 mM EDTA, 25 mM NaCl and 0.025 M Tris/HCl, pH 7.5) for 6 h to remove terminal procollagen extensions. The reaction was stopped with an equal volume of 4 M NaCl and 0.5 M acetic acid, pH 7.4, and the collagen allowed to precipitate overnight. The tubes were spun as above, the supernatant again discarded and

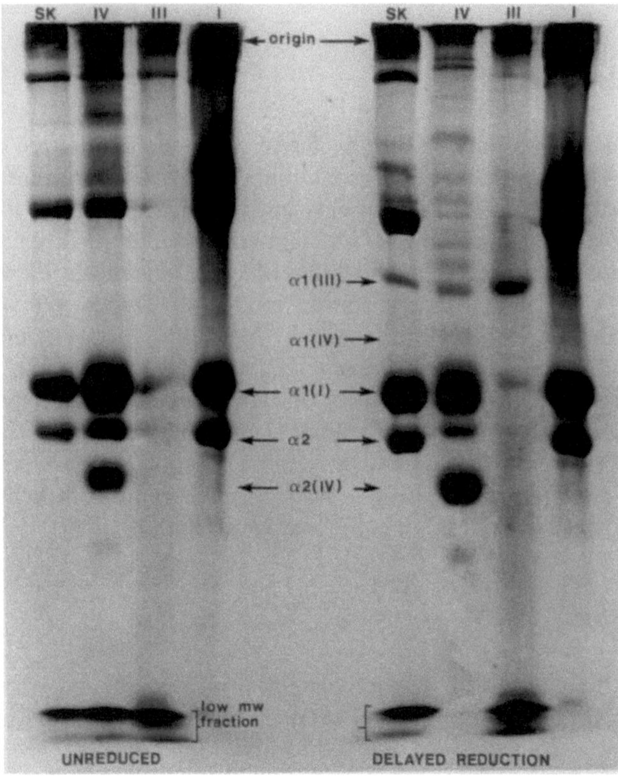

Fig. 1. Separating collagen chains by delayed reduction gel electrophoresis

the precipitate washed three more times with 1.0 ml of 75% v/v ethanol. The resulting precipitate containing radioactive collagen was dissolved in 0.5 ml of 0.5 M acetic acid, lyophilized and stored at −20°C prior to polyacrylamide gel electrophoresis. Storage time before collagen type analysis was less than 2 weeks.

Electrophoretic separation of collagen α-chains was performed on 3% w/v stacking gels and 6% w/v separation gels by delayed-reduction polyacrylamide gel electrophoresis as described by Bateman et al. (1984) and Sykes et al. (1976) (Fig. 1).

The proteins in the gel were then fixed, stained and destained and soaked in Amplify (Amersham) for 30 min prior to drying on grade 40 filter paper. The position of the radioactive bands was determined by fluorography (Bateman et al. 1984). Once the position of the radioactive bands had been determined, the bands were cut from the dried gel, immersed in distilled water, placed in a 5 ml capped vial and solubilized in 0.5 ml 90% v/v NCS (Amersham) for 2 at 50°C. Scintillation liquid (4.5 ml OCS; Amersham) was then added, the vial mixed and counted in a liquid scintillation analyzer and the results expressed as mol [³H]proline.

Collagen Production by Dupuytren's Fibroblasts

The amounts and proportions of the major fibrillar collagens were assessed in five sets of skin and palmar fascia fibroblasts from age- and sex-matched patients with and without Dupuytren's contracture. The mean of the six replicates for each cell line was compared by analysis of variance for repeated measures (Winer 1971).

Fibroblast Density and Collagen Production

The effects of cell density on collagen production was assessed by seeding 1.6 cm microwells with 8×10^4, 12×10^4, 16×10^4 and 20×10^4 fibroblasts ($n = 6$ for each group). This was the largest range possible; fewer cells yielded insufficient collagen and more cells were superconfluent. These seeding densities represent cell densities of approximately 400, 600, 800 and 1000 fibroblasts/mm^2 compared with in vivo cell densities of 162, 834, and 4150 fibroblasts/mm^2 for control palmar fascia, Dupuytren's contracture cord and nodule, respectively (Murrell et al. 1989). Statistical analysis was performed by analysis of variance (Winer 1971). In all the data analyzed, the variance between groups due to a nonlinear trend never reached statistical significance and was always less than that due to a linear trend. Hence, only the variance ratio and p values due to a linear trend are presented.

Results

Fibroblast Populations

Light and electron microscopic examinations confirmed that all cultured cells were fibroblasts and free of any contaminating cell populations.

Collagen Micromethod

The main collagen α-chains consistently recovered and identified in the cell layers and media of cultured fibroblasts were those of type III collage, α1(III), and those of type I collagen, α1(I) and α2. A linear relationship was established between the initial sample concentration of both [^{3}H]proline labelled cell layers and media and the amounts, proportions and ratios of both total, type I and type III collagen α-chains recovered. This is in contrast to the densitometric scanning method, in which Poccock and Francis (unpublished results) found that the α1(I)/α2 collagen ratio decreased in a linear fashion with an increasing concentration of [^{3}H]proline-labelled collagen. The method was also more reproducible (coefficient of variance 35% vs 47%), faster (4 vs 8 contact h, 2 vs 4 weeks for results) and permitted more samples per run (48 vs 4) than Bateman et al. (1984) method.

Table 1. Collagen α-chain distributions of cultured fibroblasts. (From Murrell et al. 1990b)

	Percent α1 (III)	Percent α1 (I)	Percent α2	Total
Cell layers				
Control skin	11 (3)	57 (2)	33 (1)[a]	58 (26)
Control palmar fascia	12 (3)	56 (4)	32 (3)	59 (13)
Dupuytren's contracture skin	11 (3)	60 (2)	29 (1)	50 (12)
Dupuytren's contracture palmar fascia	10 (3)	57 (4)	34 (2)	72 (13)
Media				
Control skin	11 (2)	58 (3)	31 (2)	62 (18)
Control palmar fascia	15 (4)	59 (4)	26 (2)	62 (21)
Dupuytren's contracture skin	12 (3)	59 (2)	29 (2)	54 (9)
Dupuytren's contracture palmar fascia	12 (3)	60 (2)	28 (1)	78 (26)

Expressed as mean (SEM) percentage of total (type I and III collagen) [³H]proline recovered from the cell layers or media. Totals are expressed as mean (SEM) $\times$ 10^{-14} mol[³H]proline/ 10^6 cells. $n = 5$ for each group. There was no statistically significant difference between types of tissue (i.e., skin v palmar fascia) or the presence or absence of Dupuytren's contracture (i.e., Dupuytren's contracture vs control palmar fascia).
[a] The percentages do not always add up to 100% because of rounding errors.

Collagen Production by Dupuytren's Fibroblasts

The amounts and proportions of type I, III and total collagen were similar for each of the five sets of the four different types of cell line, both in the cell layers and the media. Variations in distribution that did occur could not be attributed to the type of tissue from which the fibroblasts originated (i.e. skin or palmar fascia) or to the presence of Dupuytren's contracture (Table 1).

Fibroblast Seeding Density

The effects of seeding density were similar for cell lines derived from both control and Dupuytren's skin and palmar fascia. Initial seeding density of cultured fibroblasts had a significant effect on collagen production, with a dramatic fall in total collagen production per cell in the media at densities higher than 12×10^4 cells/ml. This fall was almost entirely the result of a decrease in type I collagen (Fig. 2). The fall in type I collagen production was also associated with an increase in the types III/I collagen ratio and an increase in the proportion of type III collagen at high cell density. The medium/cell layer ratio for type I collagen fell in a linear fashion from 0.70 to 0.19 for α1(I) and from 0.69 to 0.16 for α2 with increasing cell density (Fig. 3).

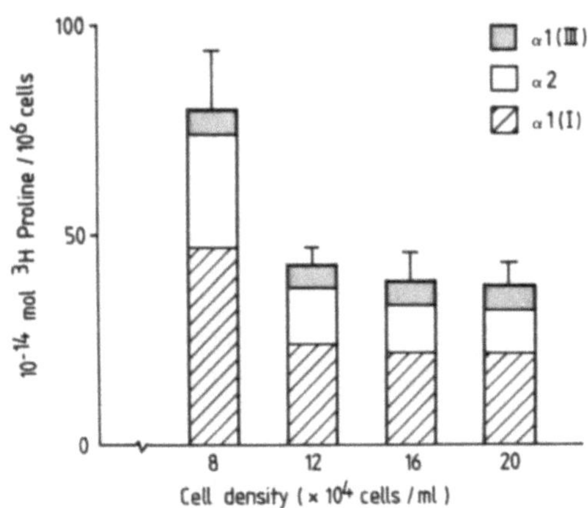

Fig. 2. The effect of cell density on collagen production by cultured fibroblasts: collagen recovered per cell in the media. Error bars represent SEM of total (type I and III collagen); $n = 6$ for each group. Probability value for variance ratio due to a linear trend between groups: *<0.025; ***<0.001. (From Murrell et al. 1990b)

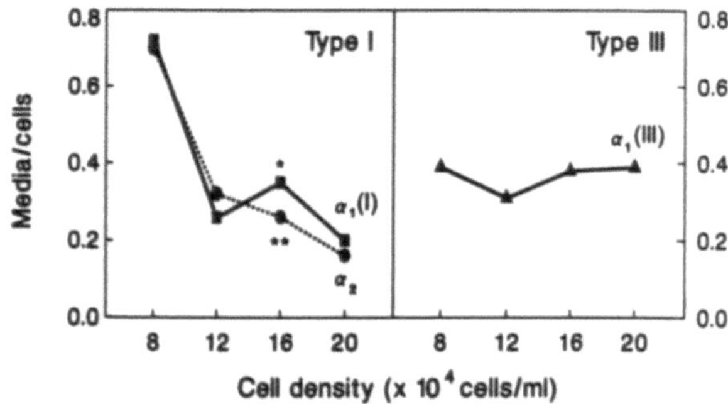

Fig. 3. Effect of cell density on collagen production by cultured fibroblasts: medium/cell layer collagen ratios expressed as mean. $n = 6$ for each group. Probability for variance ratio due to a linear trend between groups: *<0.025; **<0.005. (From Murrell et al. 1990b)

Discussion

Using a faster and more reproducible micromethod, the amounts and proportions of the major fibrillar collagen types produced by fibroblasts cultured from both skin and palmar fascia of patients with and without Dupuytren's contracture were measured. Collagen production was unaffected by fibroblast origin (skin or palmar fascia) or the presence of Dupuytren's contracture (Dupuytren's contracture or control). These results oppose an obvious genetic defect of collagen biosynthesis of the fibroblasts of patients with Dupuytren's contracture and are consistent with a preliminary gene tracking study (unpublished results) indicating no linkage of Dupuytren's contracture with the α1(I) and α2 collagen genes.

Fibroblast density did, however, have a profound effect on collagen production. An increase in the types III/I collagen ratio with increasing cell density was confirmed. Furthermore, this change in ratio was found to be secondary to an inhibition of type I collagen production. Type III collagen production was unaffected by fibroblast density. The mechanism whereby type I collagen production is inhibited at high cell density is undetermined. The results are also complementary to those of Slack et al. (1982), showing a reproduction of the glycosaminoglycan compositions found in Dupuytren's contracture by culturing fibroblasts at high density.

These and recent morphological studies by Gabbiani and Montandon (1985) indicate that the fibroblasts in Dupuytren's contracture are not abnormal. The fibroblasts merely produce less type I collagen at high cell density. As skin fibroblasts also produce less type I collagen at high cell density, the same process is likely to account for the collagen changes in keloids, hypertrophic scars, healing wounds and fetal skin (conditions associated with fibroblasts at high cell density and an increase in the III/I collagen ratio).

Further attempts to understand the processes of fibrosis and of wound healing should be directed towards the stimuli for fibroblast proliferation. One mechanism for fibroblast stimulation may be oxygen free radicals (Murrell 1987a,b, 1990a).

Acknowledgements. We thank the Rhodes Trust for support for GACM and the patients and surgeons of the Nuffield Orthopaedic Centre for tissue samples.

References

Bateman JF, Mascara T, Chan D, Cole WG (1984) Abnormal type I collagen metabolism by cultured fibroblasts in lethal perinatal osteogenesis imperfecta. Biochem J 217:103–115

Bazin S, Lelous M, Duance VC, Sims TJ, Bailey AJ, Gabbiani G, d'Andiran G, Pizzolato G, Browski A, Nicoletis C, Delaunay A (1980) Biochemistry and histology of the connective tissue of Dupuytren's disease lesions. Eur J Clin Invest 10:9–16

Brickley-Parsons D, Glimcher MJ, Smith RJ, Albin R, Adams JP (1981) Biochemical changes in the collagen of the palmar fascia in patients with Dupuytren's disease. J Bone Joint Surg [Am] 63(5):787–797

Clore JN, Cohen IK, Diegelmann RF (1979) Quantitative assay of types I and III collagen synthesized by keloid biopsies and fibroblasts. Biochim Biophys Acta 586:384–390

Epstein EH (1974) $[\alpha 1(III)]_3$ Human skin collagen: release by pepsin digestion and preponderance in fetal life. J Biol Chem 249(10):3225–3231

Epstein EH, Munderloh NH (1975) Isolation and characterization of CNBr peptides of human $[\alpha 1(III)]_3$ collagen and tissue distribution of $[\alpha 1(I)]_2 \alpha 2$ and $[\alpha 1(III)]_3$ collagens. J Biol Chem 250(24):9304–9312

Gabbiani G, Montandon D (1985) The myofibroblasts in Dupuytren's disease and other fibromatoses. In: Hueston JT, Tubiana R (eds) Dupuytren's disease, 2nd edn. Churchill Livingstone, Edinburgh, pp 86–93

Guber S, Rudolph R (1978) The myofibroblast. Surg Gynecol Obstet 146:641–649

Herrmann H, Dessau W, Fessler LI, von der Mark K (1980) Synthesis of types I III and AB_2 collagen by chick tendon fibroblasts in vitro. Eur J Biochem 105:63–74

Murrell GAC, Murrell TGC, Pilowsky E (1987a) A hypothesis for the resolution of Dupuytren's contracture with allopurinol. Specul Sci Technol 10(2):107–112

Murrell GAC, Francis MJO, Bromley L (1987b) Free radicals and Dupuytren's contracture. Br Med J 295:1373–1375

Murrell GAC, Francis MJO, Howlett CR (1989) Dupuytren's contracture: fine structure in relation to aetiology. J Bone Joint Surg [Br] 71(3):367–373

Murrell GAC, Francis MJO, Bromley L (1990a) Modulation of fibroblast proliferation by oxygen free radicals. Biochem J 265:659–665

Murrell GAC, Francis MJO, Bromley L (1990b) The collagen changes of Dupuytren's contracture. J Hand Surg [Br] (in press)

Slack C, Flint MH, Thompson BM (1982) Glycosaminoglycan synthesis by Dupuytren's cells in culture. Connect Tissue Res 9:263–269

Sykes B, Puddle B, Francis M, Smith R (1976) The estimation of two collagens from human dermis by interrupted gel electrophoresis. Biochem Biophys Res Commun 72(4):1472–1487

Uitto J, Booth BA, Polak KL (1980) Collagen biosynthesis by human skin fibroblasts. II. Isolation and further characterization of type I and type III procollagens synthesized in culture. Biochim Biophys Acta 624:545–561

Winer BJ (1971) Statistical principles in experimental design, 2nd edn. McGraw-Hill, New York, pp 319–337, 514–527

Proteoglycans and Glycosaminoglycans

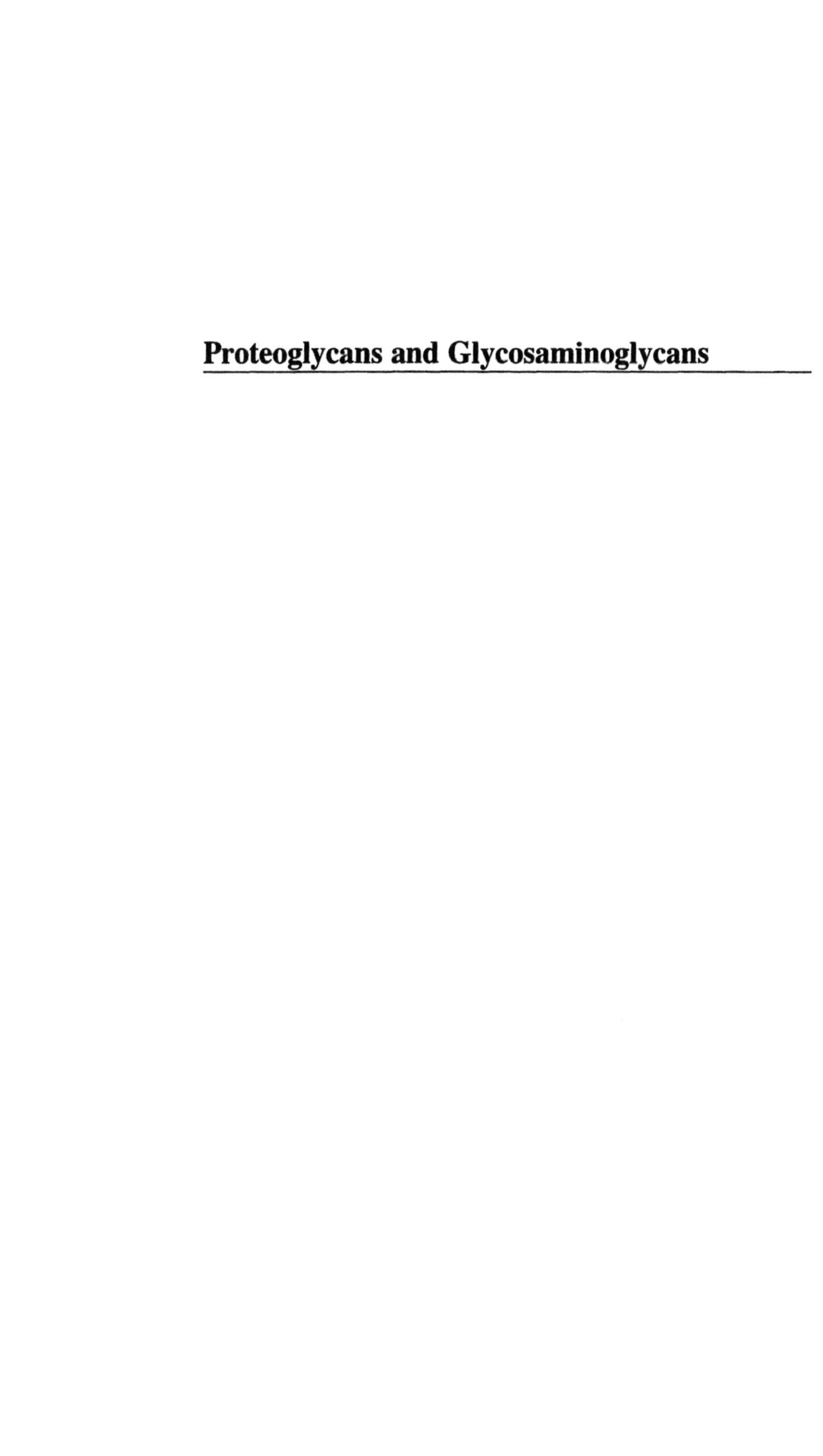

Proteoglycans in Biopsies of Dupuytren's Contracutre

E. Gurr, M. Borchert, W. Borchert, and A. Delbrück

Introduction

Proteoglycans were first described in cartilage as molecules containing chondroitin sulfate firmly bound to noncollagenous proteins (Shatton and Schubert 1954). In the following four decades intensive investigations on the structure and function of these molecules resulted in the discovery of multiple forms and families of proteoglyans. Later studies more specifically defined what proteoglycans are. In 1982 proteoglycans were stated to be a group of macromolecules consisting of a core protein to which at least one glycosaminoglycan side chain was covalently bound (Hascall and Kimura 1982). Proteoglycans occur predominantly in the extracellular matrix and as a constituent of cell membranes and within cells. However, little is currently known about these proteoglycans with respect to Dupuytren's disease.

Biochemistry of Extracellular Proteoglycans

In the extracellular matrix proteoglycans appear within the interfibrillar space and on the periphery of collagen fibrils. Most of our knowledge regarding the structure of these proteoglycans was found by investigating cartilge proteoglycans, which consist of two main families: large proteoglycans and small proteoglycans (Heinegard and Paulsson 1984). Large proteoglycans make up the interfibrillar space of the extracellular cartilage matrix. By aggregation with hyaluronan, complexes of several million daltons are built up. Small proteoglycans do not aggregate with hyaluronan. Currently, one has to assume that these proteoglycans are a distinct family rather than the result of proteolytic degradation of proteoglycan-hyaluronan complexes, which occurs during turnover of proteoglycans within the extracellular matrix.
Large aggregating proteoglycans have several domains (Dudhia et al. 1990; Paulsson et al. 1987; Doege et al. 1987). Proteoglycans and hyaluronan interact via the hyaluronan-binding region G1 (Fig. 1). G1 is located at the NH_2-terminal of the protein core and contains three kringles. Two of the three kringles (named kringle B) are structurally identical and consist of 99 amino acids. Binding to hyaluronan is stabilized by link proteins. G2, the second

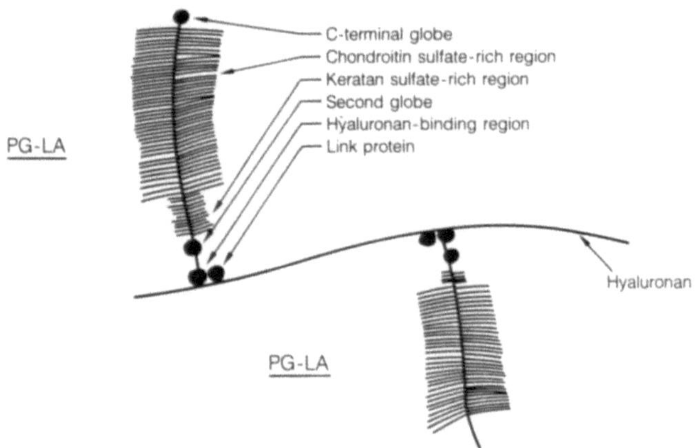

Fig. 1. Structure of large, hyaluronan aggregating proteoglycans (PG-LA)

globular domain, consists of the two B kringles known from G1. The functional role of G2 remains obscure. The third globular domain, G3, is located at the COOH-terminal of the core protein and differs from G1 and G2. G3 is found in chicken, rat, bovine, human, and pig proteoglycans and has lectin-binding properties. The core protein itself has a molecular weight of about 220 kDa; the molecular weight of the whole proteoglycan molecule is about 2000 kDa. Glycosaminoglycans are bound to the core protein in three domains: one keratan sulfate-rich region and two chondroitin sulfate regions.

Proteoglycan biosynthesis follows the well-known pathway of glycoprotein synthesis (Hardingham 1986; Poole 1986). It starts with transcription and translation of the core protein. Within the rough endoplasmic reticulum, synthesis of N-linked oligosaccharides occurs. In the Golgi apparatus, synthesis of polysaccharide side chains, including epimerization of glucuronic acid and sulfatation, takes place. This is followed by secretion of the whole molecule into the extracellular space. Hyaluronan is synthesized by a membrane linked enzyme complex (Prehm 1984). The hyaluronan-proteoglycan aggregate is formed extracellularly, after a lag phase in which modification of the binding region may occur (Bayliss et al. 1984; Plaas and Sandy 1986).

Maintenance of the extracellular matrix is the result of a balance of synthesis and degradation. Many factors are known to influence the biosynthesis of proteoglycans, e.g., somatomedin (Nevo 1982), insulin (Prins et al. 1982), insulin-like growth factors (Mitchell and Hardingham 1982), platelet-derived growth factor (Dresow and Delbrück 1986), interleukin-1 (Tyler 1986), tumor necrosis factor α (Saklatvala 1986), and transforming growth factor β (Tyler 1986). Feedback regulation has been demonstrated in chondrocyte cell cultures (Handley et al. 1986). Additionally, biosynthesis of proteoglycans is stimulated and/or inhibited by mechanical forces (Gillard et al. 1979). Mechanical forces also influence the pattern of proteoglycan expression. For example, in tendon the concentration of large proteoglycans was higher in regions with a high

Table 1. Small extracellular proteoglycans (PG-S)

	PG-S1	PG-S2	?
Alternative name	Biglycan	Decorin	Fibromodulin
Molecular weight (kDa)	120	85	?
Core potein size (kDa)	45	45	59
Side chain(s)	2 CS (bone)	1 CS (bone, nasal cartilage)	1 KS (cartilage, sclera, tendon, cornea)
	2 DS (cartilage, sclera, skin, tendon)	1 DS (articular cartilage, sclera, skin, tendon)	
Binding to	?	Collagen I/II	Collagen I/II

CS, chondroitin sulfate; DS, dermatan sulfate; KS, Keratan sulfate. The tissues in which the PG-S are found are given in parentheses.

pressure load and lower in regions which were predominantly stressed (Vogel et al. 1986). The highest concentration of large aggregating proteoglycans was found in high load-bearing hyaline cartilage, e.g., articular cartilage and the nucleus pulposus of intervertebral discs (Gurr 1986). Degradation of proteoglycans is performed mainly by intracellular metalloproteases, which degrade the core protein (Tyler 1986). As a result, hyaluronan and the binding region of the proteoglycan remain in the matrix. During the process of inflammation some additional reactants e.g., PMN elastase (Menninger et al. 1981) and oxygen radicals (Greenwold and Moak 1986), are thought to invade connective tissue compartments. In vitro experiments have demonstrated the destructive potency of these reactants.

The functional role of large proteoglycans is to confer mechanical stability, especially with respect to load-bearing and complete reformation after deformation. Large proteoglycans have a very high density of negative charges, giving the tissue a high water-binding capacity. Thus, the tissue swells until the collagen network stops swelling. Pressure load diminishes the water content, but during relaxation the displaced water is drawn back into the tissue by the negative charges (Urban and Maroudas 1980).

Small proteoglycans differ distinctly from the large ones. Small proteoglycans have core proteins with molecular weights of about $30-40$ kDa. The core proteins of the different types share structural features; however, they represent different gene products (Heinegard et al. 1990). Near the NH_2-terminal they are substituted with one or two glycosaminoglycan side chains. These may be chondroitin sulfate or dermatan sulfate, depending on the origin of the tissue and the type of proteoglycan. Three extracellular small proteoglycans have thus far been identified: PG-S1 (biglycan), PG-S2 (decorin) (Fisher et al. 1989), and fibromodulin (Oldberg et al. 1989) (Table 1). A single type of core protein can bear different types of polysaccharide side chains. Therefore it appears that the signal for the synthesis of a specific type of side chain does not depend on the core protein. It is thought that regulation depends on the availability of the epimerase in different cells.

The function of the small proteoglycans is currently unknown, although it has been shown that decorin and fibromodulin bind to collagen type I and II, via the core protein, at distinct regions of the fibril (Scott 1984) and that they appear to play a role in the regulation of collagen fibrillogenesis. It has been demonstrated that decorin limits growth of the fibrils (Vogel et al. 1984; Hedblom and Heinegard 1989). Additionally, a mechanism of platelet binding to collagen via the von Willebrand dimer and a small dermatan sulfate proteoglycan has been proposed (Neame 1990). Nothing is yet known about the function of the glycosaminoglycan side chains of small proteoglycans.

Proteoglycans in Dupuytren's Disease Fascia and Peritoneal Fascia

The extracellular matrix of the palmar fascia is altered in Dupuytren's disease. The palmar fascia, which is smooth and thin in the normal hand, shows coarse strands and nodules, which limit its function. Stretching of the hand is circumscribed depending on the stage of disease. Based on the hypothesis that proteoglycans are involved in this process, experiments were started to investigate pathological changes in the palmar fascia of Dupuytren's disease. However, the small amounts of proteoglycans which were available for analysis proved to be a significant problem. In particular chemical methods are not sensitive enough for the analysis of proteoglycans from a single normal palmar fascia. To overcome these difficulties, 42 g of peritoneal fascia were taken from two patients within 12 h post mortem and used as "normal fascia". Ten pooled biopsies from patients with Dupuytren's disease, age 28–73, with an overall wet weight of 17 g were evaluated in parallel. Isolation and analysis was performed as reported elsewere (Borchert 1992). Briefly, the pools were extracted and ultracentrifuged in a cesium chloride density gradient. Proteoglycans were isolated from these fractions by ion exchange chromatography, fractionated by gel chromatography and characterized by gel electrophoresis and amino acid chromatogrophy. The latter was performed with the support of Dr. Stuhlsatz (RWTH Aachen, Institute of Clinical Chemistry, Aachen, FRG).

Preparation of Proteoglycans

The fraction of proteoglycans extracted by $4 M$ guanidinium hydrochloride including protease inhibitors was 31% in peritoneal fascia and 35% in Dupuytren's contracture tissue, as estimated by the glycosaminoglycan content of extracts and residue. Addition of Triton $\times 100$ to the guanidinium hydrochloride solution resulted in a 4% increase in proteoglycans in Dupuytren's contracture tissue; addition of CHAPS resulted in about a 12% increase of the extraction yield in both peritoneal fascia and Dupuytren's contracture tissue. Cesium chloride density gradient ultracentrifugation of the extracts under dissociative conditions with a starting density of 1.35 g/l resulted in seven fractions. Most of the proteoglycans were found in fractions 1 and 2 (A1), the fractions with the highest density. There was no general difference in the shapes of the uronic acid, glycosaminoglycan, and protein gradients between Dupuytren's contracture tissue and peritoneal fascia.

Ion exchange chromatography was performed on DEAE-Sephacel with a solution of $7\,M$ urea in $0.05\,M$ sodium acetate buffer, pH 6.5, including sodium chloride concentrations between 0 and $2\,M$ in steps of $0.5\,M$. The proteoglycans were eluted with $0.5\,M$ sodium chloride shown by the uronic acid glycosaminoglycan, and protein peak. This peak is found not only within the A1 fraction but also in the A2 and A3 fractions. Again there are no remarkable differences between the normal and the pathological fascia.

The extracts obtained by Triton $\times 100$ and CHAPS extraction were eluted with a linear gradient of sodium chloride without alterations in the shape of the glycosaminoglycan and protein curves: the glycosaminoglycan peak appears again in the range of $0.5\,M$ sodium chloride in the eluent. In all ion exchange chromatographies these $0.5\,M$ sodium chloride peaks were pooled and used for further investigations. Ion exchange chromatography and density gradient ultracentrifugation therefore were performed as purification procedures. The results are not interpreted analytically.

Gel chromatography was performed on Sephacryl S 500 under dissociative conditions in $4\,M$ guanidinium hydrochloride with those proteoglycan fractions isolated by the ion exchange procedure. In the proteoglycan preparations obtained both from Dupuytren's contracture and from human peritoneal fascia two peaks were seen (Fig. 2): one peak with proteoglycans of large molecular size, eluted near the void volume and referred to as G1, and a second one containing smaller molecules. The latter peak was separated into two fractions, G2 and G3, with respect to the protein peak seen in the range of fraction 52 of G3. Although the shape of the curve in G1 from Dupuytren's contracture tissue is not very smooth, it is clear that this peak is shifted to a larger molecular size compared with peritoneal fascia. The preparations of A2 and A3 (not shown) also demonstrated G2 and G3 but no G1. Characterization of the molecular size by K_{av} points to a significantly larger molecular size of the large proteoglycans of Dupuytren' disease fascia (K_{av} G1: Dupuytren's fascia proteoglycans 0.18, peritoneal palmar fascia proteoglycans 0.30). In contrast there are only small differences in G2/G3. In Dupuytren's contracture tissue the K_{av} values of the respective fractions of the CHAPS and Triton $\times 100$ extracts do not differ from those of the extracts obtained by guanidinium hydrochloride solutions without chaotropic additives (not shown).

Gel Electrophoresis

The procedure most often used for characterization of proteoglycans is electrophoresis in an agarose/polyacrylamide mixed gel. All procedures reported in the literature used vertical gels requireing large amounts of proteoglycans, which were not available in Dupuytren's disease. Therefore a procedure was developed using ultrathin horizontal gels. A very sensitive two

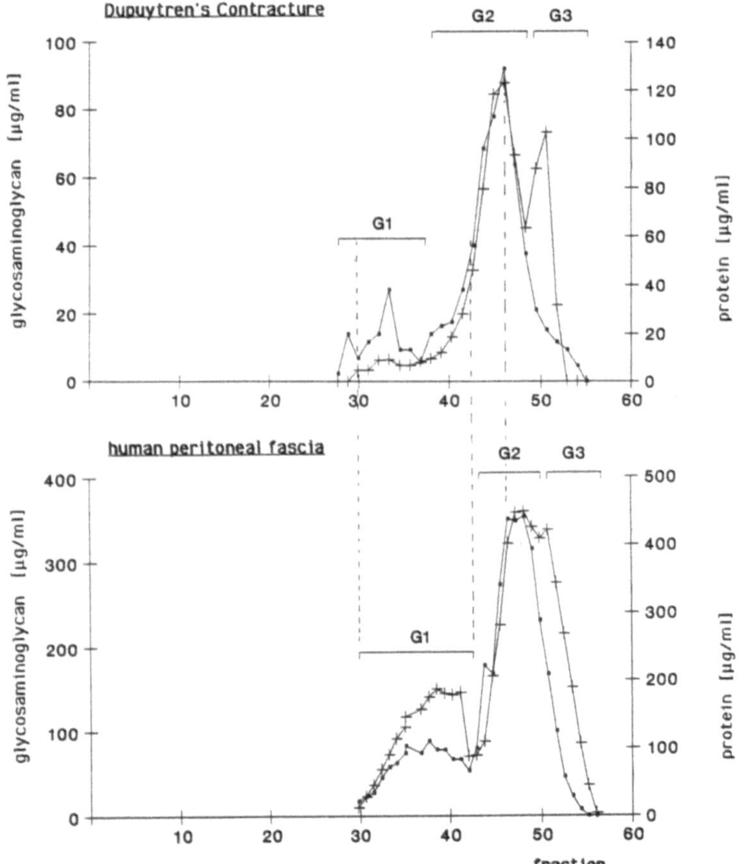

Fig. 2. Gel chromatography of isolated proteoglycan fractions from Dupuytren's contracture (*top*) and human peritoneal fascia (*bottom*). Conditions of chromatography: Sephacryl S 500, 155 × 1 cm, 4 *M* guanidinium hydrochloride in 0.05 *M* sodium acetate buffer, pH 5.8, including thymol, elution rate 4 ml/min, 4°C. --+-- glycosaminoglycan; --●-- protein

step staining procedure for proteoglycans by alcian blue followed by silver staining was also developed. With this procedure electrophoresis was performed with 5 µg proteoglycan per slot (Borchert 1992).

The electrophoretic separation of fascia proteoglycan preparations and of both pure chondroitin sulate from human intervertebral discs and large aggregating proteoglycans isolated from pig articular cartilage as standards shows three clearly separated bands (Fig. 3): (1) a slowly migrating band corresponding to the isolated proteoglycans and not seen either by protein or hyaluronan staining procedures (not shown), (2) a fast migrating band corresponding to isolated glycosaminoglycans, and (3) a band which migrates between the other two and, as will be demonstrated, contains the small proteoglycans.

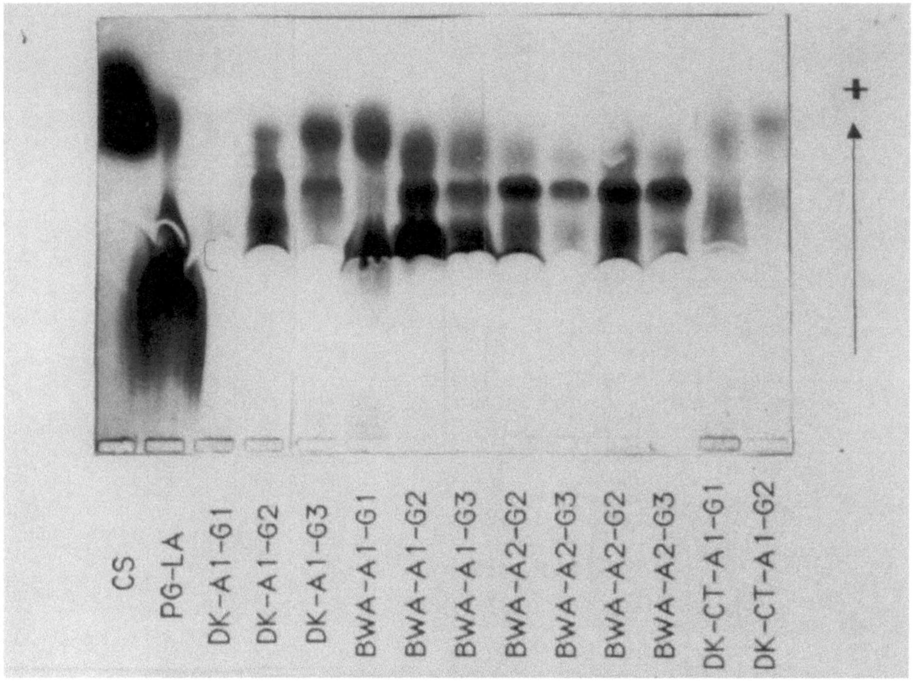

Fig. 3. Agarose-polyacrylamide gel electrophoresis of proteoglycans isolated from Dupuytren's contracture (*DK*) and healthy peritoneal fascia (*BWA*). *A1–A3*, fractions of high, middle and low density obtained after ultracentrifugation; *G1–G3*, fractions isolated by gel chromatography (for details see Fig. 2); *CS*, chondroitin sultate; *PG-LA*, large aggregating proteoglycan extracted from pig articular cartilage. Staining: toluidine blue followed by silver

The A1-G1 preparation of Dupuytren's contracture fascia mainly contains the large proteoglycan band and a smaller one at the position of the pure glycosaminoglycans. The A1-G2 preparation of Dupuytren' contracture fascia (DK A1-G2) contains mainly the small proteoglycan band and both some large proteoglycans and some isolated glycosaminoglycans (Fig. 3). The bands in preparation A1-G3 of Dupuytren's contracture fascia (DK A1-G1) correspond to the glycosaminoglycans and, for the less intensively stained band, to small proteoglycans. There are no general differences with respect to the proteoglycan preparations derived from the peritoneal fascia (BWA). The main component of fractions A2 and A3 (not shown) correspond to the small proteoglycans.

Degradation of the A1-G1 preparation from Dupuytren's disease fascia by chondroitinases AC and ABC resulted in bands which were neither alcian blue nor silver stainable (Fig. 4, DK). This demonstrates that both the glycosaminoglycan side chains of the large proteoglycans and the isolated glycosaminogylcans must be chondroitin sulfate. The A1-G2 preparation including large and small proteoglycans resulted in a single glycosaminoglycan

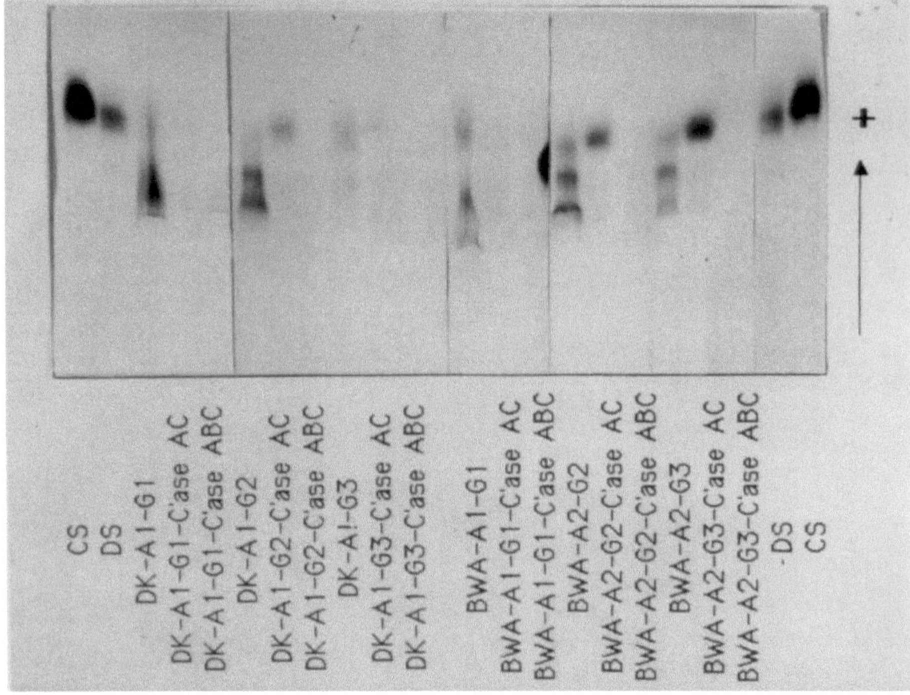

Fig. 4. Agarose-polyacrylamide gel electrophoresis of proteoglycans isolated from Dupuytren' contracture (*DK*) and healthy peritoneal fascia (*BWA*). *A1*, fraction of high density obtained by ultracentrifugation; *G1–G3*, fractions isolated by gel chromatography (for details see Fig. 2); *CS*, chondroitin sulfate; *DS*, dermatan sulfate; *C'ase AC* and *ABC*, proteoglycans degraded by chondroitinase AC and ABC. Staining by toluidine blue

band after degradation with chondroitinase AC. After degradation with chondroitinase ABC no band was seen in the gel. Therefore all glycosaminoglycans in A1-G2 must be chondroitin sulfate or dermatan sulfate with respect to the specificity of the enzymes. The appearence of the glycosaminoglycan band after chondroitinase AC degradation points to dermatan sulfate chains with glucuronic acid-containing domains near the region binding to the core protein, which could be cleaved by chondroitinase AC without degradation of the whole polysaccharide chain. The results of the appropriate preparations of peritoneal fascia proteoglycans are in accordance with those from Dupuytren's disease fascia (Fig. 4, BWA).

Analysis of the core proteins was performed in SDS-polyacrylamide gradient gels (Fig. 5). The core proteins of the large proteoglycans (DK A1-G1; BWA A1-G1) obtained by chondroitinase AC/ABC degradation smear along the high molecular end of the lane. One has to assume polydispersity, as is well known to occur with cartilage proteoglycans. However, there is one distinct band in the range of 230 kDa, not well seen in Fig. 5 but corresponding to the molecular weight of the core protein of the large aggregating cartilage

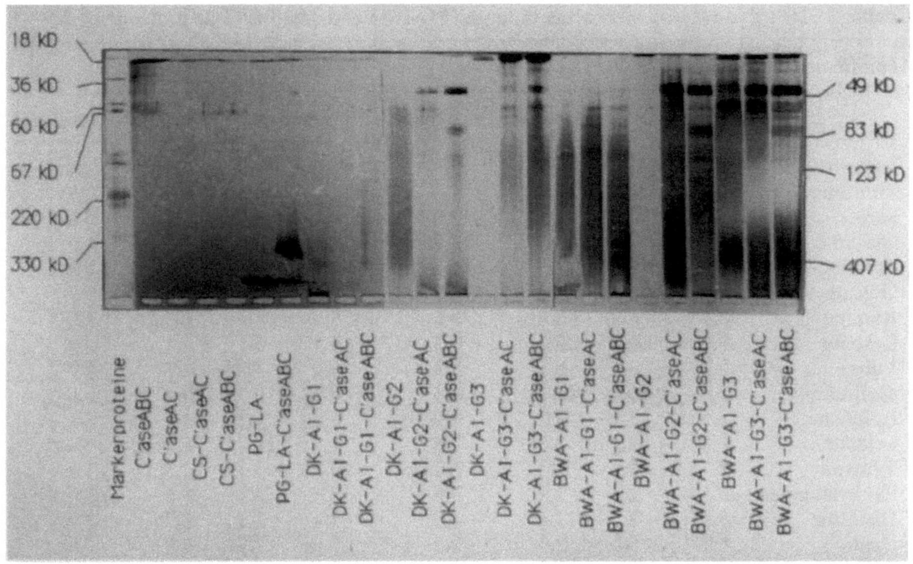

Fig. 5. SDS-polyacrylamide gel electrophoresis of proteoglycans isolated from Dupuytren's contracture (*DK*) and peritoneal fascia (*BWA*). *A1*, fraction of high density obtained by ultracentrifugation; *G1–G3*, fractions isolated by gel chromatography (for details see Fig. 2); *CS*, chondroitin sulate; *DS*, dermatan sulfate; *C'ase AC* and *ABC*, proteoglycans degraded by chondroitinase AC and ABC; *PG-LA*; large aggregating proteoglycan isolated from pig articular cartilage, Staining: silver

proteoglycan type. Chondroitinase AC degradation of the A1-G2 preparations, which include the small proteoglycans, resulted in core protein bands of about 49 kDa, as reported for small proteoglycans in the literature. After degradation with chondroitinase ABC these bands became much stronger. Therefore most of the small proteoglycans must have dermatan sulfate side chains but a small amount seems to have chondroitin sulfate side chains. After degradation with chondroitinase ABC, an additional band of 83 kDa appears which cannot be explained at the time. Again, there is no indication for differences between peritonal fascia proteoglycans and proteoglycans deriving from Dupuytren's disease fascia.

Amino Acid Analysis

The amino acid patterns are in accordance with those well known for large and small proteoglycans (Table 2). The large proteoglycan core protein in the Al-G1 preparation of peritoneal fascia (PG-LA, BWA) contains about 9% glycine and serine, which mainly occur within the chondroitin sulfate region. The core protein of the small proteoglycan A1-G2 (PG-S, BWA) contains about 9% leucine, an amino acid which is part of a region 24 amino acids in length and ten times repeated, mediating binding to collagen (Heinegard et al.

Table 2. Distribution of amino acids in large (PG-LA) and small (PG-S) proteoglycans

Amino acid	PG-LA				PG-S			
	BWA	DC	Tendon[a]	Cartilage[a]	BWA	DC	Tendon[a]	Cartilage[a]
Aspartic acid	8.6	6.7	6.8	5.8	13.0	12.8	14.5	12.6
Threonine	9.4	5.5	6.3	6.6	5.4	5.5	5.0	6.4
Serine	9.9	19.1	12.5	9.0	8.9	9.5	9.8	8.6
Glutamic acid	13.2	13.5	16.3	13.7	10.4	10.6	10.9	8.0
Proline	8.8	5.0	9.5	11.7	7.6	7.6	8.9	2.8
Glycine	8.8	16.4	12.2	12.9	8.4	9.6	8.9	9.2
Alanine	6.4	6.7	6.6	8.6	5.4	5.4	6.3	7.0
Cysteine	0.5	<0.1	<0.1	0.3	<0.1	0.1	<0.1	0.9
Valine	5.2	3.4	6.1	5.9	5.0	4.8	3.7	5.7
Methionine	0.4	<0.1	<0.1	<0.1	<0.1	0.2	<0.1	0.6
Isoleucine	3.3	2.1	4.0	3.0	4.2	4.2	3.5	7.4
Leucine	6.9	4.2	7.5	7.8	11.8	11.2	11.3	10.4
Tyrosine	2.1	<0.1	1.3	2.7	0.2	0.4	2.3	3.9
Phenylalanine	3.5	2.3	2.9	3.6	3.5	3.3	3.0	3.9
Histidine	2.9	3.1	2.8	2.9	4.4	3.1	2.7	2.9
Lysine	6.1	9.1	2.0	2.7	7.6	7.9	6.9	7.0
Arginine	4.1	2.8	3.2	2.9	4.1	3.5	2.7	6.5

[a] From Vogel and Heinegard 1987.
BWA, peritoneal fascia; DC, Dupuytren's contracture; PG-LA, large hyaluronan-aggregating proteoglycans; PG-S, small proteoglycan.
Results are given as amino acids/100 amino acids.

1990). The pattern of A1-G2 (PG-S, DC) of Dupuytren's disease corresponds well to that of peritoneal fascia; A1-G1 (PG-LA, DC) of Dupuytren's disease, however, has an increased concentration of glycine and serine. Based on these data one has to conclude that the large proteoglycans from Dupuytren's contracture have more chondroitine sulfate side chains, a fact which would explain the larger molecular size demonstrated by gel filtration.

Conclusions

Three glycosaminoglycan-containing fractions were demonstrated in peritoneal fascia and Dupuytren's contracture fascia. By the methods used in these experiments, no glycosaminoglycan population was obtained as a pure preparation. A fraction of protein-free glycosaminoglycans seen in the mixed gel electrophoresis consists of chondroitin sulfate and may include a small peptide fragment from the core protein, which could not be stained by the methods used for the electrophoresis gels. The small proteoglycans had a core protein of about 49 kDa corresponding to the results obtained for PG-S1 and PG-S2. The glycosaminoglycan side chains of the small proteoglycans consist mainly of dermatan sulfate and, to a lesser extent, of chondroitin sulfate. Some of the dermatan sulfate chains may have glucuronic acid-containing domains near the core protein. The large proteoglycans have chondroitin sulfate side chains and a polydisperse core protein. The molecular size of the Dupuytren' contracture proteoglycan seems to be larger as demonstrated by gel chromatography. Although the types and composition of the small proteoglycans were not characterized completely, there is no indication for differences between normal fascia and Dupuytren's contracture fascia. The alterations are restricted to the large proteoglycan family. The occurrence of a large proteoglycan in Dupuytren's disease fascia with an increased volume points to the more cartilage-like behavior of the altered tissue. However, these results have to be corroborated by additional experiments using palmar fascia itself.

References

Bayliss M, Ridgway G, Ali A (1984) Delayed aggregation of proteoglycans in adult human articular cartilage. Biosci Rep 4:827–833

Borchert W (1992) Doctoral thesis. Medical School, Hannover

Doege K, Sasaki M, Horigan E, Hassell JR, Yamada Y (1987) Link protein cDNA sequence reveals a tandemly repeated protein structure. Proc Natl Acad Sci USA 83:3766–3770

Dresow B, Delbrück A (1986) Growth factors and uncontrolled proliferation of chondrocytes. J Clin Chem Clin Biochem 24:940–942

Dudhia J, Fosang AJ, Hardingham TE (1990) Domain structure and sequence similarities in cartilage proteoglycans. Biochem Soc Trans 18:198–200

Fisher LW, Termine JD, Young MF (1989) Deduced protein sequence of bone small proteoglycan I (biglycan) shows homology with proteoglycan II (decorin) and several nonconnective tissue proteins in a variety of species. J Biol Chem 264:4571–4576

Gillard GC, Reilly HC, Bell-Booth PG, Flint MH (1979) The influence of mechanical forces on the glycosaminoglycan content of the rabbit flexor digitorum profundus tendon. Connect Tissue Res 7:37–46

Greenwald RA, Moak SA (1986) Degradation of hyaluronic acid by polymorph nuclear leukocytes. Inflammation 10:15–30

Gurr E (1986) Biomechanic influence on the proteoglycan synthesis of chondrocytes. J Clin Chem Clin Biochem 24:928–930

Handley CJ, McQuillan DJ, Campbell MA, Bolis S (1986) Steady-state metabolism in cartilage explants. In: Kuettner KE, Schleyerbach R, Hascall VC (eds) Aricular cartilage biochemistry. Raven, New York, pp 163–180

Hardingham TE (1986) Biosynthesis of proteoglycans by chondrocytes. J Clin Chem Clin Biochem 24:922–925

Hascall VC, Kimura JH (1982) Proteoglycans: isolation and characterisation. Methods Enzymol 82:769–800

Hedblom E, Heinegard D (1989) Interaction of a 59-kD connective tissue matrix protein with collagen I and II. J Biol Chem 264:6898–6905

Heinegard D, Paulsson M (1984) Structure and metabolism of proteoglycans. In: Piez CA, Reddi A (eds) Extracellular matrix biochemistry. Elsevier, Amsterdam, pp 277–328

Heinegard D, Hedblom E, Antonsson P, Oldberg A (1990) Structural variability of large and small chondroitin sulphate/dermatan sulphate proteoglycans. Biochem Soc Trans 18:209–212

Menninger H, Burkhardt, H, Röske W, Ehlebracht W, Hering B, Gurr E, Mohr W, Mierau HD (1981) Lysosomal elastase: effect of mechanical and biochemical properties of normal cartilage, inhibition by polysulfonated glycosaminoglycan, and binding to chondrocytes. Rheumatol. Int 1:73–81

Mitchell D, Hardingham T (1982) The control of chondroitin sulphate biosynthesis and its influence on the structure of cartilage proteoglycans. Biochem J 202:387–395

Neame P (1990) Domains in cartilage proteoglycans: do they define the structure? Biochem Soc Trans 18:201–204

Nevo Z (1982) Somatomedine as regulators of proteoglycan synthesis. Connect Tissue Res 10:109–113

Oldberg A, Antonsson P, Lindblom , Heinegard D (1989) A collagen-binding 59-KD protein (fibromodulin) is structurally related to the small interstitial proteoglycans PG-S1 and PG-S2 (decorin). EMBO J 8:2601–2604

Paulsson M, Mörgelin M, Wiedemann H, Beadmore-Gray M, Dunham D, Hardingham TE, Heinegard D, Timpl R, Engel J (1987) Extended and gloublar protein domains in cartilage proteoglycans. Biochem J 245:763–772

Plaas AHK, Sandy JD (1986) The affinity of synthesized proteoglycan for hyaluronic acid can be enhanced by exposure to mild alkali. Biochem J 234:221–223

Poole AR (1986) Proteoglycans in health and disease: structures and functions. Biochem J 236:1–14

Prehm P (1984) Hyaluronate is synthesized at plasma membranes. Biochem J 220:597–600

Prins AP, Lipman JM, Mc Devitt CA, Sokoloff L (1982) Effect of purified growth factors on rabbit articular chondrocytes in monolayer culture. II. Sulfated proteoglycan synthesis. Arthritis Rheum 25:1228–1238

Saklatvala J (1986) Tumor necrosis factor α stimulates resorption and inhibits synthesis of proteoglycan in cartilage. Nature 322:547–549

Scott JE (1984) The periphery of the developing collagen fibril. Biochem J 218:229–233

Shatton I, Schubert M (1954) Isolation of mucoproteins from cartilage. J Biol Chem 211:565–573

Tyler J (1986) Mediators of cartilage destruction. J Clin Chem Clin Biochem 24:954–955

Urban J, Maroudas A (1980) Intervertebral disc in relation to its physiological function and requirements. Clin Rheum Dis 6:51–76

Vogel KG, Paulsson M, Heinegard D (1984) Specific inhibition of type I and type II collagen fibrillogenesis by the small proteoglycan of tendon. Biochem J 223:587–597

Vogel KG, Keller EJ, Lenhoff RJ, Campbell K, Koob TJ (1986) Proteoglycan synthesis by fibroblast cultures initiated from regions of adult bovine tendon subjected to different mechanical forces. Eur J Cell Biol 41:102–112

Glycosaminoglycan Distribution Pattern in Dupuytren's Contracture Biopsies

N. Gässler

Introduction

Glycosaminoglycans consist of polysaccharide chains attached to a core protein. Together with the core protein they make up the proteoglycans. To a large extent the structure of the glycosaminoglycans was established by the work of Meyer (1970). Glycosaminoglycans are linear polymers of repeated disaccharides. The number of repeated disaccharides varies, but typical values are in the order of 50. The constituent monosaccharide residues usually show the chair C-1 conformation. The reason this conformation is favored by the D-monosaccharides lies within the position of the substituents. In the C-1 conformation, most will occupy equatorial positions and maintain the largest possible distance from one another. The length of the disaccharide unit, as measured by X-ray crystallography, varies from 0.93 to 0.97 nm for the different glycosaminoglycans (Heinegard and Paulson 1984).

Hyaluronic acid (Fig. 1) is the largest glycosaminoglycan, with a molecular weight ranging from a hundred thousand to several million. It is unbranched and contains from 50 to several thousand disaccharides units. The disaccharide consists of an *N*-acetylglucosamine linked by a β-glycosidic bond to a glucuronic acid. It does not contain any sulfate groups.

Chondroitin and chondroitin sulfate also contain only one type of uronic acid, i.e., glucuronic acid. Two types of chondroitin sulfate can be distinguished, differing in the ester group attached to carbon 4 or 6 of the *N*-acetylgalactosamine molecule. The number of repeated disaccharides within a chain varies within different preparations from 20 to 60 with an average of about 40, corresponding to a molecular weight of about 20 000. The number of sulfate groups also varies, with an average of about 0.8 sulfate groups per disaccharide.

The nomenclature of dermatan and dermatan sulfate is confusing because they can be viewed as modified chondroitin sulfate. Two different disaccharide units containing either D-glucuronic acid or L-iduronic acid, which is the C-5 epimer of D-glucuronic acid, and a hexosamine are distributed in a copolymeric fashion with several alternating segments, each containing one to several disaccharide units of either type. The number of these units in the glycosaminoglycan chain is variable, but on the average is somewhat higher than that of chondroitin

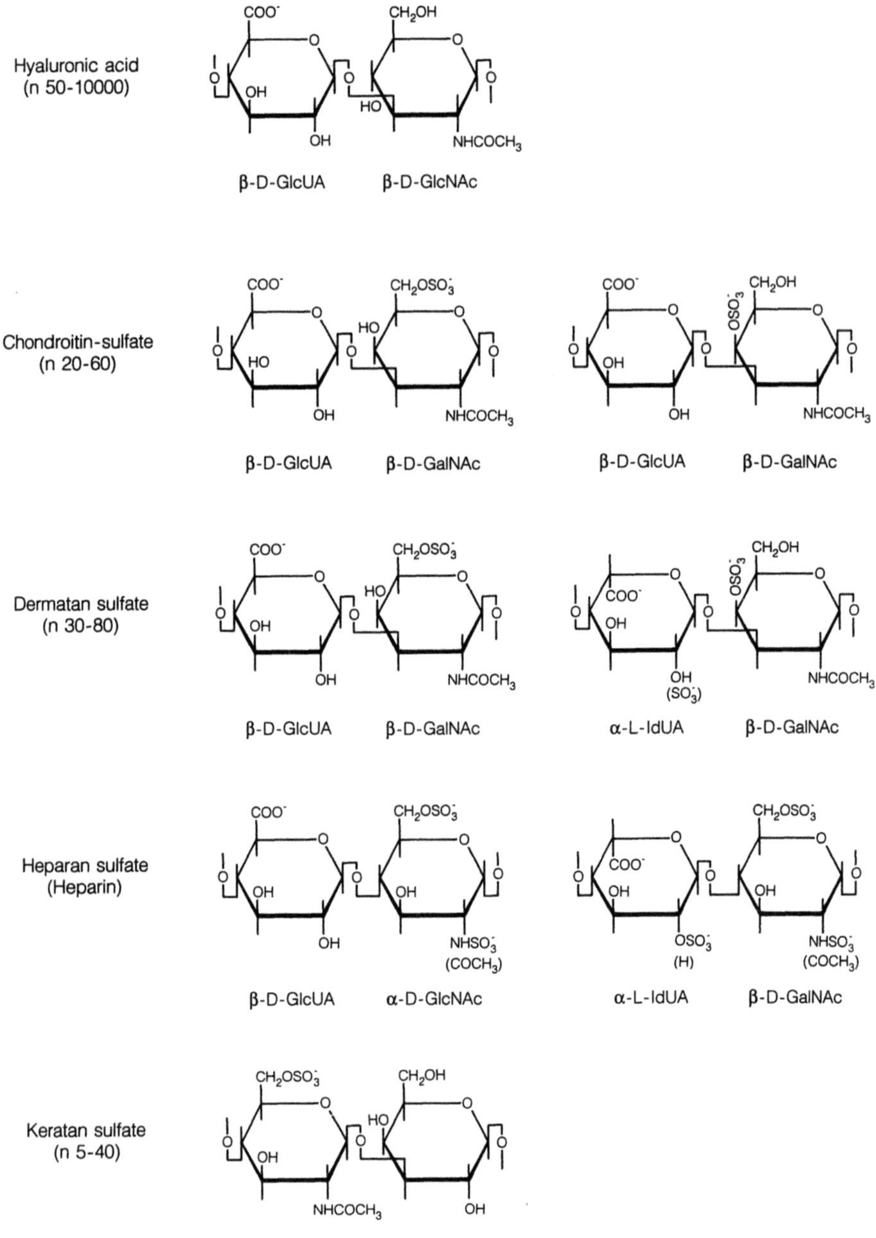

Fig. 1. Structures of repeating disaccharide units of the glycosaminoglycans (*n* denotes number of disaccharide units in the chain). *GlcNAc*, *N*-acetylglucosamine; *GlcUA*, glucuronic acid; *IdUA*, iduronic acid; *GalNAc*, *N*-acetylgalactosamin; *Gal*, galactose

sulfate (about 50–60). The proportion of L-iduronic acid-containing disaccharides in a single chain varies greatly from a few percent to almost 100%. The hexosamine contains the sulfate group at position 4 or 6.

Keratan sulfate and heparan sulfate are two other types of glycosaminoglycans with different types of disaccharides and disaccharide units. In heparan sulfate N-acetylglucosamine is linked by a β-glycosidic bond to glucuronic acid (type I) or to iduronic acid (type II). The disaccharides in keratan sulfate contain a sulfated N-acetylglucosamine linked to galactose. The molecules also contain sulfate groups at various positions.

The main purpose of pathobiochemical investigations of the pattern of glycosaminoglycans from palmar fascia tissue was to find an explanation for the limited function of tissues from individuals with Dupuytren's contracture.

Material and Methods

Biopsy specimens from patients with Dupuytren's disease of the hand were taken upon surgery and classified, according to their macroscopic appearance into four groups as:

1. Apparently normal
2. Tissue adjacent to bands or nodules
3. Bands
4. Nodules

To determine the types and amounts of various sulfated and unsulfated glycosaminoglycans of both healthy human palmar fascia and tissue from Dupuytren's contracture, a specific and reliable method, first described by Gurr et al. (1985), was used. A modification of this method now additionally allows the determination of heparan sulfate and keratan sulfate (Gässler et al. 1991, unpublished results) (Fig. 2). Specific glycosaminoglycan degrading enzymes (chondroitinase AC, -ABC and heparitinase I,II) and high performance liquid chromatography (HPLC) using a potent anion exchanger are employed for the specific and quantitative determination of the individual glycosaminoglycan fractions. The amount of the different glycosaminoglycans is calculated from the amount of the corresponding disaccharides after digestion using disaccharide standards. As the linearity and reproducibility of the HPLC analysis has been evaluated, exact and quantitative results are obtained under these conditions. Glycosaminoglycan disaccharides give HPLC peaks proportional to concentrations between 10 and 4800 µmol/l. The coefficients of variation within a series range between 1.7% and 3.4%. Coefficients of variation ranging from 2.0% to 4.0% are obtained from day to day. The uronic acid content of the glycosaminoglycans is assayed by the carbazole reaction (Bitter and Muir 1962). The sulfated glycosaminoglycan components are assayed with dimethylmethylene blue (Farndale et al. 1986).

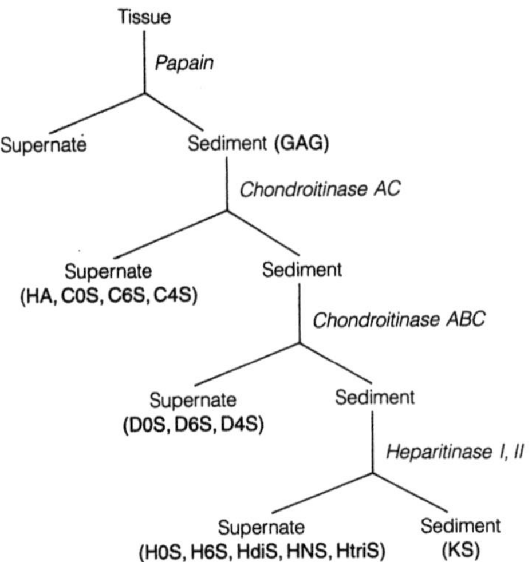

Fig. 2. Isolation and characterization of the tissue by papain, chondroitinase AC, chondroitinase ABC and heparitinase I and II. *GAG*, glycosaminoglycans (total); *HA*, hyaluronic acid; *COS*, chondroitin; *C6S*, chondroitin-6-sulfate; *C4S*, chondroitin-4-sulfate; *DOS*, dermatan; *D6S*, dermatan-6-sulfate; *D4S*, dermatan-4-sulfate; *HOS*, heparan; *H6S*, heparan-6-sulfate; *HdiS*, heparan-N,6-disulfate and heparan-N,2-disulfate; *HNS*, heparan-N-sulfate; *HtriS*, heparan-N,6,2-trisulfate; *KS*, keratansulfate

Results and Discussion

The results of the glycosaminoglycan determinations of normal palmar fascia tissue compared to the results of the four groups of abnormal tissue are described below.

The concentration of uronic acid (Fig. 3) increased with the severity of the disease, being three times higher in nodules than in normal fascia. The increase in the concentration of dimethylmethylene blue (Fig. 4) reflects an increase in the concentration of sulfated glycosaminoglycans in the abnormal tissue. The results of the glycosaminoglycan determinations of the normal palmar fascia (Fig. 5) shows that hyaluronic acid is the main constituent of the tissue. In the four groups of abnormal tissue the hyaluronate content is almost the same. Only in bands or nodules is the content slightly decreased. The content of dermatan and dermatan sulfate in nodules is significantly elevated. It is five times that of healthy fascia, whereas the fractions of chondroitin and chondroitin sulfate in bands or nodules show concentrations up to 11 times higher than those found in normal fascia. The obtained concentrations of glycosaminoglycan are in agreement with the results by Flint et al. (1982) and Tunn et al. (1988), who studied glycosaminoglycans in different parts of the tissue of Dupuytren's contracture and compared the findings with those from normal palmar fascia.

88   N. Gässler

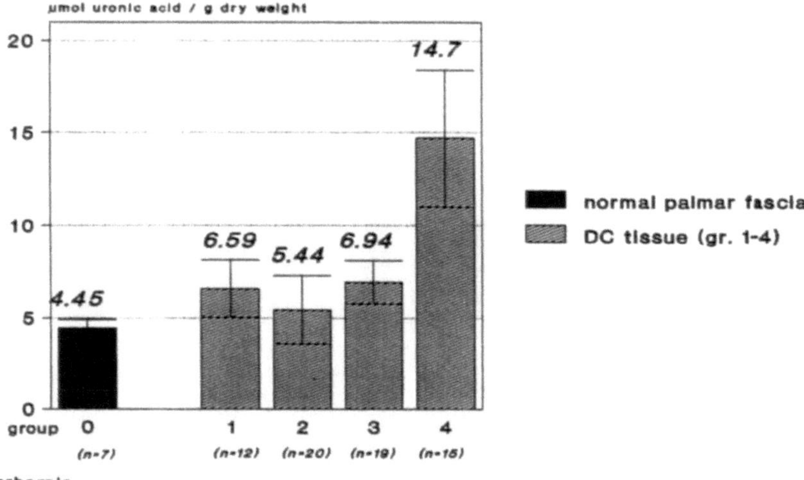

Fig. 3. Concentration of glycosaminoglycans (GAG) per gram dry weight in palmar fascia from Dupuytren's contracture and healthy palmar aponeurosis. Grouping of specimens according to their macroscopic appearances (see Table 1). Total GAG estimation by uronic acid assay using carbazole

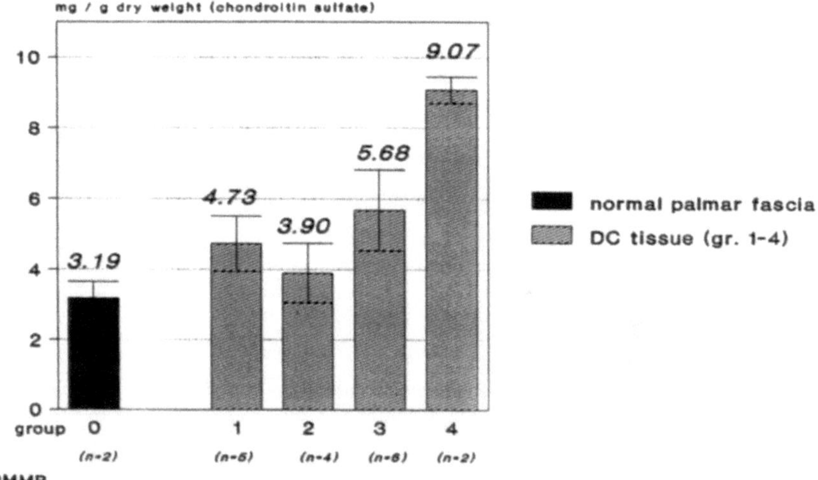

Fig. 4. Concentration of glycosaminoglycans (GAG) per gram dry weight in palmar fascia from Dupuytren's contracture and healthy palmar aponeurosis. Grouping of specimens according to their macroscopic appearances (see Table 1). Total GAG estimation by dimethylmethylene blue (*DMMB*) assay

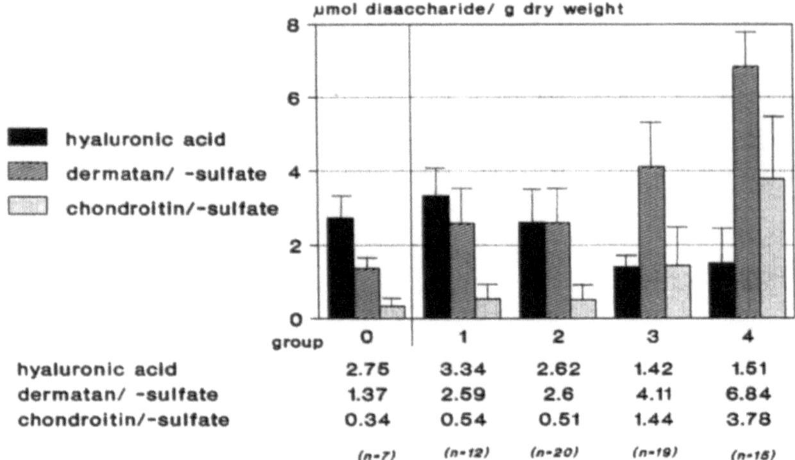

	group 0	1	2	3	4
hyaluronic acid	2.75	3.34	2.62	1.42	1.51
dermatan/ -sulfate	1.37	2.59	2.6	4.11	6.84
chondroitin/-sulfate	0.34	0.54	0.51	1.44	3.78
	(n=7)	(n=12)	(n=20)	(n=19)	(n=18)

Fig. 5. Glycosaminoglycan patterns of normal palmar fascia and in specimens from Dupuytren's disease. Grouping of specimens according to their macroscopic appearances (see Table 1)

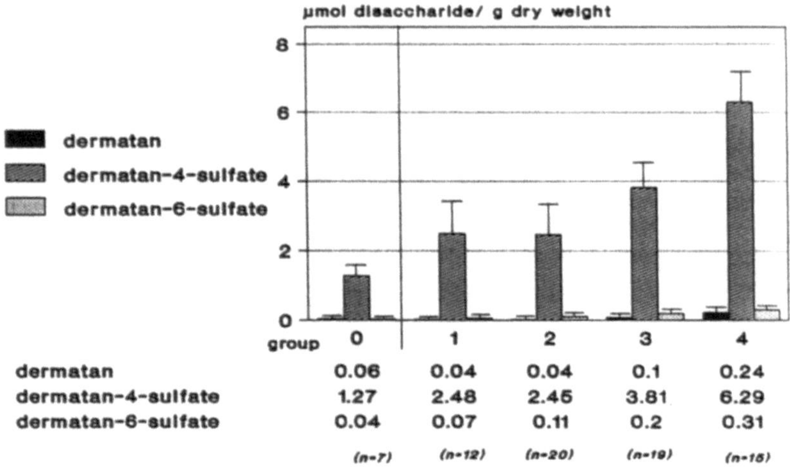

	group 0	1	2	3	4
dermatan	0.06	0.04	0.04	0.1	0.24
dermatan-4-sulfate	1.27	2.48	2.45	3.81	6.29
dermatan-6-sulfate	0.04	0.07	0.11	0.2	0.31
	(n=7)	(n=12)	(n=20)	(n=19)	(n=18)

Fig. 6. Dermatan- and dermatan sulfate isomer patterns of normal palmar fascia and in specimens from Dupuytren's disease. Grouping of specimens according to their macroscopic appearances (see Table 1)

The pattern of the 4- and 6-sulfated isomers of dermatan sulfate found in Dupuytren's contracture tissue (Fig. 6) is the same within all the macroscopically different tissues. The 4-sulfated compound is the predominant isomer, comprising about 90% of the total concentration of dermatan sulfate.

Concerning the chondroitin sulfate, three different patterns of isomers can be observed (Fig. 7). In normal palmar fascia the 4-sulfated and 6-sulfated

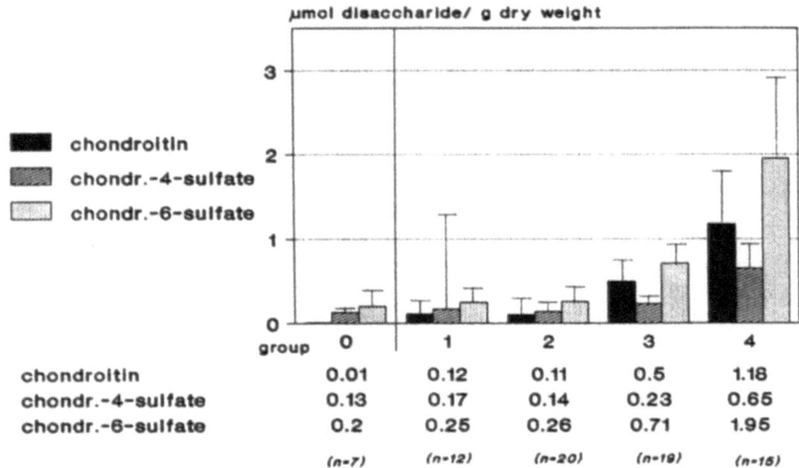

	group 0	1	2	3	4
chondroitin	0.01	0.12	0.11	0.5	1.18
chondr.-4-sulfate	0.13	0.17	0.14	0.23	0.65
chondr.-6-sulfate	0.2	0.25	0.26	0.71	1.95
	(n=7)	(n=12)	(n=20)	(n=19)	(n=15)

Fig. 7. Chondroitin- and chondroitin sulfate isomer patterns of normal palmar fascia and in specimens from Dupuytren's disease. Grouping of specimens according to their macroscopic appearances (see Table 1)

compounds occur in equal concentrations, while unsulfated chondroitin is not detectable or is detected only in traces.

In bands or nodules the content of chondroitin is markedly increased. The content of chondroitin-4-sulfate is higher than in normal palmar fascia, but smaller in relation to the total chondroitin and chondroitin sulfate concentration. As can be expected, the concentrations of the chondroitin sulfate isomers obtained from apparently normal tissue or tissue adjacent to bands or nodules lie between these two patterns.

Determination of glycosaminoglycan disaccharides in nodules (Fig. 8) shows that dermatan/dermatan sulfate and chondroitin/chondroitin sulfate are the main constituents of the tissue. The heparan sulfate and keratan sulfate compounds make up about 21% of the total content of glycosaminoglycans; hyaluronan is detectable in small concentrations.

Multivariate statistical analysis of the data (Fig. 9) yields a classification that clearly allows one to distinguish between the different specimens, whether they were taken from nodules or bands, or from apparently normal or adjacent tissue, or from normal palmar fascia. This biochemical classification is in good agreement with the macroscopic classification. Less difference is found between the tissue adjacent to bands or nodules and normal tissue. This too, however, is in agreement with the difficulties concerning classification according to macroscopic appearance.

Conclusions

Glycosaminoglycan analysis with the combined enzymatic/HPLC method allows characterization and clear classification of different biopsy specimens

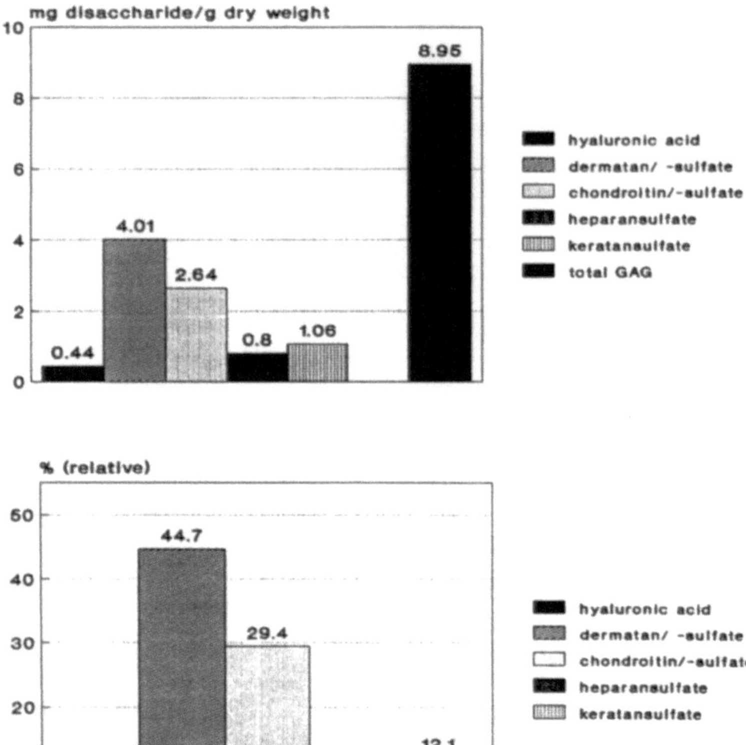

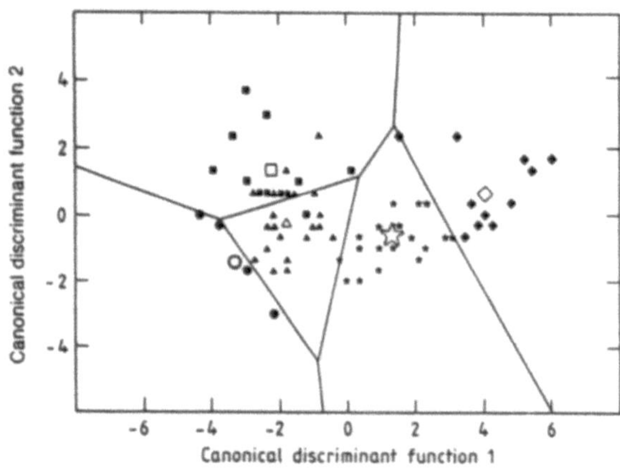

Fig. 8. Glycosaminoglycan (*GAG*) patterns of nodules in palmar fascia from Dupuytren's contracture

from Dupuytren's contracture. Therefore biochemical analysis is a useful tool, equivalent or supplementary to morphological examination. Furthermore, the differences in glycosaminoglycan content in biopsies from the various stages of Dupuytren's disease also reflect differences in the larger functional units, the proteoglycans. Electron microscopic examination, for example, revealed the presence of different proteoglycans in each of the four stages (Scott et al. 1989); thus, biochemical analysis also confirms morphological studies.

Acknowledgement. The author is greatly indebted to Miss M. Arlart and Miss S. Hartje for their skillful technical assistance and to Dr. P. Brenner of the Clinic of Plastic, Hand and Reconstructive Surgery, Hanover Medical School, for his support in acquiring biopsy material.

References

Bitter T, Muir HM (1962) A modified uronic acid carbazole reaction. Anal Biochem 4:330–334

Farndale RW, Buttle DJ, Barrett AJ (1986) Improved quantitation and discrimination of sulfated glycosaminoglycans by use of dimethylmethylene blue. Biochim Biophys Acta 883:173–177

Flint MH, Gillard GC, Reilly HC (1982) The glycosaminoglycans of Dupuytren's disease. Connect Tissue Res 9:173–179

Gurr E, Pallasch G, Tunn S, Tamm C, Delbrück A (1985) High performance liquid chromatographic assay of disaccharides and oligosaccharides produced by the digestion of glycosaminoglycans with chondroitin sulphate lyases. J Clin Chem Clin Biochem 23:77–87

Heinegard D, Paulson M (1984) Structure and metabolism of proteoglycans. In: Piez KA, Reddi AH (eds) Extracellular matrix biochemistry. Elsevier, New York, pp 277–328

Meyer K (1970) Reflections on "mucopolysaccharides" and their protein polysaccharide complexes. In: Balazs EA (ed) The Chemistry and molecular biology of the intracellular matrix, vol 1. Academic, London, pp 5–24

Scott JE, Haigh M, Nusgens B, Lapiere CM (1989) Proteoglycan: collagen interactions in dermatosporatic skin and tendon. An electron histochemical study using cupromeronic blue in a critical electrolyte concentration method. Matrix 9:437–442

Tunn S, Gurr E, Delbrück A, Buhr T, Flory J (1988) The distribution of unsulphated and sulphated glycosaminoglycans in palmar fascia from patients with Dupuytren's disease and healthy subjects. J Clin Chem Clin Biochem 26:7–14

◁ **Fig. 9.** Classification of specimens from healthy palmar fascia and Dupuytren's disease by multivariate statistical evaluation of the glycosaminoglycan patterns. *Closed circles*, healthy controls; *closed squares*, apparently normal fascia; *closed triangles*, fascia adjacent to bands and nodules; *closed stars*, bands; *closed diamonds*, nodules. The *open symbols* indicate the respective group centroid

Biochemical Parameters for the Diagnosis
of Dupuytren's Disease

N. Gässler, P. Brenner, A. Berger, and A. Delbrück

Introduction

The diagnosis of Dupuytren's disease is based on clinical rather than
serological parameters. In this study, the concentrations of several components
of connective tissue in serum/plasma have been assayed to assess their
usefulness in the diagnosis and monitoring of Dupuytren's disease.
To investigate the inflammatory genesis of Dupuytren's contracture,
polymorphonuclear granulocyte (PMN) elastase and the inhibitors α_2-
macroglobulin and α_1-antitrypsin (Lang et al. 1989) have been studied
intensively. The release of collagenase and gelatinase from phagocytic
leukocytes is associated with inflammation and the serum concentrations of
these enzymes have also been measured (Bergmann et al. 1989). In plasma, the
concentration of fibronectin, a high molecular weight glycoprotein, is increased
in inflammatory processes. Altered concentrations of fibronectin in the tissue
may lead to a change in the binding affinity between the cell surface and collagen fibers (Dati et al. 1981). Collagen type III is the most important type of
collagen in the Dupuytren's contracture tissue (Bailey et al. 1977). The NH_2-
terminal propeptide of type III collagen (PIIINP), a direct parameter of newly
synthesized type III collagen (Respondek et al. 1989), has also been assayed.
In the biosynthesis of chondroitin sulfate proteoglycans, one of the enzymes
involved is UDP-D-xylose:proteoglycan core protein β-D-xylosyltransferase (β-
D-xylosyltransferase). Previously, we have reported a significant increase in the
concentration of sulfated glycosaminoglycans in the tissue of Dupuytren's
contracture. In bands or nodules, as classified according to their macroscopic
appearance, chondroitin sulfate shows concentrations up to ten times higher
than found in normal fascia (Tunn et al. 1988). It also seemed useful to
investigate β-D-xylosyltransferase as a biochemical parameter in Dupuytren's
disease, since this enzyme is highly specific for cells able to synthesize
proteoglycans, especially chondrocytes (Kleesiek et al. 1987). Hyaluronan
(hyaluronic acid) is another high molecular weight glycosaminoglycan which
plays a key role in formation of the extracellular matrix of connective tissue
(Fraser et al. 1981). Interleukin-1β (IL-1β) and tumor necrosis factor-α (TNF-
α) are cytokines promoting antigen-specific immune responses, inflammation,
and remodeling of the extracellular matrix (Postlethwaite et al. 1989).

Material and Methods

We investigated blood samples (serum and plasma) collected from patients with manifest Dupuytrens contracture. There were 60 male patients distributed according to age as proposed by Mikkelsen (1990): 34–72 years, 45–72 years and 55–72 years. The patients were recruited from the Clinic of Plastic, Hand and Reconstructive Surgery at the Medical School of Hanover. Prior to surgery six samples were taken from each person (serum and plasma from three locations) from a dorsal vein of the hand with Dupuytren's contracture, from the cubital vein of the same extremity and from the cubital vein of the opposite extremity. For all patients, the stage of the disease was classified as stage 3 or 4, according to Millesi (1981). The serum/plasma was stored at $-70°C$ for up to 2 months until the assays were performed.

PMN elastase was measured in plasma by an immunoassay with antibody fragments (Fab) (Merck, Darmstadt) (Neumann et al. 1984). The plasma concentration of α_2-macroglobulin was determined by an immunoprecipitation assay and nephelometric detection (Beckman, Munich), and serum α_1-antitrypsin levels were determined by the method described previously (Sternberg 1977). Plasma leukocyte collagenase and gelatinase were measured by a previously described enzyme-linked immunosorbent assay (ELISA) (Bergmann et al. 1989). Plasma fibronectin was determined by an immunometric assay with specific antibodies (Behringwerke, Marburg) (Mosesson and Umfleet 1970). Plasma PIIINP was measured by a radioimmunoassay (Behring-Hoechst, Frankfurt), as described previously (Rohde et al. 1979). Serum β-D-xylosyltransferase was measured by a radiometric assay (Kleesiek et al. 1987). Hyaluronan was determined by a previously described radiometric assay (Pharmacia, Uppsala, Sweden) (Engström-Laurent et al. 1985). Serum IL-1β was measured by a solid-phase ELISA test kit with monoclonal antibodies to human IL-1β (Cistron, Pine Brook, New Jersey), and serum TNF-α was determined by an enzyme immunoassay with two clones of antibodies (Boehringer Mannheim, Mannheim) (Meager et al. 1989). Other analyses (creatinine, urea, sodium and potassium) were performed with serum by routine methods. The reference values were determined according to the literature. To distinguish differences between the locations of venopuncture, the data were evaluated using the Mann-Whitney U-test (Mann and Whitney 1947).

Results

Normal concentrations of PMN elastase, α_1-antitrypsin, α_2-macroglobulin, fibronectin, PIIIP, and hyaluronan were found in Dupuytrens subjects (Table 1). Only lower concentrations of collagenase and gelatinase were found. Compared to the mean values in healthy subjects, all three groups of gelatinase concentrations were significantly lower ($p \leq 0.001$) (Table 1). In the group of older patients with Dupuytren's contracture (≥ 55 years; $n = 13$), the lowest concentrations were found. Gelatinase in plasma from the dorsal hand vein was

Table 1. Mean concentrations/activities of extracellular matrix components in sera/plasma from patient's with Dupuytren's disease (age 34–72)

Biochemical parameter		Number of patients	Reference values	Mean concentration ($\pm$ SD)		
				Group A	Group B	Group C
PMN elastase	(μg/l)	19	22 ± 20	21.1 ± 11.4	22.6 ± 7.5	23.3 ± 8.9
α_1-Antitrypsin	(g/l)	31	0.92–2.62	1.47 ± 0.32	1.45 ± 0.33	1.48 ± 0.36
α_2-Macroglobulin	(g/l)	29	1.20–3.20	1.96 ± 0.45	1.93 ± 0.49	1.94 ± 0.51
Collagenase	(mg/l)	17	0–50	2.42 ± 1.18	2.84 ± 2.30	1.72 ± 0.75
Gelatinase	(mg/l)	17	27–94	11.6 ± 8.2	13.6 ± 11.4	19.1 ± 15.2
Fibronectin	(g/l)	41	0.25–0.40	0.31 ± 0.15	0.30 ± 0.15	0.31 ± 0.14
NH_2-terminal procollagen III peptide	(kU/l)	32	0.30–0.80	0.68 ± 0.25	0.65 ± 0.21	0.66 ± 0.21
β-D-xylosyltransferase	(kU/l)	21	–	419 ± 128	407 ± 164	438 ± 152
Hyaluronan	(μg/l)	22	7–65	34.6 ± 17.9	24.7 ± 10.5	34.9 ± 19.5
Interleukin-1β	(ng/l)	20	–	17.5 ± 8.6	20.0 ± 9.3	18.6 ± 9.9
Tumor necrosis factor-α	(ng/l)	7	–	0.51 ± 0.25	0.65 ± 0.43	0.88 ± 0.91
Sodium	(mmol/l)	39	132–155	141 ± 3.0	140 ± 3.0	140 ± 3.0
Potassium	(mmol/l)	37	3.6–5.4	4.3 ± 0.4	4.4 ± 0.4	4.4 ± 0.4
Creatinine	(mmol/l)	39	<115	85 ± 12	87 ± 13	86 ± 14
Urea	(mmol/l)	38	3.30–6.70	5.33 ± 1.66	5.21 ± 1.63	5.12 ± 1.52

Group A, blood samples from dorsal hand vein; group B, blood samples from the cubital vein of the same extremity; group C, blood samples from the cubital vein of the opposite extremity.

10.9 mg/l, in plasma from the cubital vein of the same extremity 9.5 mg/l and of the opposite extremity 14.1 mg/l (data not shown). In the group of Dupuytren's patients 45–72 years of age, ($n = 16$; data not shown) the results for gelatinase are similar to the results shown in Table 1.

Regarding the site of venopuncture, the different groups showed no significant differences with respect to the concentrations of all tested parameters. It should be noted that the concentration of hyaluronan differs between group A (blood samples from the dorsal hand vein) and group B (blood samples from the cubital vein of the same extremity) but not between group A and group C (blood samples from the cubital vein of the opposite extremity (Table 1). The differences are not significant. The concentrations of hyaluronan are similar in all three age groups.

With the possible exception of TNF-α concentration, we found no link between the age of Dupuytren's disease patients and any of the other parameters. The single exception could be concentrations of tumor necrosis factor. TNF-α concentrations among patients aged 55–72 are 1.23 ng/l ($n = 4$), 1.09 ng/l ($n = 5$) in the group 45–72 years, and 0.88 ng/l ($n = 7$) in patients 34–72 years. These findings correspond to those from normal subjects reported in the literature (Engström-Laurent et al. 1985).

Conclusions

This study was designed to develop a biochemical approach for the diagnosis of Dupuytren's disease. Most of the parameters were normal and unsuitable as markers of Dupuytren's disease. This might be due to the fact that connective tissue components are widely distributed in the body and only small amounts of these are actually involved in Dupuytren's contracture.

Whether collagenase and gelatinase could be suitable biochemical and possibly even age-dependent parameters for collagen changes in Dupuytren's disease has to be investigated in further studies. The major biochemical characteristic of Dupuytren's disease is the progressive and irreversible deposition of excess fibrous collagen (Bailey et al. 1977). A stimulating factor may produce the observed changes in the collagen in Dupuytren's disease. However, one might also presume that the low concentrations of gelatinase, and perhaps collagenase too, are direct indicators of disturbed collagen degradation.

There is no explanation why the concentrations of hyaluronan in blood samples collected from the cubital vein of the affected extremity (group B) are lower than the concentrations in the dorsal vein of the hand with Dupuytren's contracture (group A) or than the concentrations of group C. Further studies should investigate whether hyaluronan makes up part of the extracellular matrix of connective tissue in Dupuytren's disease.

Since indicators of inflammation (PMN elastase, α_2-macroglobulin, α_1-antitrypsin, human leukocyte collagenase and gelatinase, fibronectin and the cytokines IL-1β and TNF-α) were not found to be increased in severe clinical stages, Dupuytren's disease shows no serological evidence of systemic inflammatory components.

Acknowledgement. We gratefully acknowledge the measurement of leukocyte collagenase and gelatinase by Dr. Tschesche (University of Bielefeld, Department of Biochemistry). We are also grateful to Dr. Kleesiek (Centre of Heart Disease, Bad Oeynhausen) for measuring β-D-xylosyltransferase in blood samples. We thank Mrs. S. Hartje for her valuable technical assistance.

References

Bailey AJ, Sims TJ, Gabbiani G, Bazin S, LeLous M (1977) Collagen of Dupuytren's disease. Clin Sci Mol Med 53:499–502

Bergmann U, Michaelis J, Oberhoff R, Knäuper V, Beckmann R, Tschesche H (1989) Enzyme linked immunosorbent assay (ELISA) for the quantitative determination of human leucocyte collagenase and gelatinase. J Clin Chem Clin Biochem 27:351–359

Dati F, Bowen M, Cooper EH (1981) Fibronectin: Ergebnisse bei malignen Erkrankungen, entzündlichen Prozessen und Infektionen. Congress for Laboratory Medicine, May 3–8, Berlin

Engström-Laurent A, Laurent UBG, Lilja K, Laurent TC (1985) Concentration of sodium hyaluronate in serum. Scand J Clin Lab Invest 45:497–504

Fraser JRE, Laurent TC, Pertoft H, Baxter E (1981) Plasma clearance, tissue distribution and metabolism of hyaluronic acid injected intravenously in the rabbit. Biochem J 200:415–424

Kleesiek K, Reinards R, Okusi J, Wolf B, Greiling H (1987) UDP-D-xylose: proteoglycan core protein β-D-xylosyltransferase: a new marker of cartilage destruction in chronic joint diseases. J Clin Chem Clin Biochem 25:473–481

Lang H, Dreher M, Heuber A (1989) Diagnotische Spezifität der Plasma-Elastase als prädiktiver, biochemischer Marker für infektiöse bzw. entzündliche Komplikationen. Mitt Dtsch Ges Klin Chem 1:10–16

Mann HB, Whitney DR (1947) On a test of whether one of two random variables is stochastically larger than the other. Ann Math Statist 18:50–60

Meager A, Leung H, Woolley J (1989) Assay for tumor necrosis factor and related cytokines. J Immunol Methods 116:1–17

Mikkelsen OA (1990) Epidemiology of a Norwegian population. In: McFarlane RM, Flint MH (eds) Dupuytren's disease. Churchill Livingstone, Edinburgh, pp 191–200

Millesi H (1981) In: Nigst H, Buch-Gramcko D, Millesi H (eds) Handchirurgie, vol 1. Thieme, Stuttgart

Mosesson MW, Umfleet RA (1970) The cold-insoluble globulin of human plasma. J Biol Chem 245:5728–5734

Neumann S, Gunzer G, Hennrich N, Lang H (1984) "PMN-elastase assay": enzyme immunoassay for human polymorphonuclear elastase complexed with α_1-proteinase inhibitor. J Clin Chem Clin Biochem 22:693–698

Postlethwaite AE, Smith GN, Lachman LB, Endres RO, Poppleton HM, Hasty KA, Seyer JM, Kang AH (1989) Stimulation of glycosaminoglycan synthesis in cultured human dermal fibroblasts by interleukin 1. J Clin Invest 83:629–636

Respondek M, Seidel MJ, Lautenschläger J, Müller W (1989) Hyaluronsäure und N-terminales Prokollagen-III-Peptid im Urin bei entzündlichen und degenerativen Gelenkerkrankungen. J Rheumatol 48:117–122

Rohde H, Vargas L, Hahn EG, Kalbfleisch H, Bruguera M, Timpl R (1979) Radioimmunoassay for type III procollagen peptide and its application to human liver disease. Eur J Clin Invest 9:451–459

Sternberg JC (1977) A rate nephelometer for measuring specific proteins by immunoprecipitin reactions. Clin Chem 23:1456–1464

Tunn S, Gurr E, Delbrück A, Buhr T, Flory J (1988) The distribution of sulphated and unsulphated glycosaminoglycans in palmar fascia from patients with Dupuytren's disease and healthy subjects. J Clin Chem Clin Biochem 26:7–14

Pathobiochemistry of Cells
in Dupuytren's Contracture

Investigations of Cell Cultures Derived from Patients Suffering from Dupuytren's Contracture

J. Neumüller

Introduction

Comparative cell cultures derived from biopsies of healthy subjects and patients suffering from disease allow one to study permanent alterations on the cellular level. The isolation of cells and their subcultivation shock the cells and alter their behavior with respect to a transition from the resting to the cycling state of the cell cycle. This is, at least in part, due to the loss of contact inhibition by elements of the extracellular matrix (ECM) and other cells in the vicinity; nonetheless, many of the features of cultured cells still correspond to their in vivo situation. Cultured cells derived postoperatively from patients start their proliferation from a certain stage of disease, which is characterized by the distribution of different cell types and their functions.

In the case of fibromatous disorders such as Dupuytren's contracture (DC) the cells of the connective tissue can be easily studied as fibroblast cultures. Numerous scientific working groups have reported on cell cultured from DC biopsies. Alterations in collagen synthesis or in the synthesis of other elements of the ECM [1–3] and the in vitro persistence of myofibroblasts in cultures derived from nodules of the affected palmar aponeurosis [4–6] have been described.

At the Ludwig Boltzmann Institute of Rheumatology and Balneology in Vienna-Oberlaa I have been working with fibroblasts derived from biopsies of different origin, such as the synovial membrane from patients with rheumatoid arthritis or osteoarthrosis or from patients who underwent meniscectomy or who were operated on for lesions of the crucial ligament. I have also been studying synovial fibroblasts and dermal fibroblasts of the affected and nonaffected skin of patients with psoriatic arthritis. The results of these investigations have been published with regard to the light microscopical and ultrastructural morphology [7–13] as well as the growth and cell cycle parameters [14,15] of these cells.

The task of studying cultures derived from DC involved comparing these cultures with the ones just described and with others established from ligamentous tissues of other disorders such as carpal tunnel syndrome (CTS), tendopathia nodosa (TN), and hallux valgus (HV).

Table 1. Patient characteristics

Carpal tunnel syndrome			Dupuytren's contracture			Tendopathia nodosa			Hallux valgus		
Patient	Sex	Age	Patient	Sex	Age	Patient	Sex	Age	Patient	Sex	Age
1	F	41	1	M	58	1	F	65	1	F	54
2	F	59	2	F	70	2	F	70	2	F	44
3	F	52	3	M	65	3	F	53	3	F	50
4	F	52	4	M	46	4	F	41	4	F	60
5	F	62	5	M	44						
6	F	77	6	M	44						
7	F	75	7	M	44						
8	M	64									

Material and Methods

Cell Culture

Cells were cultured from small biopsy fragments ($5-10\,mm^3$) in 50 ml polystyrene flasks (Nunc) in Parker's medium 199 supplemented with 15% fetal bovine serum, 100 IU/ml penicillin and 100 µg/ml streptomycin. For subcultivation cells were detached with 0.25% trypsin in Ca^{2+}/Mg^{2+}-free phosphate-buffered saline. For all experiments only cells from passages 5–10 were used. Cultures were derived from eight CTS, seven DC, four TN and four HV biopsies. An overview of the sex and age of the patients from whom the cultures were derived is given in Table 1.

Transmission Electron Microscopy Preparation of Tissue Specimens

Tissue fragments of $5-10\,mm^3$ were fixed in 2.5% glutaraldehyde in $0.1\,M$ cacodylate buffer (pH 7.2) for 12 h, rinsed, postfixed with 1% OsO_4 for 90 min, dehydrated in several steps of ethanol and embedded in Spurr's ultraviscosity resin (Polaron) after application of propylene oxide. The polymerization of the resin was carried out at 67°C for 48 h. Semithin and ultrathin sections were performed with a Reichert ultramicrotome using a diamond knife. Semithin sections were stained for light microscopy (LM) investigation with borax/crystal violet, ultrathin sections contrasted with uranylacetate and lead citrate as usual.

Transmission Electron Microscopy Preparation of Cell Cultures

Cell cultures were grown in 6 cm diameter plastic dishes until they reached preconfluency or confluency. The cultured cells were fixed and dehydrated in

the same way as the tissue fragments. After dehydration 5 ml propylene oxide
were added to the dishes. When the polystyrene support of the monolayer
began to dissolve, the monolayer came up to the surface of the liquid as a
floating sheet [16] and could be easily transferred to the resin in a flat silicone-
embedded form. Further processing was carried out as described above.
The demonstration of acid phosphatase in lysosomes and phagolysosomes was
performed according to the method of Gomori modified by Yajima [17,18].

Transmission Electron Microscopy

Ultrathin sections from tissues and cell cultures were investigated using a Zeiss
EM 109 transmission electron microscope.

Image Analysis

In the EM study, which allows only a qualitative view of the morphology, two
criteria seemed to be altered in the cells of the DC: the irregularity of the
nucleus and the extent of the lysosomal apparatus. Using image analysis an
attempt was made to quantify these criteria in terms of morphometric
parameters.
Image analysis was performed using an image analysis computer (Vidas,
Kontron, Germany) connected to a high resolution TV camera (Cohu, Japan).
Electron micrographs of equal magnification ($\times 7000$) (negatives) were
recorded by the TV camera and stored by the computer. Image processing was
performed in the following way: (a) inversion of the negative image to a
positive one; (b) contrast enhancement; (c) fragmentation according to a
definition of limits of the upper and lower gray values and conversion to a
binary image; (d) identification of the objects to be isolated; (e) "cleaning" of
the image by removing small and disturbing particles; and finally (f)
measurement of the form factor of the cell nuclei (a parameter reflecting
irregularity) and the percentage of the area taken up by the lysosomes with
respect to the total area of cytoplasm minus the area of the cell nucleus.

Autoradiography

A total of 5×10^4 cells were plated in sterile microchambers (Bellco, USA)
with two compartments each. The left compartment was used for continuous
labeling (CL) with 0.5 µCi/ml [^{3}H]-thymidine (specific activity 49.8 Ci/mmol),
the right one for pulse labeling (PL) with 2 µCi/ml [^{3}H]-thymidine for 30 min.
CL was carried out once during cell inoculation, PL 24, 48, 72, and 96 h after
inoculation.
After PL or CL, the slides forming the bottom of the microchambers were
washed three times with PBS, fixed in 1:3 acetic acid/methanol for 3×30 min

and air dried. Pooled slides were coated with Ilford L4 emulsion and exposed in a dark box for 10 days, developed with Ilford Microphen diluted 1:1 with distilled water, washed twice with distilled water and then fixed with Ilford Hypam 1:10 for 10 min. After washing and drying, the cells were counterstained with Giemsa.

Growth Parameters

For the evaluation of plating efficiency (PE), cells were plated in 6 cm diameter plastic dishes (Nunc) at different but low densities: 100, 250, 500, 750, 1000, 2500 and 5000 cells per dish. After 10 days of growth cells were fixed in methanol for 15 min and stained with Giemsa. The colonies of at least four interconnected cells per dish were counted under a stereomicroscope and the percentage of colonies from the initial inoculum was calculated [19]. The viability (V) of the cultured cells was calculated as the percentage of living cells, using the trypan exclusion test [20].

Statistics

Because of the absence of a gaussian normal distribution of the values obtained from image analysis, autoradiography and the growth parameters, the parameter-free rank tests of Kolmogoroff [21] and Smirnoff [22,23] and Wilcoxon [24] were used for statistical evaluation.

Results and Discussion

Morphological Investigations

When viewed under the LM, fibroblasts from different sources and diseases seem at first sight to be very similar. They are spindle-like with many cell projections and bear an elliptic nucleus in the center. It is only the so-called myofibroblasts which already at the level show alterations of the nucleus: deep invaginations and indentations. Such cells occur at higher frequency in cultures derived from nodules of DC, but above all they are characteristic of the connective tissue involved in the course of fibrosis and wound healing in scar formation. Therefore, in rheumatoid synovium, in which necrosis is followed by scar formation and remodeling, myofibroblasts are also found to be increased in cell cultures derived from that tissue.

In DC not all the characteristics of myofibroblasts were completely preserved in cultures after subcultivation. As shown in Fig. 1a it was confirmed by morphometric investigation of the cell nuclei that invaginations and indentations (which result in a higher form factor) were indeed more common in DC and CTS cultures but were also present in cultures derived from TN and

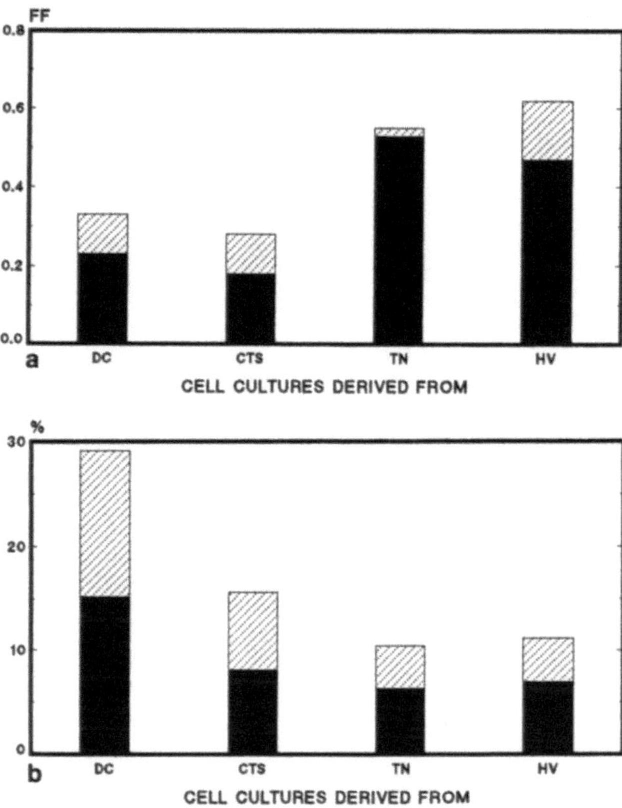

Fig. 1. a Form factor (*FF*) of cell nuclei. FF is defined as the (diameter)^2/2π × area. **b** Amount of area occupied by lysosomes with respect to the area of the cytoplasm. *Blackened area*, mean value; *hatched area*, standard deviation; *DC*, Dupuytren's contracture; *CTS*, carpal tunnel syndrome; *TN*, tendopathia nodosa; *HV*, hallux valgus

HV ($p < 0.05$). From the functional point of view this phenomenon is thought to be characteristic of cells activated with respect to DNA and protein synthesis [25].

Myofibroblasts are characterized not only by the irregularity of the cell nucleus but also by a higher representation of stress fibers, composed of actin microfilaments with electron-dense patches (dense bodies) and abundant pinocytotic and exocytotic vesicles. An increased occurrence of monocilia arising from the centrioles has also been described [15,25]. In the biopsies investigated in this study myofibroblasts with a complete range of these characteristics were found predominantly in cultures derived from DC nodules. Although tissue samples from HV and TN – but not from CTS – also contained these cells, after several passages of culture myofibroblasts partially lost some of these features.

Cells of CTS, DC and TN cultures in the states of preconfluency and confluency were connected from end to end by cell branches or laterally by gap

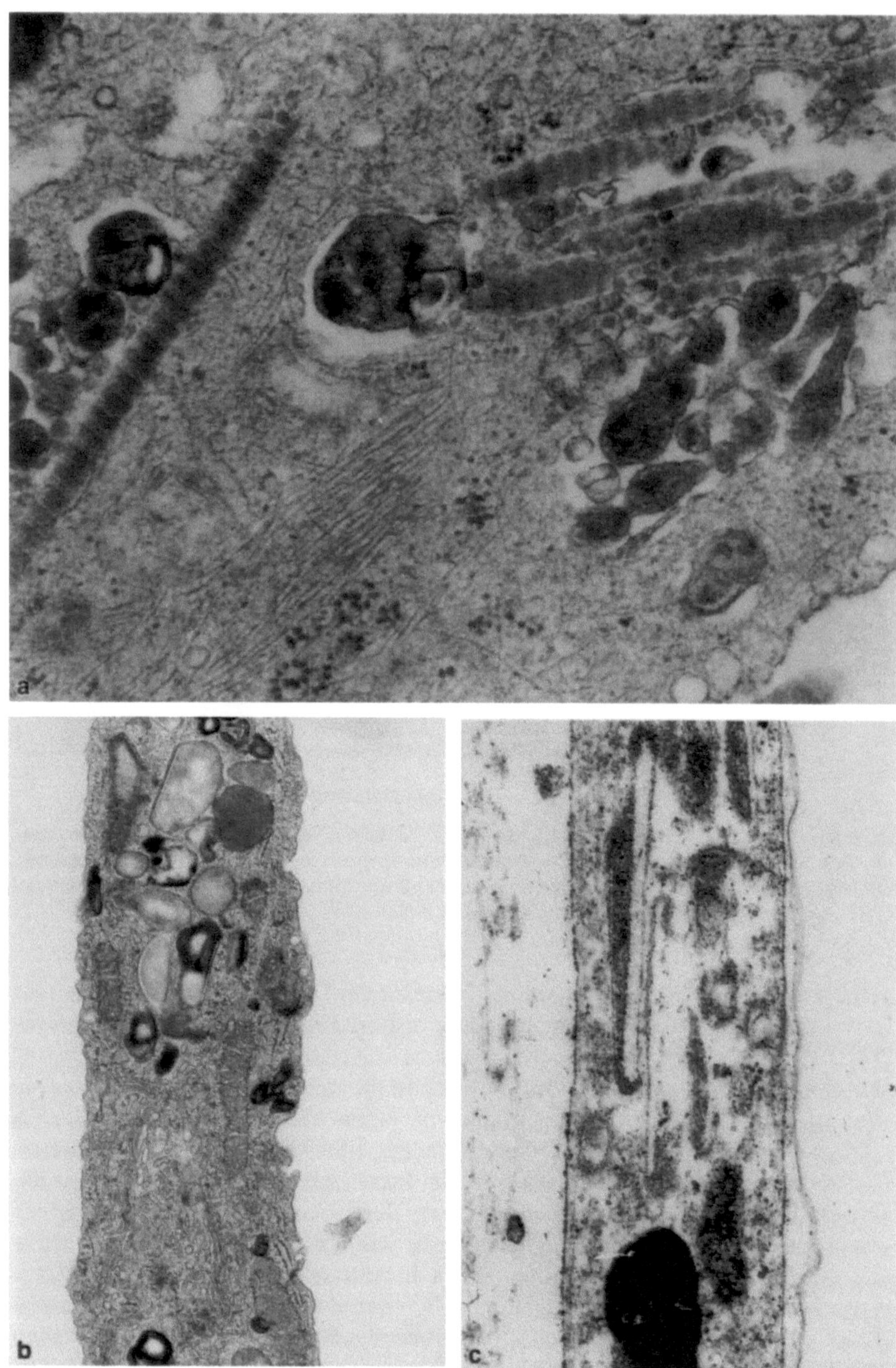

Fig. 2. a Phagocytosis of collagen fibrils. b Signs of ECM synthesis. c Phagocytosis of collagen fibrils

junctions or hemidesmosomes. In most of the CTS, TN and HV cultures the cell surface was extensively villous. The ligamentous tissues are thought to be bradytrophic. This term concerns both DNA and protein synthesis. DNA synthesis will be discussed below. Concerning protein synthesis, the ultrastructural morphology showed strong signs of ECM synthesis: many well-developed Golgi systems, an abundant rough endoplasmic reticulum, and numerous free ribosomes and polyribosomes (Fig. 2b).

Although it is known it is not well documented that the ECM in DC is altered, with subsequent increased degradation. Already in the early stages of the disease, fusion of collagen fibers can be observed by EM [26,27]. EM also reveals disintegration of elastic fibers. Fibroblasts in the connective tissue are able to degrade ECM by secretion of collagenases and elastases [28–30]. In addition, it has been demonstrated [31] that a part of the procollagen molecule never reaches the extracellular space but is already degraded intracellularly. Fibrillar collagen is not completely degraded extracellularly by proteases; instead, fragments of collagen fibrils have to be removed by phagocytotic cells. In ligament biopsies no increase in the number of phagocytes was found but, as has been shown already in other tissues and also in fibroblast cultures [32–34], fibroblasts are able to phagocytose collagen fibrils and degrade them completely inside of phagolysosomes (Fig. 2c).

This phenomenon of phagocytosis of collagen fibrils could also be demonstrated in cultures derived from DC and CTS. In some cells the fibrils were inserted in deep recessus of the cell membrane; in other cells they appeared to be completely inside the cytoplasm. In such cases the fibrils were not always surrounded by a membrane (Fig. 2a). Therefore it was not possible to judge from the micrograph whether, in the particular case, production (as described in tendon morphogenesis [35]) or degradation of fibrils was occurring. The supply of exocytotic vesicles at the intracellular end of the recessus and the branching of some fibrils in the middle of the recessus speak for the former conclusion. In order to prove the latter hypothesis, demonstration of acid phosphatase, an important lysosomal enzyme, was necessary. It was indeed possible to show with this method that degradation of collagen fibrils was taking place inside phagolysosomes (Fig. 2c). Therefore it cannot be ruled out that in both cultures and in tissues production and phagocytosis of collagen (and perhaps also of elastic) fibers can occur side by side.

Autophagocytosis was observed particularly in cultures derived from TN and HV. Although the V was higher than 98%, autophagocytosis and increased fat vacuolization were signs of the poor condition of the cells in culture.

In order to find out whether the enhanced ECM turnover in DC and CTS is followed by an increased rearrangement of the lysosomal apparatus, a morphometric investigation of the percent extension of this system was carried out using image analysis. As shown in Fig. 1b, the percentage of the area occupied by lysosomes (contrasted with lead for acid phosphatase according to the method of Gomori) is higher in DC and CTS than in TN and HV. The smallest cytoplasmic area occupied by lysosomes was found in TN ($p < 0.05$ between CTS and DP compared to TN and HV).

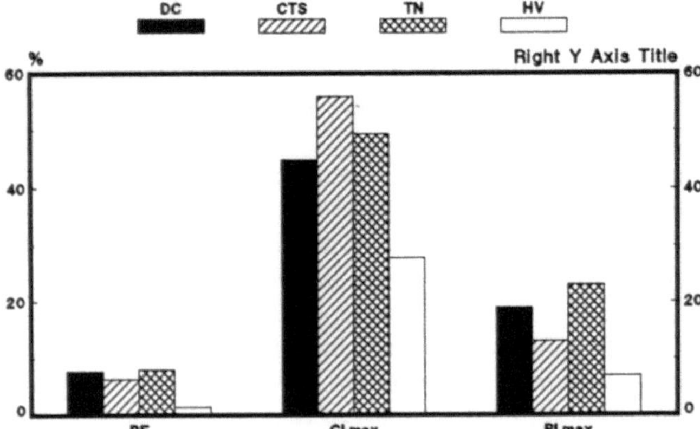

Fig. 3. Plating efficiency (*PE*), maximal continuous labeling (*CL$_{max}$*), and maximal pulse labeling (*PL$_{max}$*) of cell cultures. *DC*, Dupuytren's contracture; *CTS*, carpal tunnel syndrome; *TN*, tendopathia nodosa; *HV*, hallux valgus

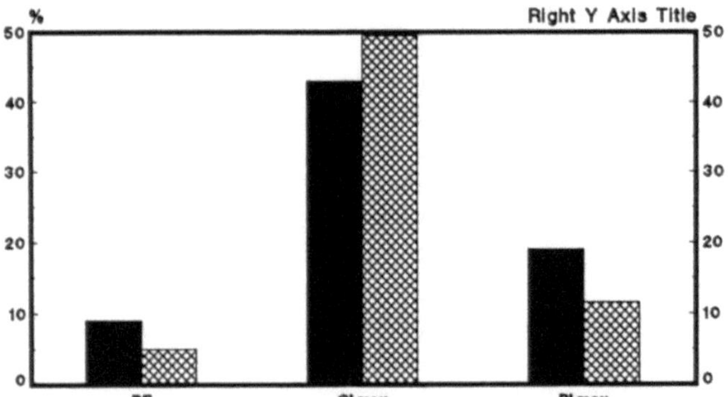

Fig. 4. Plating efficiency (*PE*), maximal continuous labeling (*CL$_{max}$*), and maximal pulse labeling (*PL$_{max}$*) from proliferative and bradytrophic tissue. *Black columns*, proliferative tissue; *cross-hatched columns*, bradytrophic tissues

Growth and Cell Cycle Parameters

The percentages of PE, CL$_{max}$ and PL$_{max}$ are summarized in Fig. 3 and 4. V is not indicated because it was quite similar in all of the cultures (between 98% and 99%). All other parameters were significantly decreased in cultures derived from HV ($p < 0.01$). PL$_{max}$ was significantly higher in cultures from TN than in those from DC ($p < 0.02$).

The influence that the source of biopsies exerted on the behavior of the cell cultures with respect to the criteria bradytrophic or proliferative (tissues with capillarization and abundant fibroblasts) was also investigated. Cultures from proliferative tissues exhibited a significantly higher PE than cultures from bradytrophic tissues ($p < 0.05$).

Many cell cultures from proliferative tissues showed signs of aging. As in other diseases (e.g., rheumatoid arthritis) induced proliferation of connective tissue cells during inflammation causes accelerated biological aging, which can be recognized in vitro by decreased growth parameters.

In this study no significant qualitative alterations in DC cultures could be demonstrated. Yet quantitative differences were found regarding indentations of the nuclei, the production and degradation of collagen fibrils, and differences in growth parameters.

References

1. Brickley-Parsons D, Glimcher MJ, Smith RJ, Albin R, Adams JP (1981) Biochemical changes in the collagen of the palmar fascia in patients with Dupuytren's disease. J Bone Joint Surg [Am] 63:787–797
2. Bartal AH, Stahl S, Karev A, Lichtig C (1987) Dupuytren's contracture studied with monoclonal antibodies to connective tissue differentiation antigens. Clin Exp Immunol 68:457–463
3. Józsa L, Demel S, Pintér T, Renner A, Réffy A, Sántha A, Salamon A (1988) Immunopathological study on palmar aponeurosis in Dupuytren's disease. Acta Histochem (Jena) 83:153–158
4. Józsa L, Salamon A, Réffy A, Renner A, Demel S, Donhöffer A, Pintér T, Thöring J (1988) Fine structural alterations of the palmar aponeurosis in Dupuytren's contracture. Zentralbl Allg Pathol 134:15–25
5. Gabbiani H, Majno G (1972) Dupuytren's contracture: fibroblast contraction. An ultrastructural study. Am J Pathol 66:131–138
6. Salamon A, Hámori J (1980) Die Rolle der Myofibroblasten in der Pathogenese der Dupuytren'schen Kontraktur. Handchirurgie 12:113–117
7. Squier CA, Kremenak CR (1980) Myofibroblasts in healing palatal wounds of the beagle dog. J Anat 130:585–594
8. Schürch W, Seemayer TA, Lagacé R (1981) Stromal myofibroblasts in primary invasive and metastatic carcinomas. Virchows Arch [Pathol Anat] 391:125–139
9. Callea F, Mebis J, Desmet VJ (1982) Myofibroblasts in focal nodular hyperplasia of the liver. Virchows Arch [Pathol Anat] 396:155–166
10. Bhawan J (1981) The myofibroblast. Am J Dermatol 3:73–78
11. Ohtani H, Sasano N (1980) Myofibroblasts and myoepithelial cells in human breast carcinoma. Virchows Arch A [Path Anat] 385:247–261
12. Ohtani H, Sasano N (1983) Stromal cell changes in human colorectal adenomas and carcinomas. Virchows Arch [Pathol Anat] 401:209–222
13. Squier CA (1981) The effect of stretching on formation of myofibroblasts in mouse skin. Cell Tissue Res 220:325–335
14. Mohr W, Vossbeck G (1985) Untersuchungen zur Proliferation und ^{3}H-Prolin-Inkorporation von Zellen der Palmarfibromatose (Morbus Dupuytren). Z Rheumatol 44:226–230
15. Neumüller J, Tohidast-Akrad M, Ammer K, Hakimzadeh A, Stransky G, Weis S, Partsch G, Eberl R (1988) Ultrastructural and autoradiographic investigations of cell cultures derived from tendons or ligamentous material from patients with fibromatous disorders. Exp Cell Biol 56:113–130
16. Arnold JR, Boor PJ (1986) Improved transmission electron microscopy (TEM) of cultured cells through a 'floating sheet' method. J Ultrastruct Mol Struct Res 94:30–36
17. Yajima T (1986) Acid phosphatase activity and intracellular collagen degradation by fibroblasts in vitro. Cell Tissue Res 245:253–260
18. Yajima T (1988) Localization of acid phosphatase activity in collagen-secreting and collagen-resorbing fibroblasts. Histochemistry 90:245–253
19. Adams RLP (1983) Cell culture for biochemists. Elsevier, Amsterdam, p 99

20. Paul J (1970) Cell and tissue culture. Churchill Livingstone, Edinburgh, p 357
21. Kolmogoroff AN (1933) Sulla determinazione empirica di una legge di distribuzione. G Inst Ital Attuari 4:83–91
22. Smirnoff NW (1939) On the estimation of the discrepancy between empirical curves of distribution for two independent samples. Bull Univ Moskov Ser Int Sect A 2: 3–8
23. Smirnoff NW (1948) Tables for estimating the goodness of fit of empirical distributions. Ann Math Statist 19:279–281
24. Wilcoxon F (1945) Individual comparisons by ranking methods. Biometrics 1:80–83
25. Ghadially FN (1982) Ultrastructural pathology of the cell and matrix. Butterworths, London
26. Martini AK, Puhl W (1980) Mikromorphologische Untersuchungen bei Morbus Dupuytren. Z Orthop 118:291–299
27. Legge JWH, Finlay JB, McFarlane RM (1981) A study of Dupuytren's tissue with the scanning electron microscope. J Hand Surg 6:482–492
28. Pelletier-Lebon P, Hornebeck W, Dachet C, Jacotot B, Robert L (1988) Effect of lipoproteins on the elastase activity expressed by human skin fibroblasts in culture. Cell Biol Int Rep 12:449–457
29. Asuwa N (1988) Collagen degradation in the rabbit skin during short-term tissue culture. Virchows Arch [B] 55:345–354
30. Yoffe JR, Taylor DJ, Woolley DE (1984) Mast cell products stimulate collagenase and prostaglandin E production by cultures of adherent rheumatoid synovial cells. Biochem Biophys Res Commun 122:270–276
31. Laurent GJ (1986) Dynamic state of collagen: pathways of collagen degradation in vivo and their possible role in regulation of collagen mass. Am J Physiol 251:C1–C9
32. Eyden BP (1989) Collagen secretion granules in reactive stromal myofibroblasts, with preliminary observations on their occurrence in spindle cell tumours. Virchows Arch [A] 415:437–445
33. Everts V, Beertsen W (1987) The role of microtubules in the phagocytosis of collagen by fibroblasts. Coll Relat Res 7:1–15
34. Michna H (1988) Intracellular collagen fibrils: evidence of an intracellular source from experiments with tendon fibroblasts and fibroblastic tumour cells. J Anat 158:1–12
35. Birk DE, Trelstad RL (1986) Extracellular compartments in tendon morphogenesis: collagen fibril, bundle, and macroaggregate formation. J Cell Biol 103:231–240

Fibroblast Gel Culture: A Model for Biochemical Investigations of Dupuytren's Contracture

A. Delbrück and H. Schröder

Introduction

In Dupuytren's contracture a more or less heterogeneous cell population proliferates and infiltrates the palmar fascia. To investigate the biochemistry and metabolism of a distinct cell population involved in the pathogenesis of Dupuytren's contracture, cell culture systems offer the opportunity to study metabolism independent of local or exogenous factors interfering with the regulation of cell functions. Monolayer cell cultures are widely used to study reaction mechanisms on the cellular level, in particular in fibroblasts. However, the morphologic phenotype of fibroblasts, their arrangement within the extracellular matrix, and their metabolic characteristics differ in monolayer cultures compared to in connective tissues in situ. In monolayer cultures, fibroblasts are confluent with extensive side to side contacts without the appropriate extracellular matrix between the cells. By contrast, in situ, fibroblasts are embedded in and surrounded by a specific matrix and the cells have cell to cell contact via thin processes which extend into the matrix, touching the neighboring cells with their tips. Therefore, a culture system which offers all the requirements mentioned above would be useful. A fibrin gel culture system proved to be the most suitable system for growing fibroblasts in an in vivo like fashion.

Methods

Isolation of Cells from Human Connective Tissue. The cells were incubated with collagenase for varying times corresponding to the age of the donor ($3 \times 30{-}40\,$h, 37°C), filtered through glass fibers, centrifuged and washed with minimum essential medium (MEM) containing 10% fetal calf serum (FCS). They were then resuspended in MEM/FCS and counted in a cell counter.

Fibrin Gel Preparation. A suspension containing 1.5 mg/ml human fibrinogen, 6.0 µg/ml human fibronectin, 1 U/ml factor XIII, 2 mmol/l calcium, MEM/FCS 10%, and 150 000 cells/ml was dispensed into culture dishes coated with a thin film of high temperature agarose. Coagulation was started by adding 0.1 U/ml of thrombin.

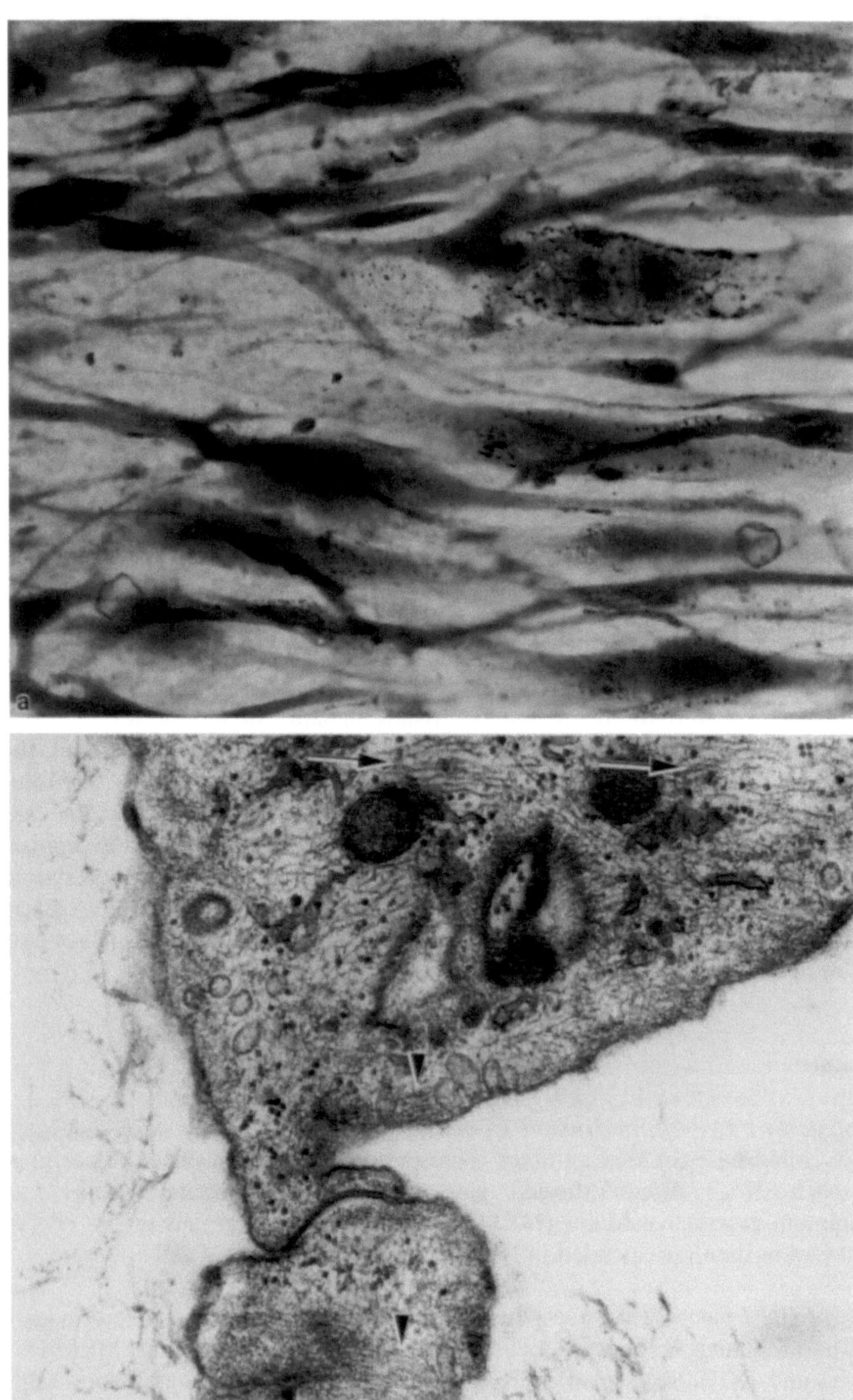

Incubation. The cell/fibrin gel system was incubated at 37°C under 5% CO_2/ 95% air, with a medium change every third day.

Results

Using collagenase to free the cells gives a high yield of viable cells. Suspending the cells in a fibrinogen-MEM solution is necessary to get an equal three-dimensional distribution of cells in the gel. Gel formation is initiated by the addition of thrombin, immediately after dispensing the fibrinogen/cell suspension, and completed by factor XIII, present in the suspension. The gel is stable and easy to handle for medium changes, etc. The protein gel matrix facilitates reisolation of the fibroblasts or separation of glycosaminoglycans for further analysis.

Figure 1a shows a fibroblast gel culture taken at the 110th day of culture, Fig. 1b an electron micrograph of the cells in culture. The figure clearly demonstrates the in vivo like three-dimensional arrangement of the Dupuytren's contracture cells embedded within the extracellular matrix. The cells exhibit all the morphological characteristics of viable fibroblasts including gap junctions between the tips of the cell extensions and contractile microfilaments. The fibroblasts have been continuously cultured without subculturing for more than 130 days. Reisolation of the cells after 80 days and reestablishing the gel culture allowed continuation of the cell culture with the still viable cells.

Employing labeled precursors it could be shown that the cultured fibroblasts synthesize glycosaminoglycans and collagen at a considerable rate (Fig. 2). Incorporation of label into DNA reflects the growth activity of the cells. After a growth period of about 50 days, [³H]thymidine incorporation reaches a steady state, indicating that cell replacement rather than proliferation is occurring. Proteoglycan and collagen synthesis remain unchanged, as demonstrated by the incorporation rates of the respective precursors [³⁵S]sulfate and [³H]-hydroxyproline. Therefore, we conclude that, as in connective tissues in vivo, fibroblasts in gel culture reach a steady state of cell growth and death but continue to synthesize extracellular matrix. Thus, the fibrin gel culture system affords a preincubation time of at least 50 days before the cells reach steady state and experiments can be started. Due to the limited number of experiments carried out so far, a result of the lengthy culture times and labor intensive handling involved, it is not possible to interpret the data as to possible metabolic differences between Dupuytren's contracture cells and

◁ **Fig. 1a,b.** Culture of cells from Dupuytren's contracture in a fibrin gel (110th day of culture). The cells were fixed with glutaraldehyde in sodium cacodylate buffer and then with osmium tetroxide in the same buffer. **a** The myofibroblasts form a three-dimensional network. **b** Gap junctions connect the cells which contain, beside organelles, abundant thin (*arrowheads*) and intermediate (*arrows*) filaments. **a** ×310; **b** ×40 000

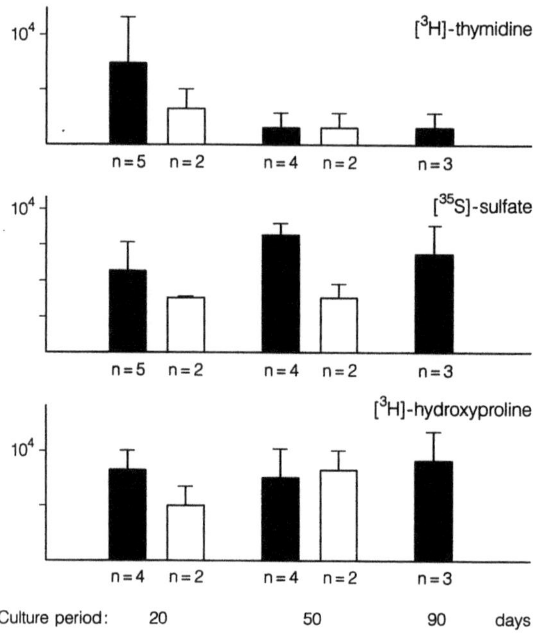

Fig. 2. Labeled precursor incorporation into extracellular components and DNA in fibrin gel cell culture of cells (90 days continuous culture) from Dupuytren's contracture. *Filled columns*, Dupuytren's contracture cells; *open columns*, palmar fascia cells

controls. It may be that Dupuytren's contracture cells show a slightly higher [³⁵S]sulfate incorporation than palmar fascia cells.

As shown by Flint et al. [1] and our laboratory [2], the glycosaminoglycan pattern in palmar fascia undergoes characteristic changes during development of the contracture. In comparing the glycosaminoglycans in biopsies from Dupuytren's contracture, from healthy palmar fascia (Fig. 3), and in the respective cell culture matrices prepared according to Gurr et al. [3], the glycosaminoglycan distribution in the gel culture matrix differs from that found in the tissues of both Dupuytren's contracture and palmar fascia. Thus, cells in fibrin gel culture express a unique phenotype, determined solely by the experimentally provided extracellular matrix. Cells from healthy palmar fascia and Dupuytren's contracture exhibit almost the same pattern of glycosaminaglycan expression (Fig. 4).

The pattern of glycosaminoglycan expression in cells in culture resembles that occurring in fetal connective tissues and in the early stages of wound healing. The remarkably small proportion of dermatan sulfate more or less indicates the absence of small proteoglycans in the extracellular matrix of the respective cell cultures. This may be due to the lack of an appreciable amount of collagen fibers synthesized at this stage of culture, as shown in the electron microscopic examinations. However, preliminary data from our attempts to isolate proteo-

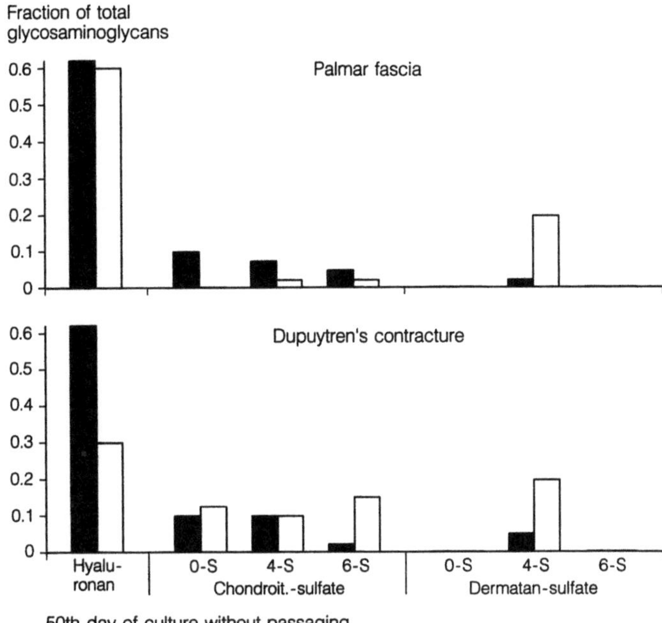

Fig. 3. Glycosaminoglycan patterns in fibroblast gel culture (*filled columns*) and tissue biopsy (*open columns*)

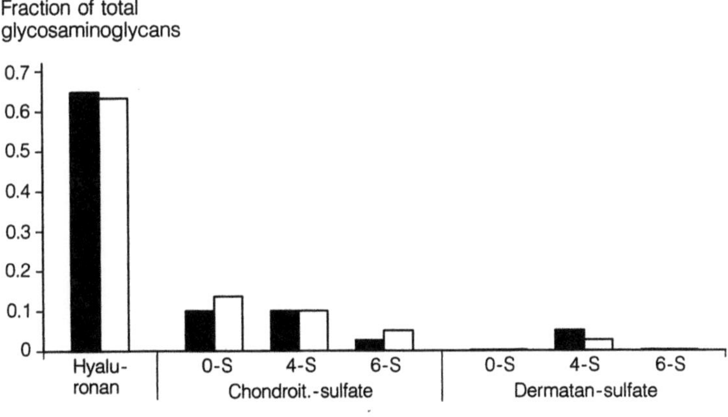

Fig. 4. Glycosaminoglycan patterns in fibroblast gel cultures and biopsies of healthy palmar fascia and Dupuytren's contracture. *Open columns*, Dupuytren cells; *filled columns*, palmarfascia cells

glycans from the gel culture matrices suggest the presence of both large and small proteoglycans.

Discussion

In the experimental extracellular matrix, the cells are surrounded by and under the influence of a large amount of fibrin, some fibronectin and factor XIII, beside the fetal calf serum. The former three components are known to stimulate proliferation of fibroblasts, thus providing an environment for the cells which is very close to the one found at the early stage of wound healing. In addition to the proliferation stimulating activity of fibrin, fibronectin and factor XIII, other, so far unknown modulating activities, may contribute to the expressed phenotype. Factors present in fetal calf serum act on the cells in a similar way. The result of the multifactorially determined interaction between extracellular matrix and the cells under investigation in this system is, among others, aberration of glycosaminoglycan synthesis, as demonstrated in the expression pattern observed in these experiments. If this is indeed true, then cells isolated from Dupuytren's contracture biopsies have not undergone permanent alterations of their metabolic and morphological characteristics in vivo. Instead, they remain able to express a different phenotype depending on the environment they are allowed to grow in.

Further investigations should answer the numerous questions emerging from these findings and further characterize this model for studies on the cellular level in connective tissue research. A variation in the composition of the experimental gel matrix should provide an improved in vivo like model for growing cells from Dupuytren's contracture and, at the same time, yield more information about mediators which actually determine the phenotype of these cells in situ and in vitro.

Acknowlegdements. Our group is indebted to Dr. G. Brandes (Laboratory for Electron Microscopy of the Hannover Medical School) for providing the morphologic examinations and figure.

References

1. Flint MH, Gillard GC, Reilly HC (1982) Connect Tissue Res 9:173–179
2. Tunn S, Gurr E, Delbrück A (1988) J Clin Chem Clin Biochem 26:7–14
3. Gurr E, Pallasch G, Tunn S, Tamm C, Delbrück A (1985) J Clin Chem Clin Biochem 23:251–253

Reactivity of Cells in Nodules of Dupuytren's Contracture with Monoclonal Antibodies Recognizing Leukocyte Antigens and von Willebrand's Factor

C. Sachse and P. Brenner

Introduction

In populations of Scandinavian or Celtic origin Dupuytren's contracture belongs to the most frequent disorders of connective tissue (Hill 1985). The most significant symptoms of this disease are the development of nodules in the palmar aponeurosis and progressive irreversible contractures involving one or more fingers (Luck 1959: McFarlane 1983).

The etiology and pathogenesis of Dupuytren's contracture are still poorly understood. By ultrastructural studies a peculiar cell type has been identified in the nodules which are widely thought to represent the active phase of the disease. These cells, which were termed "myofibroblasts," posess characteristics of both fibroblasts and smooth muscle cells and seem to be responsible for the contractile forces leading to the clinical deformities (Gabbiani and Majno 1972; James and Odom 1980; Brickley-Parsons et al. 1981; McFarlane 1983; Tomasek et al. 1987). The cells of Dupuytren's contracture differ from normal palmar fibroblasts with respect to their morphologic, cytogenetic and metabolic features (Azzarone et al. 1983; Delbrück and Schröder 1983; Mohr and Vossbeck 1985; Wurster-Hill et al. 1988). Immunologic studies of the cytoskeleton and the extracellular matrix of myofibroblasts revealed that these cells are a nonmuscle type (Azzarone et al. 1983; Tomasek et al. 1986), but their exact origin remains unclear. They may develop from resident palmar fibroblasts or perivascular cells (James and Odom 1980; Kischer et al. 1982; Kischer and Speer 1984; Mohr and Vossbeck 1985), but even the possibility of them deriving from peripheral blood leukocytes or endothelial cells cannot fully be ruled out. Immunostaining with antibodies to connective tissue differentiation antigens showed a considerable variability of antigen expression in the cells of Dupuytren's contracture (Bartal et al. 1987).

Monoclonal antibodies have proven to be useful tools to identify different subsets of leukocytes and other cell types based on the presence of cell surface antigens. Therefore, the reactivity of cells in nodules of Dupuytren's contracture was examined with a panel of antibodies marking the cell types possibly playing a role in the pathogenesis of the disease.

Materials and Methods

Tissue

Twenty patients with Dupuytren's contracture underwent partial or total fasciectomy. The age of the patients (all male) was 32–69 years (median: 53.5 years) and the duration of the disease 1–20 years (median: 6 years). The palmar fascia was transported to the laboratory immediately after excision; there, a large nodule (defined as a hard fusiform thickening of the palmar fascia) was dissected from the surrounding tissue, which was then fixed in 5% formalin for routine hematoxylin-eosin staining to confirm the diagnosis. The nodule was cut into pieces 1–2 mm in diameter and frozen to −70°C. Later, the pieces were covered with OCT compound (Ames, Indiana, USA), and cryostat sections of 4–5 µm thickness were prepared and mounted on glass slides. The slides were stored at −70°C until the indirect immunofluorescence assay. Small strips of normal palmar fascia were obtained from five patients operated on for carpal tunnel release. They were treated and stored as described above to serve as controls.

Antibodies

The monoclonal antibodies for cell type characterization are listed in Table 1. In all immunofluorescence assays IgG-specific affinity-purified goat anti-mouse immunoglobulin, conjugated with dichlorotriazinylaminofluorescein (Dianova, Hamburg, FRG), served as secondary antibody.

Table 1. Primary monoclonal antibodies

Monoclonal antibody (clone)	CD designation	Major specifities	Working dilution	Source
Anti-LCA	CD 45	Peripheral blood cells, tissue macrophages, histiocytes	1:100	1
27 E 10	None	Granulocytes, monocytes, macrophages in acute inflammation	1:100	2
25 F 9	None	Macrophages of chronic stage inflammation	1:100	2
EBM 11	CD 68	Monocytes, wide range of macrophages	1:50	3
MT 310	CD 4	T helper lymphocytes, monocytes, some macrophages	1:100	3
DK 25	CD 8	Suppressor/cytotoxic T lymphocytes	1:100	3
F 8/86	None	Endothelial cells, megakaryocytes	1:50	3
V 3260	None	All mesenchymal cells including endothelium, fibroblasts, macrophages and histiocytes	1:100	1

1, Merck, Darmstadt, FRG; 2, Dianova, Hamburg, FRG; 3, Dakopatts, Glostrup, Denmark.

Immunofluorescence Staining

To run the indirect immunofluorescence assays the slides were thawed and air dried for 20 min. The sections were fixed for 10 min in acetone at room temperature; to control antigen degradation during fixation, for every primary antibody used some additional unfixed slides were also examined. A washing step was performed (15 min in phosphate-buffered saline, PBS, $0.01 M$ phosphate, $0.15 M$ NaCl, pII 7.2), and a monoclonal antibody in a dilution predetermined to be appropriate (Table 1) was placed on the slides. After incubation (1 h at room temperature) the slides were washed with PBS for 30 min, incubated (1 h) with the secondary antibody in a 1:20 dilution and washed again, this time for 90 min. Finally the sections were mounted in a buffered glycerol solution (nine parts glycerol, one part PBS). Routine controls for staining specifity were carried out in parallel sections by omitting the primary antibody and incubating with normal mouse serum. These control treatments consistently resulted in no detectable staining except for the autofluorescence of elastic fibers, which because of their yellowish color are easily distinguishable from the specific fluorescence. Additionally, for all antibodies to leukocyte and macrophage antigens, cytosmears of peripheral blood cells or cultured monocytes were used to control antibody reactivity.

Evaluation

Even within a single nodule of Dupuytren's contracture cell density may vary considerably. In this study preliminary experiments were performed to select areas with high cell densities, which are best suited for the examination of cell surface antigens. The grade of cellularity was measured by reaction with anti-vimentin antibody, which according to its known specifity immunostains all mesenchymal cells and thereby every cell type possibly present in Dupuytren's contracture. The reactivity of one of the other monoclonal antibodies to the cells was judged by comparison with the binding of anti-vimentin antibody. A reaction was determined to be strongly positive if the extent of immunostaining was comparable to the result with anti-vimentin. It was judged weakly positive if only scattered cell clusters or small parts of the tissue reacted leaving distinct areas within the section unstained. All nonstaining tissues were judged as negative.

Results

With anti-vimentin antibody it was possible to identify regions of high cellularity in every specimen examined. Anti-vimentin antibody was able to immunostain the cells of Dupuytren's contracture and of normal palmar fascia, while the extracellular matrix remained negative. As expected from light microscopy, the cell density generally was higher in Dupuytren's contracture

Table 2. Reactivity of interstitial cells in nodules of Dupuytren's contracture with monoclonal antibodies recognizing leukocyte antigens and von Willebrand's factor

Patient	Grade of reactivity with monoclonal antibody						
	Anti-LCA (CD 45)	27 E 10	25 F 9	EBM 11 (CD 68)	MT 310 (CD 4)	DK 25 (CD 8)	F 8/86
1	−	−	++	++	−	+	E
2	−	−	++	+	−	−	E
3	−	−	++	+	−	−	E
4	+	+	+	+	−	+	E
5	−	−	+	−	−	−	E
6	−	−	++	+	−	−	E
7	−	−	++	+	−	+	E
8	−	−	+	−	−	−	E
9	−	−	++	+	−	−	E
10	−	−	++	++	−	−	E
11	−	−	++	+	−	−	E
12	−	−	++	+	−	−	E
13	−	−	+	+	−	+	E
14	+	+	++	+	−	+	E
15	−	−	++	+	−	−	E
16	−	−	++	++	−	−	E
17	−	+	+	−	−	+	E
18	−	−	+	+	n.t.	−	E
19	−	−	++	−	−	−	E
20	−	−	++	+	−	−	E

Reactivity: ++, strongly positive reaction (comparable to anti-vimentin); +, weakly positive reaction; −, negative reaction; E, positive reaction restricted to endothelial cells; n.t., not tested.

than in normal palmar fascia. The reactions of the other monoclonal antibodies with preselected areas of high cell density are summarized in Table 2.

With antibody to leukocyte common antigen and with monoclonal antibody (MoAb) 27 E 10, in the majority of cases no immunostaining was observed. Isolated antibody binding cells could be seen in the tissue or occurring as small scattered clusters in 2 and 3 patients and no and one control, respectively.

In contrast the myofibroblasts of Dupuytren's contracture were stained strongly by MoAb 25 F 9, while normal palmar fascia fibroblasts did not react (Fig. 1). In 14 of the 20 tissue sections of Dupuytren's contracture nearly all of the cells present in the specimen bound MoAb 25 F 9, while in six cases a more regional pattern of immunostaining was observed, with some parts of the section remaining negative. MoAb 25 F 9 bound intensely to the cytoplasm of the cells leaving the cell nuclei and the surrounding extracellular matrix unstained. Most sections of Dupuytren's contracture bound MoAb EBM 11, too. Nevertheless, with this antibody focal or regional patterns of positive cells dominated, and diffuse immunostaining was restricted to three patients. Moreover, four patients' specimens did not react at all with MoAb EBM 11. Of the five sections of normal palmar fascia four were negative, while the fifth reacted weakly positive with widely scattered stained cells.

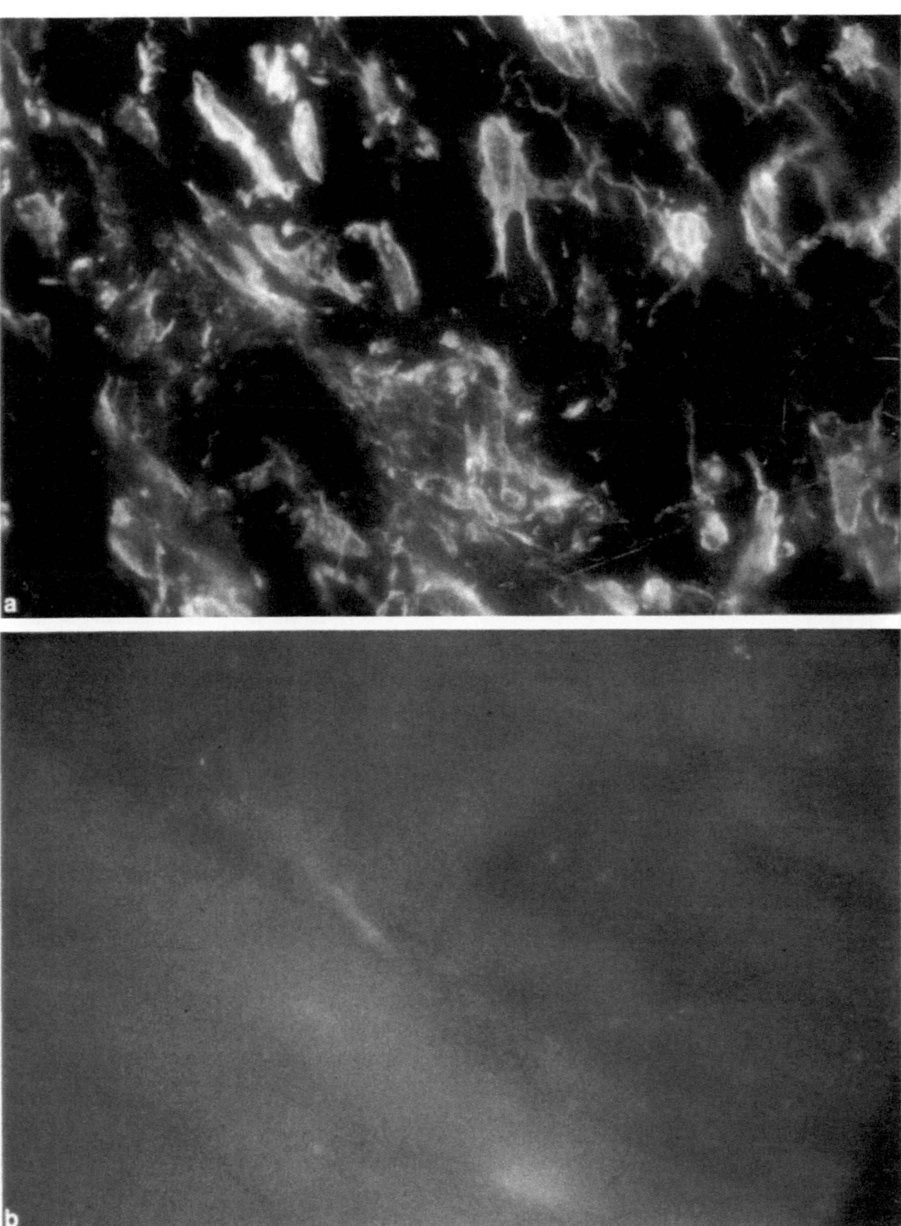

Fig. 1a,b. Photomicrographs of indirect immunofluorescence with MoAb 25 F 9. In nodules of Dupuytren's contracture (**a**) diffuse and intense immunostaining is observed, while in normal palmar fascia (**b**) there is nearly no reaction (patient 16; see Table 2). ×400

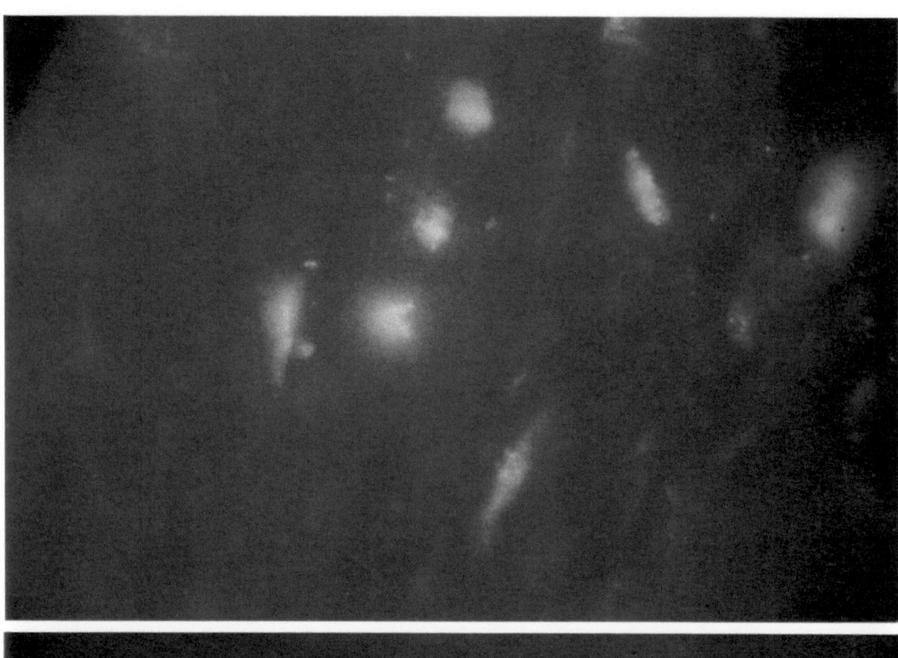

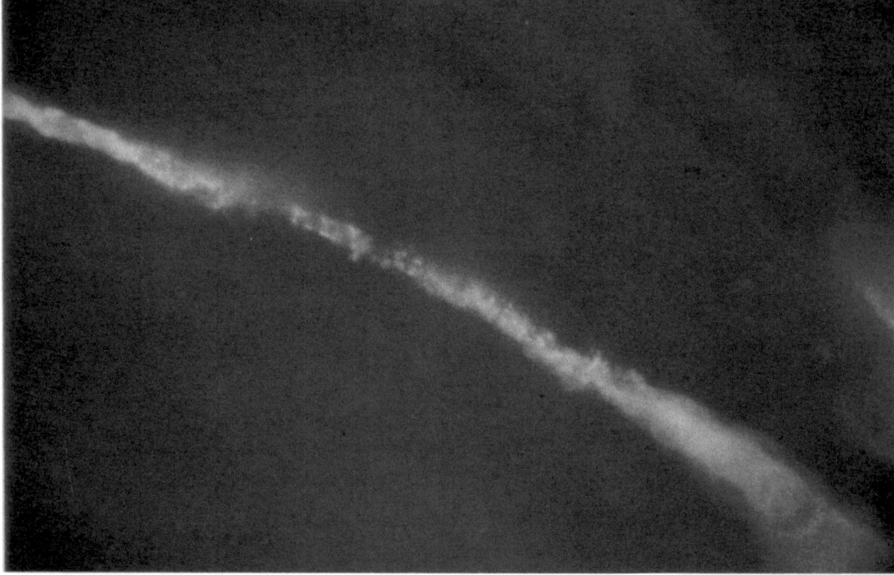

Fig. 2 *(above)*. Photomicrograph of a cluster of cells stained by MoAb DK 25 (anti-CD 8) in a nodule of Dupuytren's contracture (patient 7; see Table 2). ×400

Fig. 3 *(below)*. Photomicrograph of indirect immunofluorescence produced by MoAb F 8/86 (anti-von Willebrand's factor). The course of a small vessel is marked with all other parts of the nodule remaining negative (patient 2; see Table 2). ×400

Neither patient nor control sections showed any binding of MoAb MT 310 (anti-CD 4). In contrast, with MoAb DK 25 (anti-CD 8) weakly positive reactions with isolated clusters of immunostained cells were observed in six of 20 patient samples examined (Fig. 2). On retesting with parallel sections this finding could be reproduced in five of the six cases, while the majority of patients remained consistently negative. None of the normal palmar fascia sections bound MoAb DK 25.

MoAb F 8/86 (anti-von Willebrand's factor) was found to bind strongly to the vessel endothelium marking the course of small vessels throughout the normal or diseased palmar fascia (Fig. 3). Nevertheless, the reactivity to MoAb F 8/86 was strictly confined to endothelial cells, since this antibody does not immunostain the other cell types of the fascia or any part of the extracellular matrix.

Discussion

Dupuytren's contracture is characterized by the development of nodular structures in the palmar fascia and consecutive contractures of one or more fingers (Luck 1959; McGrouther 1982; McFarlane 1983). The highly cellular nodules appearing early in the disease process seem to play an important role in the pathogenesis of the contracture. In the nodules most cells have been converted into myofibroblasts, which are widely thought to be responsible for the contractile forces resulting in the clinical deformations (James and Odom 1980; Brickley-Parsons et al. 1981; Hill 1985). Myofibroblasts are not specific to Dupuytren's contracture, but can be found in various other conditions, many of them involving some kind of contraction (Bhatal 1972; Ryan et al. 1974; Baur et al. 1975, Churg and Kahn 1977). Ultrastructural studies revealed the morphologic features of myofibroblasts, but their origin remains unknown. The immunological properties of these cells have been examined with respect to their cytoskeleton, their attachment to the extracellular matrix and their expression of connective tissue differentiation antigens (Azzarone et al. 1983; Tomasek et al. 1986; Bartal et al. 1987).

In the last few years there has been increasing evidence that, under certain circumstances, leukocyte differentiation antigens are shared by connective tissue cells generally not considered to be directly involved in immunological processes (Malejczyk and Romaniuk 1989; Skjodt et al. 1989; Castagnoli et al. 1990). Although autoimmunological and immunopathological mechanisms in the pathogenesis of Dupuytren's contracture have repeatedly been discussed (Millesi 1959; Gay and Gay 1972; Busse et al. 1983; Jozsa et al. 1988), little is known about the possible role of myofibroblasts in such processes. The monoclonal antibody technique represents an important tool both for recognizing different cell types and for analyzing functionally different subsets of morphologically identical cells. Therefore the reactivity of cells in Dupuytren's contracture to a panel of monoclonal antibodies – recognizing different markers of blood leukocytes, tissue macrophages or endothelium – was examined.

The antibody to leukocyte common antigen (CD 45) was named as such because it immunostains all cells of myeloid or lymphoid origin with the exception of plasma cells, but including tissue macrophages. MoAb 27 E 10 reacts with more than 20% of freshly isolated monocytes and granulocytes. The corresponding antigen is strongly expressed on macrophages in acutely inflamed tissues (Zwadlo et al. 1986; Topoll et al. 1987), but is absent on nonmacrophage tissue cells and on normal resident mononuclear phagocytes in healthy tissues. Cells binding anti-CD45 or MoAb 27 E 10 were found very rarely in either Dupuytren's contracture or normal palmar fascia. Thus, in the nodules of Dupuytren's contracture there is no evidence of a major invasion of blood cells into the tissue or of an acute inflammatory process involving macrophages. These results correspond well with the known light microscopy findings in Dupuytren's contracture.

MoAbs 25 F 9 and EBM 11 (anti-CD 68) are able to stain mature tissue macrophages. The cells of Dupuytren's contracture, but not of normal palmar fascia, reacted strongly with both antibodies. Generally, using MoAb 25 F 9 (positive on resting mature macrophages and in many models of chronic stage inflammation, negative on blood monocytes; Hume et al. 1985; Zwadlo et al. 1985) the specimens were stained more thoroughly than with MoAb EBM 11 (a general monocyte and macrophage marker; Esiri and McGee 1986; Franklin et al. 1986). Nevertheless, with both antibodies there was considerable variation of immunostaining within the patient group. It is not clear why some markers (as those detected by MoAbs 25 F 9 and EBM 11) typical for macrophages should be expressed on the myofibroblasts of Dupuytren's contracture. Other antigens present on most tissue macrophages, such as leukocyte common antigen (CD 45) or CD 4, were not found on the cells of the nodules. Thus, these cells represent a cell type immunologically distinct both from normal resident palmar fibroblasts and from typical tissue macrophages but sharing some antigens with both cell species. The origin of the myofibroblasts remains unknown; they could originate from normal fibroblasts or be descendants (perhaps via pericytes) of blood monocytes, having invaded the palmar fascia at the very beginning of the disease. Nonetheless, since myofibroblasts bear antigens typical for macrophages, the possibility of them being able to produce or react to mediators of immune response, e.g., interleukins, should be considered. If myofibroblasts are sensitive to immunological signals or interactions, this could be of major importance for our understanding of the pathogenesis of Dupuytren's contracture.

In about a third of the examined nodules small clusters of CD 8-positive cells (probably lymphocytes) were seen. These cannot just represent unselective invasion of blood cells, since CD 4-positive cells – which are more frequent in peripheral blood – were not detected in any of the specimens of Dupuytren's contracture. The significance of this finding remains unclear.

With several antibodies, especially with those to the macrophage antigens, the intensity of reaction varied considerably in the patient collective. In different patients, but sometimes even within a single nodule, there seemed to exist several functional states of the cells recognized by immunological methods. This finding may be important with respect to the clinical course of Dupuytren's contracture, but it may explain, too, the difficulties encountered in investigation of the pathogenesis.

References

Azzarone B, Failly-Crepin C, Daya-Grosjean L, Chaponnier C, Gabbiani G (1983) Abnormal behavior of cultured fibroblasts from nodule and nonaffected aponeurosis of Dupuytren's disease. J Cell Physiol 117:353

Bartal AH, Stahl S, Karev A, Lichtig C (1987) Dupuytren's contracture studied with monoclonal antibodies to connective tissue differentiation antigens. Clin Exp Immunol 68:457

Baur PS, Larson DL, Stacey TR (1975) The observation of myofibroblasts in hypertrophic scars. Surg Gynecol Obstet 141:22

Bhatal PS (1972) Presence of modified fibroblasts in cirrhotic livers in man. Pathology 4:139

Brickley-Parsons D, Glimcher, MJ, Smith RJ, Albin R, Adams JP (1981) Biochemical changes in the collagen of the palmar fascia in patients with Dupuytren's disease. J Bone Joint Surg [Am] 63:787

Busse E, Nilius R, Busse HJ (1983) Immunologische Aspekte der Pathogenese der Dupuytrenschen Kontraktur. Zentralbl Chir 108:855

Castagnoli C, Stella M, Magliacani G, Teich-Alasia S, Richiardi P (1990) Anomalous expression of HLA class II molecules on keratinocytes and fibroblasts in hypertrophic scars consequent to thermal injury. Clin Exp Immunol 82:350

Churg A, Kahn LB (1977) Myofibroblasts and related cells in malignant fibrous and fibrohistiocytic tumors. Hum Pathol 8:205

Delbrück A, Schröder H (1983) Metabolism and proliferation of cultured fibroblasts from specimens of human palmar fascia and Dupuytren's contracture. J Clin Chem Clin Biochem 21:11

Esiri MM, McGee, J O'D (1986) Monoclonal antibody to macrophages (EBM/11) labels macrophages and microglial cells in human brain. J Clin Pathol 39:615

Franklin WA, Mason DY, Pulford K, Falini B, Bliss E, Gatter KC, Stein H, Clarke LC, McGee J O'D (1986) Immunohistological analysis of human mononuclear phagocytes and dendritic cells by using monoclonal antibodies. Lab Invest 54:322

Gabbiani G, Majno G (1972) Dupuytren's contracture: fibroblast contraction? An ultrastructural study. Am J Pathol 66:131

Gay S, Gay B (1972) Ist die Dupuytrensche Kontraktur eine Autoimmunerkrankung? Zentralbl Chir 97:728

Hill A (1985) Dupuytren's contracture. J Bone Joint Surg [Am] 67:1439

Hume DA, Allan W, Golder J, Stephens RW, Doe WF, Warren HS (1985) Preparation and characterization of human bone marrow-derived macrophages. J Leucocyte Biol 38:541

James WD, Odom RB (1980) The role of the myofibroblast in Dupuytren's contrcture. Arch Dermatol 116:807

Jozsa L, Demel S, Pinter T, Renner A, Reffy A, Santha A, Salamon A (1988) Immunopathological study on palmar aponeurosis in Dupuytren's disease. Acta Histochem (Jena) 83:153

Kischer CW, Speer, DP (1984) Microvascular changes in Dupuytren's contracture. J Hand Surg 9:58

Kischer CW, Thies AC, Chvapil M (1982) Perivascular myofibroblasts and microvascular occlusion in hypertrophic scars and keloids. Hum Pathol 13:819

Luck JV (1959) Dupuytren's contracture. A new concept of the pathogenesis correlated with surgical management. J Bone Joint Surg [Am] 41:635

Malejczyk J, Romaniuk A (1989) Reactivity of normal rat epiphyseal chondrocytes with monoclonal antibodies recognizing different leucocyte markers. Clin Exp Immunol 75:477

McFarlane RM (1983) The current status of Dupuytren's disease. J Hand Surg 8:703

McGrouther DA (1982) The microanatomy of Dupuytren's contracture. Hand Surg 14:215

Millesi H (1959) Neue Gesichtspunkte in der Pathogenese der Dupuytrenschen Kontraktur. Bruns Beitr Klin Chir 198:1

Mohr W, Vossbeck G (1985) Untersuchungen zur Proliferation und ^{3}H-Prolin-Inkorporation von Zellen der Palmarfibromatose (Morbus Dupuytren). Z Rheumatol 44:226

Ryan GB, Cliff WJ, Gabbiani G, Irle C, Montandon D, Statkov PR, Majno G (1974) Myofibroblasts in human granulation tissue. Hum Pathol 5:55

Skjodt H, Moller T, Freiesleben SF (1989) Human osteoblastlike cells expressing MHC class II determinants stimulate allogeneic and autologous peripheral blood mononuclear cells and function as antigen-presenting cells. Immunology 68:416

Tomasek JJ, Schultz RJ, Episalla CW, Newmann SA (1986) The cytoskeleton and extracellular matrix of the Dupuytren's disease "myofibroblast": an immunofluorescence study of a nonmuscle cell type. J Hand Surg [Am] 11:365

Tomasek JJ, Schultz RJ, Haaksma CJ (1987) Extracellular natrix-cytoskeletal connections at the surface of the specialized contractile fibroblast (myofibroblast) in Dupuytren's disease. J Bone Joint Surg [Am] 69:1400

Topoll HH, Zwadlo G, Lange DE, Sorg C (1987) Analyse des entzündlichen Infiltrates verschiedener Entzündungsstadien der marginalen Gingiva mittels monoklonaler Antikörper. Zahnärztl Z 42:467

Wurster-Hill DH, Brown F, Park JP, Gibson SH (1988) Cytogenetic studies in Dupuytren's contracture. Am J Hum Genet 43:285

Zwadlo G, Bröcker E, von Bassewitz D, Feige U, Sorg C (1985) A monoclonal antibody to a differentiation antigen present on mature human macrophages and absent from monocytes. J Immunol 134:1487

Zwadlo G, Schlegel R, Sorg C (1986) A monoclonal antibody to a subset of human monocytes found only in the peripheral blood and inflammatory tissues. J Immunol 137:512

Demonstration of Myofibroblasts Using a Novel Murine Monoclonal Antibody, 3C2G10.7 Raised from Proliferating Cells in Dupuytren's Disease

D.T. Shum, G. Pringle, B. Hasegawa, J.S. Botz, and R.M. McFarlane

Introduction

The concept of the existence of a type of connective tissue cell that has properties of fibroblasts and smooth muscle cells is not new. The presence of such cells in chicken and rat aorta [7,21,25] was initially demonstrated, using the electron microscope, some 30 years ago. These cells have subsequently been described in tissues including the capsules of the adrenal gland [32] and testicle [12] and granulation tissue of rat [9] and human [34]. The dual functions as fibroblasts and smooth muscle cells have been studied by in vivo autoradiographic techniques [26,31], in vitro contractile response [23], and comparative cell modulation and growth dynamics [41]. In 1974, the term "myofibroblast" was coined [34], the ultrastructural features of this differentiated fibroblast defined, and the cells purported to be the basic locomotive units in wound contraction. The discovery of the myofibroblast was soon followed by a multitude of ultrastructural studies of the cells in a great number of pathologic fibrocontractive conditions and fibrous neoplasms [22]. Significantly, fibrogenesis in aortic atherosclerosis [15,16,28], hypertrophic scar, [3,4] and Dupuytren's disease [5,8,19] have been attributed to the presence of myofibroblasts, and their uniform presence in tumors, e.g., atypical fibroxanthoma of skin [42,43] and malignantfibrous histiocytoma [6,40], raises important questions concerning the histogenesis of these fibrohistiocytic tumors.

The use of electron microscope to study the myofibroblasts is often hindered by its very restrictive sample size. Apart from documenting the presence of such a cell, it is difficults to appreciate the spatial relationship between the myofibroblasts and other cell types within the tissue. Similarly, the use of light microscope is not without its problems. Despite the distinctive ultrastructural appearance, the nuclear irregularities are hard to appreciate by light microscopy. The cytoplasmic microfilaments and special cell to cell and cell to stroma connections are beyond the normal light microscopic resolution. In fact, myofibroblasts are probably underdetected because of their rather nondescript light microscopic appearance, and they are often confused with fibroblasts. It is of interest to note, for example, that myofibroblasts are seldom mentioned in surgical pathology reports despite their ubiquitous presence in many pathologic conditions.

Confronted by the difficulties with the traditional morphologic approach in our studies of myofibroblasts and Dupuytren's disease, we embarked upon raising a monoclonal antibody that could be used immunohistochemically on routine paraffin sections to differentiate myofibroblasts from fibroblasts and other connective tissue cells. The murine monoclonal antibody that was raised, designated as clone 3C2G10.7, appears to fulfil the requirements as a specific marker for myofibroblasts.

Experimental Design

A monoclonal antibody which identifies myofibroblasts was produced from a hydridoma created by the fusion of mouse plasmacytoma cells and spleen cells of mice immunized with a cell suspension of profilerative stage Dupuytren's tissue [24,30] rich in myofibroblasts. The functional activity of the antibody was determined immunohistochemically by the avidin – biotin peroxidase technique [26] using fresh-frozen and formalin-fixed tissue.

Methods

Antibody Preparation

Specimens of palmar fascia were obtained at the time of surgery and the sample was dissected free of surrounding fibrofatty tissue in the operating room. Active stage of the disease in nodular tissue was confirmed by frozen tissue section stained with hematoxylin. Disaggregation of the remaining nodular tissue, which has been placed in sterile Hank's solution (Gibco, Grand Island, New York) for transport to the laboratory, was achieved by first cutting the sample into fine pieces with scissors. A single cell suspension was attained by gently agitating the pieces at 37°C in a solution of RPMI 1640 with 25 mM hepes buffer 10% fetal calf serum (Gibco), collagenase type 1A (10 mg/ml) (Sigma, St. Louis, Missouri) and DNase (1.5 mg/ml) (Sigma) for about 4 h or until no clumps of tissue were visible. The cells were washed and pelleted twice in a solution of RPMI 1640 and 20% fetal calf serum in order to deactivate the enzymatic activity. Aliquoits of 1×10^7 cells/ml were frozen in fetal calf serum and 5% dimethyl sulfoxide (DMSO) and stored at $-80°C$ until required. Six week old female Balb/c mice (Harlan-Spagrue-Dawley, Indiana) were primed with 1×10^7 thawed, washed cells suspended in an emulsion of 0.1 ml RPMI 1640 medium and 0.1 ml Freund's complete adjuvant by two subcutaneous injections in the back. The mice were subsequently boosted intraperitoneally with the same number of cells suspended in RPMI 1640 and Freund's incomplete adjuvent 9 days later. Three days after the last injection, using the hydridoma technique previously described [29], the mice spleen cells were mixed with the plasmacytoma cell line 315.43 in a 5:1 ratio and fusion initiated using 40% polyethylene glycol (PEG) (Sigma). The fused cells were cultured in HAT restriction media supplemented with whole Balb/c mouse blood in 24-well plates seeded at 2×10^5 cells/well until the hydridomas were macroscopically visible. Supernantants from all wells were initially screened at 10–14 days postfusion and selected positive hydridomas were cloned and subcloned by the method of limiting dilution.

The immunoglobulin class was identified by using an alkaline phosphatase immunoassay kit (Innogenetics N.V., Belgium). In this procedure, strips, coated with separate bands of rat monoclonal antibodies against different mouse subclasses, were incubated with the supernant. The murine antibody in the sample reacted with the corresponding isotype band and was detected using rate anti-mouse Ig kappa, labeled with alkaline phosphatase. A dark band, proportional to the amount of specific antibody in the sample, was revealed after incubation with the substrate (5-bromo-4-elboro-3 indoyl phosphate in dimethyl formamide) and was interpreted visually.

Screening

All supernatants were initially screened against formalin-fixed tissue "sausages" which were assembled by juxtaposing previously diagnosed samples from individual patients into paraffin blocks [2]. Three of these sausages were formed from the palmar fascia of nine patients with Dupuytren's contracture and active stage disease [36]. A wide variety of normal adult and fetal tissue in three sausages and 21 individual paraffin blocks were screened. Once the selected clone was established, the supernantant was extensively screened against additional cases of Dupuytren's disease and myofibroblast-rich lesions. Slides for immunohistochemistry, subbed with chromatin, were prepared by using deparaffinized tissue sections cut 4 µm thick which did not require enzymatic predigestion. Pretreatment included 7 min in 3% hydrogen peroxide in methanol to elimate endogenous peroxidase activity and 20 min in 3% goat serum (Cederlane, Ontario, Canada) to quench nonspecific protein reactions. The avidin-biotin peroxidase method (Vector Laboratories, California) was followed by overnight incubation with the supernatnant diluted 1:2 with RPMI at room temperature [18]. Ten samples of Dupuytren's nodules were snap frozen and stored at −80°C. Prior to the avidin-biotin peroxidase technique, glass slides were coated with 0.05% polylysine to facilitate adherence of the 4 µm thick tissue sections. Pretreatment consisted of fixing the tissue in acetone and leaving it in 3% goat serum for 20 min to block nonspecific proteins.

Results and Discussion

The cells of a typical proliferative Dupuytren's nodule had elongated vesicular nuclei; irregularities of the nuclear membrane were barely visible at ×400 magnification. The cytoplasm was eosinophilic but microfilaments and cell connections were not seen (Fig. 1). By transmission electron microscope, the

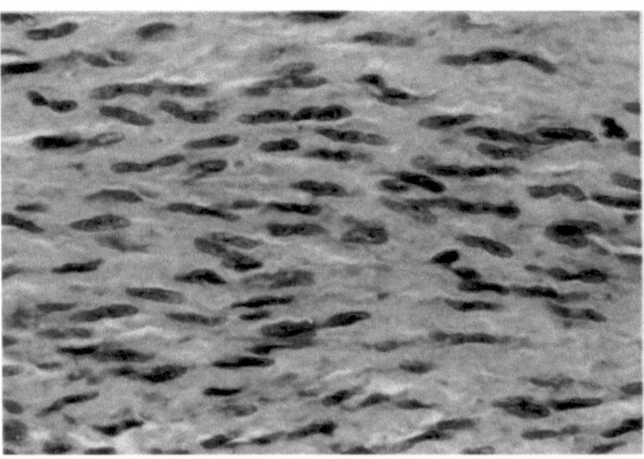

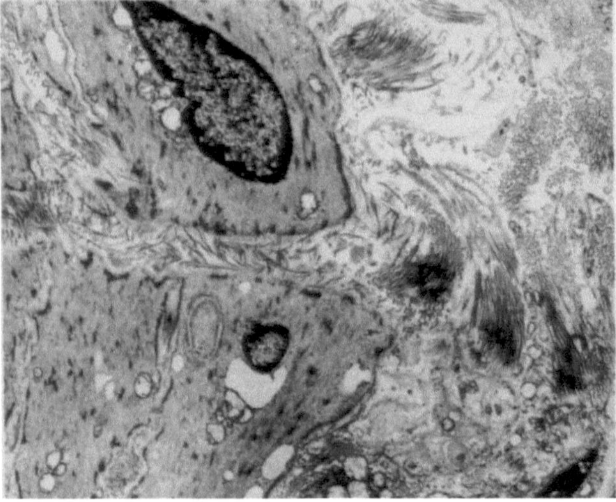

Fig. 1 *(above).* Myofibroblasts in proliferative Dupuytren's nodule showing irregular nuclear membrane. Cytoplasmic filaments with densities are not discernible. Hematoxylin and eosin, ×400

Fig. 2 *(below).* Transmission electron micrograph illustrating cells in proliferative Dupuytren's nodule. The cytoplasmic filaments with densities and cell to cell and cell to stromal connections are features typical of a myofibroblast

cytoplasmic microfilaments with densities and the cell to cell and cell to stroma connections were easily discernible. These ultrastructural features were typical of myofibroblasts (Fig. 2).

Using the 3C2G10.7 antibody, which was an IgM kappa immunoglobin, the cytoplasm of most of the cells in the Dupuytren's nodules was stained positively. The reaction was more intense with fresh, frozen unfixed tissue, but otherwise the pattern was identical to that observed in formalin-fixed, paraffin-embedded tissue, which revealed superior histologic and cytologic details.

130   D.T. Shum et al.

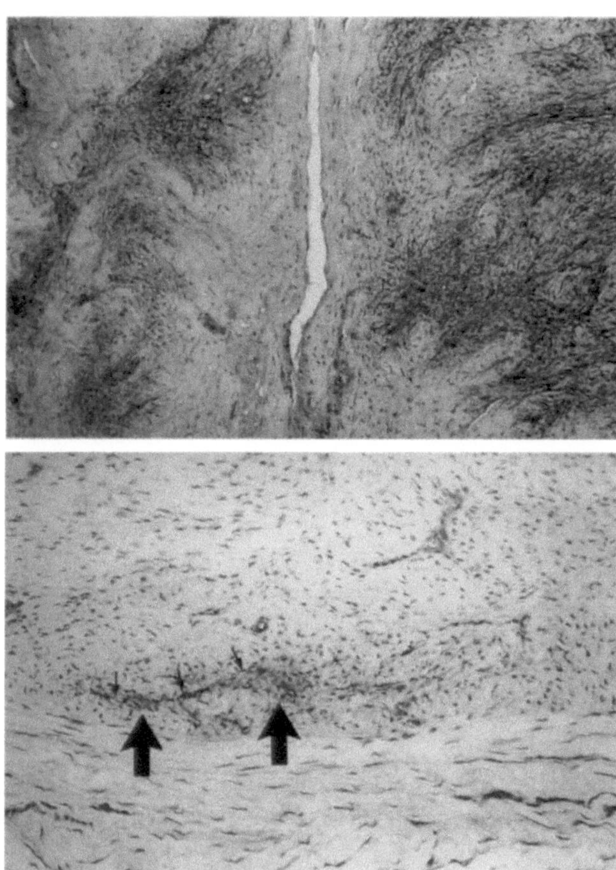

Fig. 3 *(above)*. Immunohistochemical staining of a proliferative Dupuytren's nodule, using 3C2G10.7 monoclonal antibody. Most cells in the nodule show positive cytoplasmic staining. Foci of positive cells are also noted peripheral to the main nodule *(right)*. ×25

Fig. 4 *(below)*. A focus of positive cells *(large arrows)* peripheral to a Dupuytren's nodule, as demonstrated by immunohistochemical staining using 3C2G10.7 monoclonal antibody. Positive cells surround a capillary *(small arrows)*. ×40

Microscopic foci of positively stained cells were observed peripheral to the main nodules in most of the Dupuytren's lesions (Fig. 3). In these areas, the cells had smaller nuclei and they appeared to be circumferential to capillaries that had a single layer of endothelial cells. (Fig. 4) The angiocentric arrangement of reactive cells was especially interesting in view of the fact that normal pericytes around capillaries were nonreactive to 3C2G10.7. These foci were inconspicuous under routine hematoxylin and eosin stain but we wondered if these were representative of incipient Dupuyren's nodules and propose that antigenic alteration of perivascular cells (possible pericytes or perivascular mesenchymal cells) could be an early detectable event with our antibody.

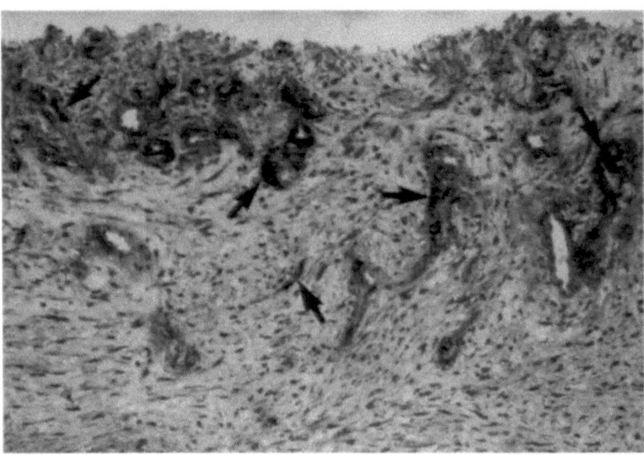

Fig. 5. Immunohistochemical staining of acute granulation tissue using 3C2G10.7 monoclonal antibody. Positive cells (*arrows*) are predominantly perivascular in location. ×40

Table 1. Immunohistochemical staining reaction with monoclonal antibody 3C2G10.7 on reactive and neoplastic lesions of myofibroblasts

Lesion	Results	Cases studied (n)
Dupuytren's disease	Staining of most cells in proliferative nodule; "satellite lesions" peripheral to the main nodule	30
Granulation tissue	Staining of pericapillary spindle cells in acute granulation tissue; positive cells found in fibrous base of chronic skin ulcer	10
Hypertrophic scar	Positive cells between collagen fibers	5
Colonic adenocarcinoma	Staining of occasional spindle-shaped stromal cells; positive cells surround neoplastic glands	2
Breast carcinoma	Staining of occasional spindle-shaped stromal cells	4
Desmoid	Staining of most tumor cells	2
Malignant fibrous histiocytoma	Staining of most tumor cells	4
Atypical fibroxanthoma	Staining of most tumor cells	2

Table 1 lists the results of immunohistochemical staining of additional pathologic conditions in which myofibroblasts have been reported as the principal cell component. In accordance with the original report of myofibroblasts in human granulation tissue [34], the 3C2G10.7 antibody revealed positively stained cells concentrated especially in the perivascular location in acute granulation tissue (Fig. 5). This was in contrast to the reaction with chronic skin ulcers and hypertrophic scars which demonstrated reactive cells oriented parallel to the skin surface throughout the fibrotic dermis (Fig. 6). The different location of myofibroblasts in acute granulation tissue and dermal scars concurred with suggestions of myofibroblasts being derived from

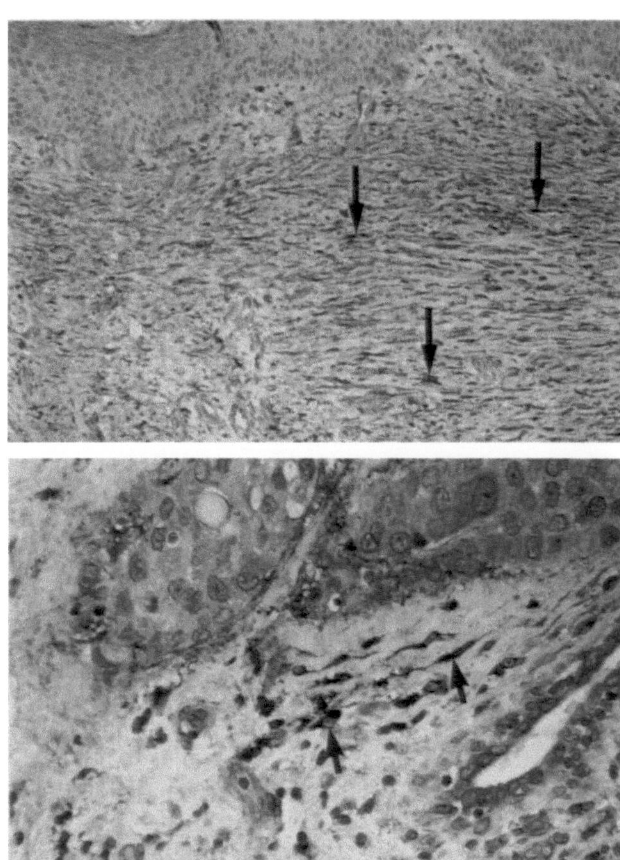

Fig. 6 *(above)*. Immunohistochemical staining of a dermal scar using 3C2G10.7 monoclonal antibody. Positive cells *(arrows)* are found throughout the fibrotic dermis and arranged parallel to the skin surface (epidermis on *top*). ×40

Fig. 7 *(below)*. Immunohistochemical staining of an invasive breast carcinoma using 3C2G10.7 monoclonal antibody. Positive spindle cells *(arrows)* are seen in the stroma surrounding nests of neoplastic cells. ×100

perivascular cells and providing fibrocontractive functions during wound healing [20]. It was significant to note that fibroblasts distant from the ulcer base were nonreactive. Examination of invasive breast and colonic adenocarcinomas showed reactive cells especially in the cellular desmoplastic stroma surrounding neoplastic glands (Fig. 7). Only a few positive cells were noted in the relatively acellular hyaline stroma of the breast carcinomas and there appeared to be staining of the collagen focally. In both types of malignancies, the results confirmed previous ultrastructural reports [10,27] and reflected the presence of myofibroblasts in the stroma of invading carcinomas. An abdominal desmoid tumor, atypical fibroxanthomas of the skin, and malignant fibrous histiocytomas were other fibroproliferative conditions that

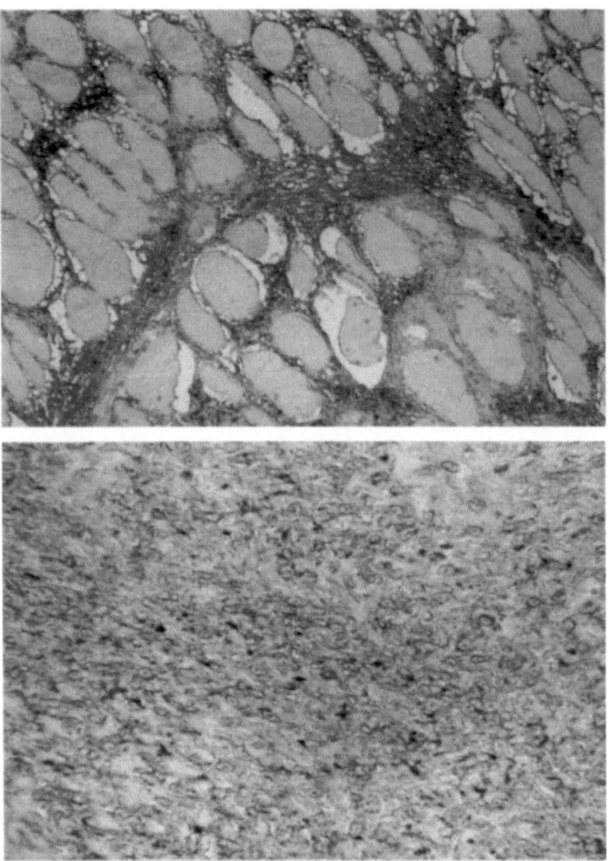

Fig. 8 *(above)*. Immunohistochemical staining of an abdominal desmoid tumor using 3C2G10.7 monoclonal antibody. Darkly stained positive tumor tissue is seen infiltrating nonstaining striated muscle fibers. ×25

Fig. 9 *(below)*. Immunohistochemical staining of a malignant fibrous histiocytoma using 3C2G10.7 monoclonal antibody. Many tumor cells show positive cytoplasmic staining. ×100

we screened for reactivity with the antibody. Most tumor cells, including morphologically atypical and giant cells in these lesions, were uniformly positive (Figs. 8, 9). In view of the prominence of myofibroblasts reported in previous ultrastructural studies [6,11,38,42] and the specific staining reaction of 3C2G10.7 on Dupuytren's nodules, granulation tissue, and dermal scars, a myofibroplastic lineage for these fibroproliferative tumors is strongly implicated.

On screening normal tissue with 3C2G10.7 (Table 2), reactive cells were noted in the tunica media of the aorta, medium size muscular artery, and coronary atherosclerotic plaque (Fig. 10). Such observations were again consistent with previous reports of the presence of myofibroblasts in these sites [13,15,16]. The remaining "control" sections tested negative with the exception of staining of

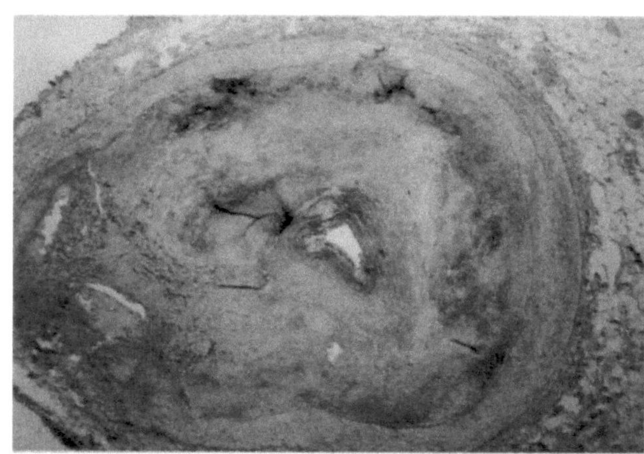

Fig. 10. Immunohistochemical staining of atherosclerotic coronary artery using 3C2G10.7 monoclonal antibody. Darkly stained positive cells are in the thickened tunica intima. There is marked luminal stenosis. ×12

Table 2. Immunohistochemical staining reaction with monoclonal antibody 3C2G10.7 on normal and fetal tissue

Tissue	Results
Myocardium	Negative
Lung	Negative
Liver	Negative
Aorta (atherosclerotic)	Positive cells in tunica media and atherosclerotic plaque
Coronary artery (atherosclerotic)	Positive cells in tunica media
Adrenal	Negative
Pancreas	Staining of islet cells
Striated muscle	Negative
Parotid	Negative
Testis	Negative
Skin and subcutaneum	Positive cells in eccrine sweat gland
Nerve	Negative
Thyroid	Negative
Spleen	Negative
Kidney	Negative
Fetal tissue (12–14 weeks)	Staining of chondrocytes and perichondral mesenchymal cells
Cartilage	Staining of chondrocytes
Bone	Negative
Plasma cells	Positive
Mast cells	Positive

mast cells, plasma cells, chondrocytes, pancreatic islet cells, eccrine sweat glands, and occasional epithelial cells. There was no explanation for this extraneous reactivity except to assume a nonspecific cross reaction that would not have untowards effects or influence on the practical use of 3C2G10.7 to identify myofibroblasts in tissue sections.

Myofibroblasts in Dupuytren's disease have been studied in the past with antibodies against vimentin, cytokeratin, desmin, actin isoforms [14,35,36,37,40], and connective tissue differentiation antigens [1]. The conclusions from these investigations were that myofibroblasts possess varied heterogenous cytoskeletal and actin compositions and that the antigenic constituent depends upon the basic pathologic process. Reactive myofibroblasts, for example, were found to be different from myofibroblasts of pathologic contractile conditions in their content of action isoforms [37]. Alternatively, the existence of phenotypic "subtypes" of myofibroblasts has been explained by theorizing that various nonmuscle connective tissue cells could modulate into a "myofibroblastic" state when contraction of local tissue was needed [13,20].

Our novel monoclonal antibody 3C2G10.7 has the capacity to react with myofibroblasts in a variety of reactive and neoplastic conditions, thereby defining an antigen common to cells showing myofibroblastic features and differentiation. The action of this antibody on Dupuytren's nodule revealed previously unrecognized early satellite lesions peripheral to the main nodule. The close proximity of these early lesions to vessels and studies on granulation tissue further suggested that early emerging myofibroblasts were located perivascularly. These results added credence to previous hypotheses that myofibroblasts were histogenetically associated with vascular smooth muscle cells [8,33,36]. Besides their unique ultrastructural features, we have concluded that myofibroblasts are antigenically distinct, and this cellular state of differentiation can be identified by the murine monoclonal antibody 3C2G10.7 at the light microscopic level using conventional immunohistochemical techniques.

Acknowledgements. The authors wish to thank Ms. Marnie Snowsell and Ms. Linda Venoit for their excellent secretarial and technical assistance.

References

1. Bartal AH, Stahl S, Karev A, Lichtig C (1987) Dupuytren's contracture studied with monoclonal antibodies to connective tissue differentiation antigen. Clin Exp Immunol 68:457
2. Battifora H (1986) Methods in laboratory investigation. The multitumor (sausage) tissue block: normal method for immunohistochemical antibody testing. Lab Invest 55:244
3. Baur PS, Larson PL, Stacey TR (1975) The observation of myofibroblasts in hypertrophic scars. Surg Gynecol Obstet 141:22
4. Dyer RF, Enna CD (1975) Ultrastructure of a keloid: an unusual incident involving lipomatous leprosy. Int J Dermatol 14:743
5. Chiu HF, McFarlane R (1978) Pathogenesis of Dupuytren's contracture: A correlative clinical – pathological study. J Hand Surg 3:1
6. Churg AM, Kahn LB (1977) Myofibroblasts and related cells in malignant fibrous and fibrohistiocytic tumors. Hum Pathol 8:205
7. Cliff WJ (1967) The aortic tunica media in growing rats studied with the electron microscope. Lab Invest 17:599
8. Gabbiani G, Majno G (1972) Dupuytren's contracture: fibroblastic contraction? An ultrastructural study. Am J Pathol 66:131

9. Gabbiani G, Ryan GB, Magno G (1971) Presence of modified fibroblasts in granulation tissue and their possible role in wound contracture. Experimentia 27:549
10. Ghosh L, Ghosh BC, Das Gupta YK (1980) Ultrastructural study of stroma in human mammary carcinoma. Am J Surg 139:229
11. Goellner JR, Soule EH (1980) Desmoid tumors. An ultrastructural study of eight cases. Hum Pathol 11:43
12. Gorgors K, Bock P (1974) Myofibroblasts in the rat testicular capsule. Cell Tissue Res 154:533
13. Gown, AM (1990) The mysteries of the myofibroblast (partially) unmasked (Editorial). Lab Invest 63:1
14. Hasegawa T, Hirone T, Kudo E, Abe J-I, Hizawa K (1990) Cytoskeletal characteristics of myofibroblasts in benign neoplastic and reactive fibroblastic lesions. Virchows Arch [A] 416:375
15. Haust MD, More RH (1966) Mechanism of fibrosis in white atherosclerotic plaques of human aorta: an electron microscopic study. Circulation 34 Suppl 3:14
16. Hinek A, Thyberg J (1977) Electron microscopic observations on the formation of elastic fibers in primary cultures of aortic smooth muscle cells. J Ultrastruct Res 60:12
17. Hirose T, Kudo E, Hasegawa T, Abe J, Hizawa K (1989) Expression of intermediate filaments in malignant fibrous histiocytoma. Hum Pathol 20:871
18. Hsu SM, Raine L, Fanger H (1981) The use of avidin-biotin peroxidase complex (ABC) in immunoperoxidase technique: a comparison between ABC and unlabelled antibody (PAP) procedures. J Histochem Cytochem 29:577
19. Hueston JT, Hurley JV, Whittingham S (1976) The contracting fibroblast as a clue to Dupuytren's contracture. Hand 8:10
20. Jester J, Rodrigues MM, Herman IM (1987) Characterization of avascular corneal would healing fibroblasts. New insights into the myofibroblasts. Am J Pathol 127:140
21. Karrer HE (1960) Electron microscope study of developing chick embryo aorta. J Ultrastruct Res 4:420
22. Lipper S, Kahn LB, Reddick RL (1990) The myofibroblast. In: Sommers SC, Rosen PP (eds) Pathology annual. Appleton-Century-Crofts, New York, p 409
23. Majno G, Gabbiani G, Hirschel BJ, Ryan GB, Statkov PR (1971) Contractions of granulation tissue in vitro: similarity to smooth muscle. Science 173:548
24. McFarlane RM (1983) The current status of Dupuytren's disease. J Hand Surg 8:703
25. Moss NS, Benditt EP (1970) Spontaneous and experimentally induced arterial lesions. I. An ultrastructural survey of the normal chicken aorta. Lab Invest 22:166
26. Neumuller J, Tohidast-Akrad M, Ammer K, Hakimzadeh A, Stransky G, Weis S, Parsh G, Eberl R (1988) Ultrastructural and autoradiographic investigations of cell cultures derived from tendons or ligamentous material from patients with fibromatous disorders. Exp Cell Biol 56:113
27. Ohtani H, Sasano N (1980) Myofibroblasts and myoepithelial cells in human breast carcinoma: An ultrastructural study. Virchows Arch [Pathol Anat] 385:247
28. Parker F, Odland GF (1966) A light microscopic histochemical and electron microscopic study of experimental atherosclerosis in the rabbit coronary artery and a comparison with rabbit aorta atherosclerosis. Am J Pathol 48:451
29. Pringle GA, Dodd CM, Pearson CH, Osborn JW, Mosmann TR (1985) Production and characterization of monoclonal antibodies to bovine skin protodermatan sulfate. Coll Relat Res 5:23
30. Rombouts JJ, Noel H, Legrain Y, Munting E (1989) Prediction of recurrence in the treatment of Dupuytren's disease: evaluation of a histologic classification. J Hand Surg 4:644
31. Ross R, Klebanoff SJ (1971) The smooth muscle cell. I. In vivo synthesis of connective tissue proteins. J Cell Biol 50:159
32. Rossouw DJ, Chase CC (1978) Ultrastructure of the capsule of the rabbit adrenal gland. Acta Anat (Basel) 100:538
33. Ryan GB, Cliff WJ, Gabbiani G (1973) Myofibroblasts in an avascular fibrous tissue. Lab Invest 29:197
34. Ryan GB, Cliff WJ, Gabbiani G, Irle C, Montandon D, Statkov PR, Majno G (1974) Myofibroblasts in human granulation tissue. Hum Pathol 5:55

35. Schurch W, Seemnayer TA, Lagace R, Gabbiani G (1984) The intermediate filament cytoskeleton of myofibroblasts: an immunofluorescence and ultrastructural study. Virchows Arch [A] 403:323
36. Shum DT, McFarlane RM (1988) Histogenesis of Dupuytren's disease: an immunohistochemical study of 30 cases. J Hand Surg 1:61
37. Skalli O, Schurch W, Seemayer T, Lagance R, Montandon P, Pittet B, Gabbiani G (1989) Myofibroblasts from diverse pathologic settings are heterogenous in their content of actin isoforms and intermediate proteins. Lab Invest 60:275
38. Stiller D, Katenkamp D (1975) Cellular features in desmoid fibromatosis and well-differentiated fibrosarcomas. An electron microscopic study. Virchows Arch [Pathol Anat] 369:155
39. Taxy JB, Battifora H (1977) Malignant fibrous histiocytoma. An electron microscopic study. Cancer 39:1044
40. Tsukada T, McNutt MA, Ross R, Gown AM (1987) HHF 35, a muscle actin-specific monoclonal antibody. II. Reactivity in normal, reactive and neoplastic human tissues. Am J Pathol 127:389
41. Vande Berge JS, Rudolph R, Poolman WL, Disharoon DR (1989) Comparative growth dynamics and action concentration between human cultured fibroblasts from granulating wounds and dermal fibroblasts from normal skin. Lab Invest 61:532
42. Weedon J, Kerr JFR (1975) Atypical fibroxanthoma of skin: an electron microscopic study. Pathology 7:173
43. Woyke S, Domagala W, Olszewoki W, Korabieu M (1975) Pseudosarcoma of the skin. Cancer 33:970

Reactivity of Nodular Cells in Vitro: A Guide to the Pharmacological Treatment of Dupuytren's Contracture

I.L. Naylor, D.J. Coleman, R.A. Coleman, S.E. Cross, and I.T.H. Foo

Introduction

Since the time of Dupuytren attempts have been made to use drugs to either alleviate the symptoms or stop the progression of Dupuytren's contracture. In Dupuytren's *leçons orales* (1832) one reads: "M. Dupuytren in treating several cases of contraction of the ring fingers employed one after the other vapourised fumigation, first of an emollient and then of a sedative character, plasters ... leeches, friction with resolvent ointments and calomel, alkaline, simple sulphurous and saponaceous douches at various temperatures and all without the slightest effect."

Such treatments reflected perhaps a desire to avoid surgical correction of the disease with its associated risks. In the intervening years many drugs of a similar diversity as used by Dupuytren have been employed in an attempt to (a) reduce an existing contracture, (b) inhibit a developing contracture, (c) facilitate resection of tissue during surgery and (d) prevent or delay the recurrence of the disease after surgery. A list of drugs used during the last 100 years of clinical practice for all these kinds of therapy is shown in Table 1. Most of these drugs have passed into history, at least as far Dupuytren's contracture is concerned. Nevertheless an assessment of their place in therapy merits consideration, since such an assessment has not previously been reported and it provides a perspective of the pharmacological approach which has been taken towards the disease.

One major problem in any discussion of the pharmacological treatment of this disease is the lack of objective, multicentre, controlled trials of potentially beneficial drugs. Most studies have included limited numbers of patients of varying ages, different sexes, and at various stages of the disease. In addition some of the subjects used in these studies have had previously unsuccessful treatments, which may complicate interpretation of any later results. Consequently, the variability in the intensity of the disease between individuals, the differences in the rate of progression of the disease and possible periods of quiescence all contribute to great difficulties in assessing whether a drug does or does not have a beneficial effect. Thus, it is not surprising that the usefulness of drug treatment in Dupuytren's contracture is so controversial.

Table 1. Drugs used to treat Dupuytren's contracture

Thiosinamin (Rhodallin)
Thiosinamin-sodium salicylate
Thiosinamin-ethyl iodide
Iodine ointment
Thyroid extract
Copper sulphate solution
Pepsin
Parathyroid extract
5% salicylic acid ointment
Humanol (human sterilised fat)
Vitamin E/tocopherols
Hydrocortisone
Trypsin/α chymotrypsin/hyaluronidase
Potassium para-aminobenzoate (PABA)
Dimethlysulphoxide (DMSO)
Procarbazine (Natulan)
Trypsin/chymotrypsin/hyaluronidase
6-Methyl predisolone
Aprotinin (Trasylol)
α-Mercaptopropionylglcine (Thiopronin)
Allopurinol

A century ago there were many theories concerning the aetiology of the disease, the majority of which are no longer tenable. In contrast, the histology of the palmar nodules and cords was precisely known. Fibroblast proliferation in the palmar nodules and alterations in the appearance of the collagen fibres of the aponeurosis led to this disease being classified as belonging to the fibromatoses. This had an influence in deciding possible treatments, since a treatment applied to any of the allied conditions, such as Peyronie's disease, was thought appropriate to try in Dupuytren's contracture. It is true to say that no drug has ever been specifically produced for Dupuytren's contracture; rather, their use has been extrapolated from experience with other diseases.

One of the early aetiological factors were thought to be a hormonal imbalance which was responsible for the fibromatoses. So, to correct this imbalance thyroid extract was given (Gilbert 1913; Leopold-Levi 1913, cited by Wainwright 1926). The results were said to be encouraging but it was not widely used. In a similar way the contracture was compared with muscles in tetany and this was believed to be due to hypocalcaemia and so this led to the introduction of parathyroid extract. The results were not encouraging (Leriche and Jung 1930, cited by Powers 1934).

A more systematic approach to treatment began when fibrolysin was introduced. This drug and its derivatives were used in Dupuytren's contracture after its reported success in the treatment of scleroderma and scar remodelling. It was said to exert its effect by softening and improving the elasticity of sclerodermatous and scar tissues. In addition to these in vivo effects the drug was found in in vitro experiments to convert collagen into gelatin. The combination of its use in one of the allied conditions and its effect on collagen in vitro led to its application in Dupuytren's contracture. It was tried over many years and by many workers; its last reported use being in 1946 by Noix, who used the drug electroiontophorectically but its effectiveness in all these studies is perhaps best summarised in the conclusion of Black in as early as 1915: "Thiosinamin has been tried but the results cannot on the whole be regarded as encouraging". Nevertheless, this was an example of a drug in which both the in vivo and in vitro findings were applied to the treatment of Dupuytren's contracture. Such a combination of in vivo and in vitro approach in drug evaluation was very rare in the treatment of this condition in those days.

In contrast to the mere softening of collagen with thiosinamin the degradation of collagen was the objective in the use of pepsin (Hesse 1931) and later in the use of trypsin, α chymotrypsin and hyaluronidase (Bassot 1969; Hueston 1971). The effects of this mixture of enzymes were pronounced and clearly did effect an improvement in the condition but the treatment has not found widespread usage.

With the introduction of steroids the therapeutic objective was to induce a restraining effect on the formation of fibrous tissue. Several groups of investigators hoped that it would have the success seen in the treatment of other fibromatoses such as Peyronie's disease (Bodner et al. 1954; Desanctis and Furey 1967; Furey 1957; Rothfeld and Murray 1967) and keloids (Conway and Stark 1951; Ketchum et al. 1974; Kill 1977; Vallis 1967). Despite initial optimism the results for hydrocortisone (Zachariae and Zachariae 1955) and later more powerful derivatives such as 6-methyl prednisolone were disappointing (Kaufhold 1962). The drugs appeared to have little effect on an existing contracture (Baxter et al. 1952) and certainly did not cause a regression of the disease (Ritchey 1952). The most significant successes were when steroid was used postoperatively when it reduced oedema and facilitated mobility and rehabilitation of the hand (Bernstein 1954).

The subsequent introduction of dimethylsulphoxide (DMSO), which was said to dissolve pathologically formed collagen but leave normal collagen intact (Rosenbaum et al. 1965; Vuopala and Kaipainen 1971), and paraaminobenzoate (PABA) proved to be of questionable effectiveness. This was surprising since both agents had previously had some degree of success in treating Peyronie's disease and scleroderma (Zarafonetis 1964; Zarafonetis and Horrax 1959).

Perhaps the most investigated drug to treat Dupuytren's contracture is vitamin E. Its reported successful use in Peyronie's disease (Burford and Burford 1957; Scardino and Scott 1949) and other fibromatoses was followed by trials in Dupuytren's contracture. The results of high dose (300 mg per day) long-term therapy were extremely variable. Conclusions as to the effectiveness of the drug ranged from a good success rate (Steinberg 1946, 1951; Thomson 1949) to total ineffectiveness (King 1949; Langston and Badre 1949; Oldfield 1954; Parsons 1948; Richards 1952). The lack of its use today perhaps indicates that time has proved it to be ineffective.

Chance findings are very common in most types of therapy in which a drug given for one disease was unexpectedly found to be beneficial for another disease. This was the case for procarbazine which Aron (1968), on giving it to a patient with Hodgkin's disease, also noted that it not only cured the lymphoma but also the patient's Dupuytren's contracture. This led to clinical trials in both Dupuytren's and Peyronie's diseases but the incidence of side effects and questionable effectiveness precluded its widespread use (Morgan and Pryor 1978; Oosterlinck and Renders 1975). However, it did establish that an antiproliferative agent had an effect on the cells present in the nodule and thereby reduced the rate of contracture.

This anti-proliferative approach was followed by drugs designed to inhibit the formation of collagen, namely the lathyrogens. An example of this class of drugs is mercaptopropionylglycine (Bray and Galeazzi 1980; Cimmino et al. 1982). These agents are the first of their type to be used clinically to treat the condition. Their promise is yet to be fully determined but on theoretical grounds they may well have a beneficial effect on the disease and prevent its progression to a fixed contractured state (Fuller 1981).

The last drug which has been used is allopurinol (Murrell et al. 1987). Again its effectiveness in Dupuytren's contracture was found by accident and its exact mode of action in improving the condition of the disease awaits elucidation. It is at present unclear how the prevention of free radical generation decreases the contracture of the disease. This topic is dealt with in much greater details elsewhere in these proceedings.

In summary, the pharmacological treatment of Dupuytren's contracture over the last 100 years has been controversial and often empirical. Many treatments are clearly ineffective, some of the more promising ones are potentially toxic and perhaps the overall position is best summarised in the statement of Wesson (1943): "Whenever a variety of treatments are recommended for any disease we know that none is specific and that the symptoms are merely being treated while waiting for Nature to bring about a cessation of advancement if not regression." Unfortunately in Dupuytren's disease regression does not occur!

The Background to the Current Study

From the list of drugs given in Table 1 it is clear that there is a lack of basic knowledge as to the nature of the factors which induce the cellular proliferation in the palmar aponeurosis and to the nature of contractility in these cells which eventually produce the fixed contracture. The nodular cell generally considered to be responsible for the process of contraction is the myofibroblast (Gokel and Hubner 1977; Tomasek et al. 1987). It would be logical to attempt to antagonise the contractility of this cell type since if contraction was inhibited the deformity would be reduced and recurrence after surgical intervention could be minimised. None of the drugs in Table 1 have the property of modifying the contractile activity of the cell. This is surprising since in 1959 Luck suggested that: "The ideal form of therapy would be a method that could be employed with the first appearance of the nodules that would cause a prompt evolution of the nodules without the nodule undergoing contracture."

The question is of course what is the best procedure to use in order to find this "method" which in our terms would be a drug to inhibit myofibroblast contractility. Consequently, a study of myofibroblasts is needed in which the cells can be studied by a reproducible method and the experimental conditions can be varied so as to detect drugs which can modify myofibroblast contractility. Perhaps the most obvious way would be to culture the cells and then assess their contractility. Although the cells have been cultured (Vande Berg and Rudolph 1985) the assessment of contractility using conventional culture techniques is complex (Badalamente et al. 1988) and easier alternatives are not very precise. For example one study measured the wrinkles formed on a silicone sheet placed beneath the culture. In addition the normal cell to cell contacts and cell to stroma contacts may be different from those found in the in vivo state.

In contrast to the complexities of the tissue culture approach the pharmacological procedure would be either (a) to utilise an in vivo model or (b) to select an isolated tissue containing myofibroblasts and use it in a classical organ bath technique. However, Dupuytren's disease has never been reported in any animal species (Davis 1965) and the work of Gabbiani et al. (1973) seemed to suggest that strips of Dupuytren's nodules when used in organ bath studies did not respond as did strips of tissues containing myofibroblasts such as granulation tissue. Thus the position appeared to be that there is no animal model and isolated strips of Dupuytren's nodular tissue did not respond.

However, it was noticed that Gabbiani et al. (1973) used an unusual auxotonic transducer (Kapanci et al. 1974) which studies in our laboratory had found to be unsuitable for in vitro work on myofibroblasts (Illingworth and Naylor 1981). If an isometric transducer was substituted for the auxotonic type then strips of Dupuytren's nodules were found to contract in vitro.

To further enhance the sensitivity and reproducibility of the method several other changes were incorporated and found to provide a stable and sensitive system. The physiological solution used in the original method was Tyrode and this was replaced by Krebs-Henseleit solution which is more generally used for the study of human tissues. The technique of superfusion (Gaddum 1953) was used in addition to the conventional immersion bath arrangements since superfusion has the major advantages of continuously washing the tissue and so provides a very stable baseline on which to accurately assess any contractile effect. In addition the tissue was connected to the transducer with braided stainless steel wire and the anchorage point in the tissue was a barbless bronze fish hook so as to avoid any loss of a response due to the compliance of the cotton thread that is normally employed. These simple changes provided a sensitive and reproducible in vitro preparation.

To contract the tissue a range of agonists were tested some of which other authors had shown to produce myofibroblast contraction in tissues such as croton oil induced granulation tissue (Gabbiani et al. 1972; Garcia-Valdecasas et al. 1981; Majno et al. 1971). These included angiotensin, noradrenaline,

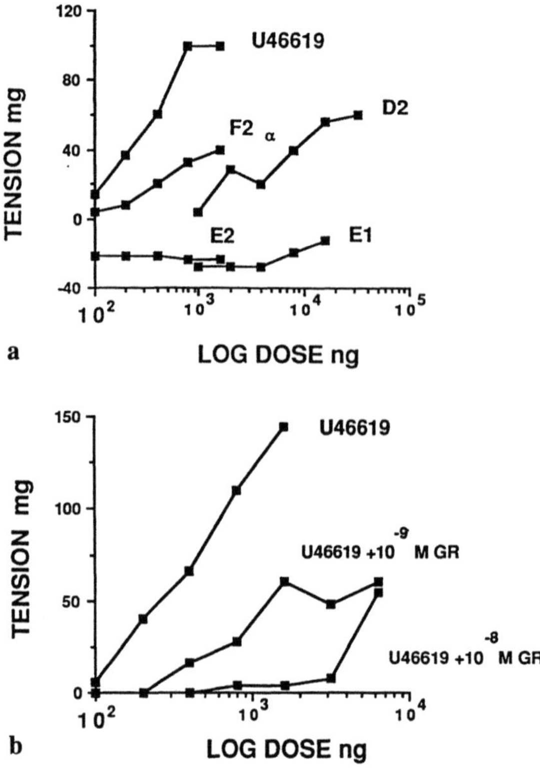

Fig. 1. a The response of Dupuytren's nodular strips to prostanoids. **b** The response to U46619 in the presence of GR 32191

histamine and 5-hydroxytryptamine (5-HT). Unexpectedly, when used in our studies with Dupuytren's nodules all these agonists proved ineffective. When prostaglandins, namely PGE_1, PGF_1, PGD_2, PGE_2 and $PGF_{2\alpha}$, were used they produced a range of effects (Fig. 1a). PGD_2, PGE_2 and $PGF_{2\alpha}$ were contractile whereas PGE_1 and PGF_1 were relaxatory. A stable form of the prostaglandin endoperoxide U46619, which acts on thromboxane receptors, was also found to be contractile. Indeed it proved to be the most potent contractile agonist of the group. The H_1 antagonist mepyramine also exerts a contractile response in these preparations. All the contractile responses were slow in onset and prolonged even in the superfusion experiments. In contrast to these effects on nodular tissues all studies on samples of cords were unresponsive to the prostanoids. It should be stressed that all the responses were fully reversible and this allowed antagonism studies to be carried out. Using the immersion baths the responses to U46619 were capable of being selectively antagonised by a specific, selective thromboxane antagonist GR32191 in a concentration-dependent manner. Over the concentration range of U46619 used, $10^{-7} M$ GR32191 completely abolished the responses whereas 10^{-8} and $10^{-9} M$ exerted a concentration-dependent antagonism (Fig. 1b). The

Induced
  Dupuytren's nodules
  Dupuytren's cords
  Tissue expander capsule
  Tissue implant capsule
  Hypertrophic scar
  Keloids
  Granulation tissue
Structural
  Postauricular skin
  Breast skin (reduction)
  Placenta
  Whartons jelly
  Endocervical canal

response to mepyramine is unaffected by GR32191 which indicates that mepyramine does not act on thromboxane receptors (Coleman et al. 1989).

We have therefore shown that certain prostanoids are potent contractile agents on human myofibroblasts found in the palmar nodules of Dupuytren's contracture, and evidence obtained with the thromboxane receptor blocking drug GR32191 suggests that thromboxane receptors are involved. Although it is not clear whether prostanoids are involved in the aetiology of the disease further studies using agents such as GR32191 may provide the answer. Certainly the in vitro studies of Dupuytren's nodules showed that stable and sensitive preparations can be obtained from nodular tissue which give reproducible responses to prostanoids. It is clear that agonist-antagonist studies can be performed with such a tissue and potential anticontractile agents can be assessed.

Unfortunately there is a problem with such studies in that large numbers of specimens are required to determine the effect of an agonist and antagonist. Tissues are simply not available in the quantities required to carry out methodical studies and so other types of tissues were investigated (Table 2).

Human tissues from keloids, hypertrophic scars and granulation tissues were investigated as was tissue formed around tissue expanders when they were removed prior to the insertion of an implant. These we classify as "induced" tissues and the presence of myofibroblasts has been documented in all of them. The most suitable tissue was found to be the tissue expander capsule as it had a range of sensitivity comparable to Dupuytren's nodules – for example it is insensitive to 5-HT but responsive to U46619.

Again this tissue is in limited supply so other tissues in which myofibroblasts occur as structural elements were investigated in the in vitro superfusion system. Post-auricular skin was used as a control for the keloids and not unexpectedly was insensitive to all the agents used. The skin from breast reduction procedures, placentae, Wharton's jelly and endocervical canal tissue were found to have limitations due to their content of smooth muscle which masked the much weaker contractile abilities of the myofibroblasts. As an

Table 3. Rat tissues used in vitro

Structural
Testicular capsule
Ovarian capsule
Placenta
Lung
Uterus
Splenic capsule
Adrenal capsule
Induced
Wound granulation tissue[a]
Implant capsular tissue
Croton oil granuloma pouch
Tissue expander capsule[b]
Oestrogen stimulated immature uterus

[a] Also from minipig.
[b] Also from pig.

alternative, animal tissues (Table 3) were investigated to see if there were any which could provide a spectrum of sensitivities similar to that of Dupuytren's nodules. For the induced myofibroblasts wound granulation was suitable especially that of the minipig. The capsules which formed around both the perspex cylinder and tissue expander in the rat were insensitive. This contrasted with the reactivity of the tissue expander capsule in the pig. Oestrogen stimulated immature rat uterus was insensitive. The croton oil induced granuloma tissue widely used as a model for myofibroblast studies was certainly sensitive but its abnormally high responsiveness to 5-HT suggest that it is atypical of other tissues containing myofibroblasts. For the structural sources of myofibroblast containing tissues testicular capsule proved useful but the others, due to the complications of smooth muscle being present, were found to be of limited usefulness. It is clear that the ideal alternative tissue to Dupuytren's nodule, either human or animal, for investigating the activity of anticontractile drugs is still to be found.

Future Possibilities

A recent series of experiments has been carried out using Dupuytren's nodules to determine if the endogenous contractile mediator(s) can be characterised in a simple in vitro system.

If a strip of nodular tissue is left in an immersion bath for a prolonged period of time (>1 h) without changing the bath fluid several events occur (Fig. 2). There is an initial decrease in tension as the tissue relaxes and if the tissue is not retensioned but left alone this is followed by a "plateau" period in which the tension remains constant. At some time after the plateau period is reached, ranging from 25–45 min, the tension slowly and steadily increases until the tissue is washed. After washing the tension slowly falls towards the baseline but

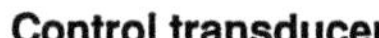

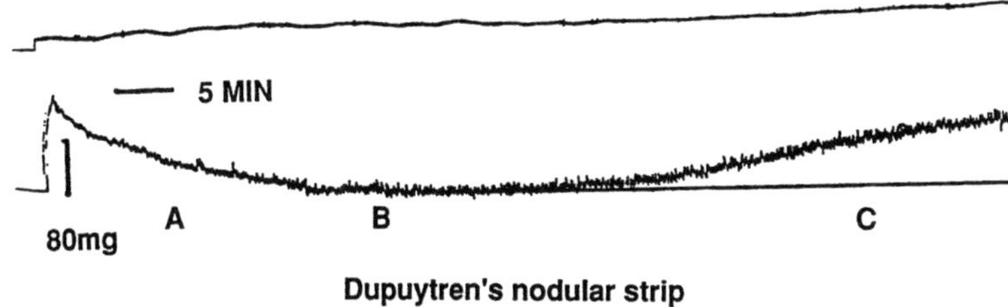

Fig. 2. The tension recorded in a strip of a Dupuytren's nodule. *A* The period of relaxation; *B* the period of maintenance of a constant tension, and *C* the period of a gradual increase in tension

never actually achieves it. Consequently it remains in a partially contracted state. This suggests that a substance(s) is released by the nodular tissue into the bathing fluid which exerts a powerful contractile effect upon itself. An analysis of the bath fluid is underway to determine the nature of this contractile substance.

Perhaps this simple experiment indicates another possible avenue of in vitro research to pursue in developing specific anticontractile agents for modulating the activities of myofibroblasts in Dupuytren's contracture.

Acknowledgements. The authors thank Doctors D. Sharpe, M. Timmons, J. Palmer, A. Batchelor and S. Kay for tissue samples. C.L. Chander, I. Osman, M. Ahmed for some of the experimental results and J. Lees for his graphics. The financial contribution of Glaxo Group Research is gratefully acknowledged as are the efforts of T.C. Teo without whom the manuscript would have been impossible.

References

Alexander DA (1923) Dupuytren's contraction (Letter). Br Med J 1:794

Anderson W (1891) Lectures on contractions of the fingers and toes; their varieties, pathology and treatment. Lancet 2:1–5, 57–59

Aron E (1968) Le traitement medical de la maladie de Dupuytren par un agent cytostatique (methylhydrazine). Presse Med 76:1956

Badalamente MA, Hurst LA, Sampson SP (1988) Prostaglandins influence myofibroblast contractility in Dupuytren's disease. J Hand Surg [Am] 13:867–871

Bassot J (1969) Traitement de la maladie de Dupuytren par exerèse pharmacodynamique bases pysio-biologiques-technique. Statistique de 34 interventions. Gaz Hop 16:557–563

Baxter H, Schiller C, Johnson LH, Whiteside JH, Randall RE (1952) Cortisone therapy in Dupuytren's contracture. Plast Reconstr Surg 9:261–273

Bernstein H (1954) Current status of cortisone in postoperative treatment of Dupuytren's contracture. NY J Med 54:90–92

Black K (1915) Dupuytren's contracture. Br Med J 1:326–328

Bodner H, Howard AH, Kaplan JH (1954) Peyronie's disease: cortisone-hyaluronidase-hydrocortisone therapy. J Urol 72:400–403

Bray E, Galeazzi M (1980) First results in the treatment of Dupuytren's disease. Arthritis Rheum 23:1408

Burford EH, Burford CE (1957) Combined therapy for Peyronie's disease. J Urol 78:265–268

Chesney J (1963) Plastic induration of the penis; Peyronie's disease. Br J Urol 35:61–66

Chesney J (1975) Peyronie's disease. J Urol 47:209–218

Cimmino MA, Cutolo M, Beltrame F (1982) Local injections of tiopronin in Dupuytren's contracture. Arthritis Rheum 25:1505

Coleman DJ, Coleman RA, Cross SE, Naylor IL (1989) Prostanoid-induced contraction of myofibroblasts; effect of the thromboxane (TP) receptor antagonist GR 32191. Br J Pharmacol 96:65P

Comtet J-J, Migne J, Fischer L (1972) Intérêt d'un inhibiteur d'enzymes dans la cicatrisation. Ann Chir Plast 17:145–149

Conway H, Stark RB (1951) ACTH in plastic surgery. Plast Reconstr Surg 8:354–377

Davis AA (1932) The treatment of Dupuytren's contracture–a review of 31 cases, with an assessment of the comparative value of different methods of treatment. Br J Surg 19:539–547

Davis JE (1965) On surgery of Dupuytren's contracture. Plast Reconstr Surg 36:277–314

Desanctis PN, Furey CA (1967) Steriod injection therapy for Peyronie's disease; a ten year summary and review of 38 cases. J Urol 97:114–116

Dupuytren G (1832) Leçons orales de clinique chirurgicale, vol 1. Bailliere, Paris

Fuller GC (1981) Perspectives for the use of collagen synthesis inhibitors as antifibrotic agents. J Med Chem 24:651–658

Furey CA (1957) Peyronie's disease; treatment by the local injection of meticortelone and hydrocortisone. J Urol 77:251–265

Gabbiani G, Hirschel BJ, Ryan GB, Statkov PR, Majno G (1972) Granulation tissue as a contractile organ. J Exp Med 135:719–734

Gabbiani G, Majno G, Ryan GB (1973) The fibroblast as a contractile cell: the myofibroblast. In: Kulonen E, Pikkarinen J (eds) Biology of fibroblast. Academic, New York, pp 139–154 (4th Sigrid Juselius Foundation Symposium, August 1972, Turku)

Gaddum JH (1953) The technique of superfusion. Br J Pharmacol Chemother 8:321–326

Garcia-Valdecasas JC, Garcia-Valdecasas FG, Pera C (1981) Pharmacological reactivity of granulation tissue. J Pharm Pharmacol 33:650–654

Gibson HRB (1952) Dupuytren's contracture. Br Med J 2:446

Gilbert M (1913) Abstract. Meeting of the Academy of Medicine, Paris. Lancet 1:1041

Gokel JM, Hubner G (1977) Occurence of myofibroblasts in the different phases of morbus Dupuytren (Dupuytren's contracture). Beitr Pathol 161:166–175

Hesse (1931) Zur Behandlung der Dupuytren'schen Krankheit. Zentralbl Chir 24:1532–1533

Hueston JT (1971) Enzymic fasciotomy. Hand 3:38–40

Illingworth DR, Naylor IL (1982) An improved, ultrasonic auxotonic transducer for use with isolated tissues. J Pharmacol Methods 8:59–71

John H (1965) Therapeutische Erfahrungen mit Dimethlysulfoxyd in der orthopadischen Praxis. Arzneimittelforschung 15:1298–1305

Kapanci Y, Assimacopoulos A, Irle C, Zwahlen A, Gabbiani G (1974) "Contractile interstitial cells" in pulmonary alveloar septa: a possible regulator of ventilation/perfusion ratio? J Cell Biol 60:375–392

Kaufhold N (1962) Die örtliche Behandlung mit 6-Methyl-Prednisolon (Urbason). MMW 104:2252–2253

Ketchum LD, Cohen IK, Masters FW (1974) Hypertrophic scars and keloids "a collective review". Plast Reconstr Surg 53:140–154

Kiil J (1977) Keloids treated with topical injections of triamcinolone acetonide (Kenalog). Scand J Plast Reconstr Surg 11:169–172

King RA (1949) Vitamin E therapy in Dupuytren's contracture; examination of claim that vitamin therapy is successful. J Bone Joint Surg [Br] 31:443

Kirk JE, Chieffi M (1952) Vitamin studies in middle aged and old individuals. IX. Tocopherol administration to patients with Dupuytren's contracture; effect on plasma tocopherol levels and degree of contracture. Proc Soc Exp Biol Med 80:565–568

Knavel AB, Koch SL, Mason ML (1929) Dupuytren's contraction with a description of the palmar fascia, and a report of 29 surgically treated cases. Surg Gynaecol Obstet 48:145–190

Lagier R, Rutishauser E (1956) Anatomie pathologique et pathogénie de la maladie de Dupuytren. Presse Med 64:1212–1216

Langston RG, Badre EJ (1948) Dupuytren's contracture. Can Med Ass J 58:557–561

Luck JV (1959) Dupuytren's contracture. A new concept of the pathogenesis correlated with surgical management. J Bone Joint Surg [Am] 41:635–665

Majno G, Gabbiani G, Hirschel BJ, Ryan GB, Statkov PR (1971) Contractions of granulation tissue in vitro; similarity to smooth muscle. Science 173:548–550

Morgan RJ, Pryor JP (1978) Procarbazine (Natulan) in the treatment of Peyronie's disease. Br J Urol 50:111–113

Murrell GAC, Pilowsky E, Murrell TGC (1987) A hypothesis on the resolution of Dupuytren's contracture with allopurinol. Specul Sci Technol 10:107–112

Noix M (1946) Traitement de la maladie de Dupuytren par la thiosinamin. J Radiol Electrol 27:476–477

Oldfield MC (1954) Dupuytren's contracture. Proc R Soc Med 47:361–365

Oosterlinck W, Renders G (1975) Treatment of Peyronie's disease with procarbazine. Br J Urol 47:219–220

Parsons AR (1948) Dupuytren's contracture treatment by massive doses of vitamin E. Ir J Med Sci 270:272–275

Powers H (1934) Dupuytren's contracture one hundred years after Dupuytren; its interpretation. J Ment Dis 80:386–409

Richards HJ (1952) Dupuytren's Contracture treated with Vitamin E. Br Med J 1:1328

Ritchey SJ (1952) The use of cortisone in Dupuytren's contracture. US Armed Forces Med J 3:811–818

Rosenbaum EE, Herschler RJ, Jacob SW (1965) Dimethyl sulphoxide in musculoskeletal disorders. JAMA 192:309–313

Ross JA (1952) Dupuytren's contracture (Letter). Br, Med J 1:232

Ross JA, Annan JH (1951) Dupuytren's contracture – a clinical review. Ann Sug 134:186–194

Rothfeld SH, Murray W (1967) The treatment of Peyronie's disease by ionophoresis of C 21 esterified glucocorticoids. J Urol 97:874–875

Scardino PL, Scott WW (1949) The use of tocopherols in the treatment of Peyronie's disease. Ann NY Acad Sci 52:390–396

Stahnke E (1927) Zur Behandlung der Dupuytren'schen Fingerkontraktur. Zentralbl Chir 54:2438–2442

Steinberg CL (1946) A new method of treatment of Dupuytren's contracture – A form of fibrositis. Med Clin North Am 30:221–231

Steinberg CL (1951) Tocopherols in treatment of primary fibrositis Arch Surg 63:824–832

Thomson GR (1949) Treatment of Dupuytren's contracture with vitamin E. Br Med J 2:1382

Tomasek JJ, Schultz RJ, Haaksma CJ (1987) Extracellular matrix-cytoskeletal connections at the surface of the specialized contractile fibroblast (myofibroblast) in Dupuytren's disease. J Bone Joint Surg [Am] 69:1400–1407

Trumper WA (1931) A case of Dupuytren's contracture. Lancet 2:17

Tubby AH (1913a) Dupuytren's contracture successfully treated by open incision and (thiosinamin) fibrolysin. Br Med J 2:1203–1204

Tubby AH (1913b) A new method of dealing with scars by multiple incision and thiosinamin. Br Med J 2:1138–1139

Vallis CP (1967) Intralesional injection of keloids and hypertrophic scars with the Dermo-jet. Plast Reconstr Surg 40:255–262

Vande Berg JS, Rudolph R (1985) Cultured myofibroblasts; a useful model to study wound contraction and pathological contracture. Ann Plast Surg 14:111–120

Vuopala LU, Kaipainen WJ (1971) DMSO in the treatment of Dupuytren's contracture – a therapeutic experiment. Acta Rheumatol Scand 17:61–62

Wainwright L (1926) Dupuytren's contracture. Practioner 117:263–265

Weaver RG, Berliner DL (1970) The action of fluocinolone acetonide upon scar tissue. J Urol 104:591–595

Wesson MB (1943) Peyronie's disease (plastic induration) cause and treatment. J Urol 49:350–355

Zachariae L, Zachariae F (1955) Hydrocortisone acetate in the treatment of Dupuytren's contracture and allied conditions. Acta Chir Scand 109:421–431

Zarafonetis CJD (1964) Antifibrotic therapy with Potaba. Am J Med Sci 248:550–561

Zarafonetis CJD, Horrax TM (1959) Treatment of Peyronie's disease with potassium para-aminobenzoate (Potaba). J Urol 81:770–772

Extracellular Matrix Components and Macromolecular Interactions

Stromal-Epithelial Cell Interactions in the Mechanisms of Hepatocyte Injury, Liver Cell Regeneration and Fibrogenesis

A.M. Gressner

Introduction

Fibrotic lesions encompass a wide spectrum of tissue and organ disorders ranging from the milder forms, as seen with keloid formation (hypertrophic scars) and Dupuytren's disease, to acquired, more life-threatening diseases; such as interstitial pulmonary fibrosis, liver fibrosis/cirrhosis, glomerulosclerosis, and even atherosclerosis. All of these disorders share common pathogenetic elements typically involving an inappropriate proliferation of mesenchymal cells, accumulation of extracellular matrix components, contraction, and obliterative alterations of the architecture of the affected tissues and organs. Some of the steps in the pathogenesis of tissue fibrosis are found in normal wound healing [1,2], but the latter process is, by some not yet clearly defined reasons, self-limiting, whereas in the exaggerated fibrogenic response certain stop signals operating in normal tissue repair are not produced, not recognized, or antagonized. In general, there are four distinct, yet interrelated phases of the fibrotic response discernible: (1) cell injury, (2) inflammation, (3) cell proliferation (regeneration), (4) extracellular matrix production and remodeling.

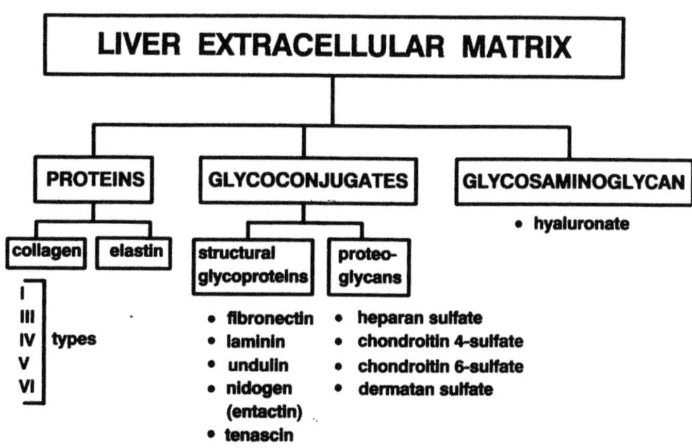

Fig. 1. The main components of liver extracellular matrix

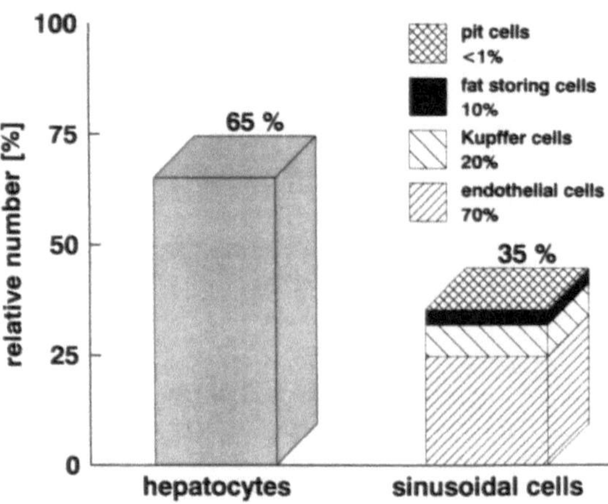

Fig. 2. Quantitative distribution of parenchymal (hepatocytes) and resident nonparenchymal (sinusoidal) cells in normal liver

This sequence of events is seen very typically in the development of liver fibrosis (fibrogenesis), probably the most abundant form of organ fibrosis [3,4]. The pathogenesis of liver fibrosis exemplifies the principal mechanisms and routes along which tissue injury is converted to an excess deposition and histologic redistribution of connective tissue (fibrosis). In this organ, fibrogenesis is initiated by acute and perpetuated by chronic hepatocyte injury. This is followed by (a) an influx of inflammatory cells (neutrophils, monocytes, lymphocytes) and activation of resident macrophages (Kupffer cells), (b) proliferation, migration and transformation of connective tissue producing cell types (mainly perisinusoidal fat storing cells, termed also Ito cells, lipocytes, vitamin A-storing cells), and (c) exaggerated production of an altered spectrum of collagens, proteoglycans, hyaluronan, and structural glycoproteins such as laminin, fibronectin, tenascin, and nidogen/entactin, which make up the fibrotic extracellular matrix [4,5] (Fig. 1). Refinement of cell isolation procedures and culture conditions have allowed in vitro studies, which suggest that in each phase of the fibrogenic sequence extensive bidirectional interactions between mesenchymal (stromal) and epithelial (hepatocytes) cells occur. Four types of mesenchymal (sinusoidal) cells, Kupffer cells, endothelial cells, fat storing cells, and pit cells, cooperate with each other and with the hepatocyte (liver parenchymal cell) (Fig. 2). The collaboration of these cells might operate physically by cell-to-cell contact (e.g., by membrane contacts between hepatocytes and perisinusoidal lipocytes located in the immediate proximity) or chemically by production (in effector cells) of cellular signals (cytokines) which induce responses in neighboring or more distant cells (target cells) (Fig. 3). A further means of stromal-epithelial communication is mediated by matrix-hepatocyte interactions, which have been shown to be important for gene activation and maintenance of a differentiated phenotype (see below). Examples (albeit not complete) of mesenchymal-hepatocyte

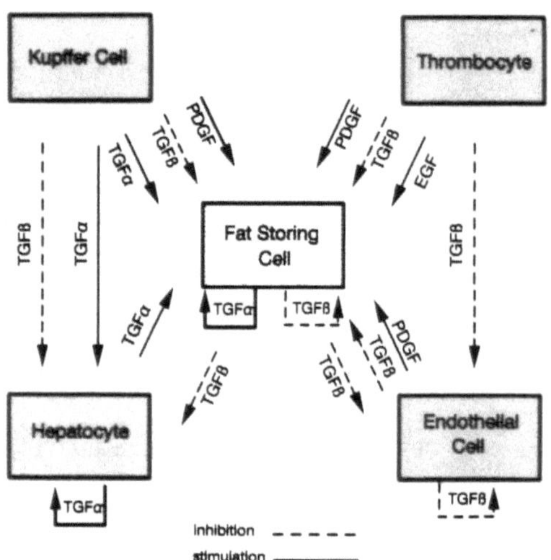

Fig. 3. The main types of cytokines involved in signal transfer between parenchymal and sinusoidal cells during hepatic fibrogenesis

interactions in the various phases of the liver fibrogenic response are summarized below, but the extensive cooperations among sinusoidal cells, e.g., between Kupffer cells and fat storing cells, will be not discussed here.

Cell-Cell Communication

Cell Injury

Hepatocyte injury is the primary event in the cascade of mechanisms leading to fibrosis. There is evidence that Kupffer cells can modulate the toxicity of injurious agents. The pool of macrophages in injured tissue is greatly enhanced by local proliferation of resident Kupffer cells and an influx of blood monocytes. By phagocytosis and endotoxin challenge macrophages are activated and secrete a large number of mediators [6,7] some of which may have deleterious effects on the integrity of hepatocytes. The conversion of molecular oxygen into superoxide anion radicals, hydrogen peroxide, and hydroxyl radicals (oxidative burst) [7] is an important adjunct in the pathogenesis of liver cell necrosis. In the model of D-galactosamine hepatitis the oxygen-derived free radical-generating capacity of isolated hepatic macrophages is several-fold enhanced [8]. If production was suppressed by prior administration of latex particles [8] or lipoxygenase inhibitors [9], hepatotoxicity and lipid peroxide level were significantly reduced. Furthermore, superoxide dismutase supplementation protected against liver injury induced by D-galactosamine [8]. Tumor necrosis factor-α (TNF-α) is another mediator of hepatocyte necrosis generated by activated macrophages (Table 1). When injected in mice, TNF can cause liver cell necrosis [10]. The

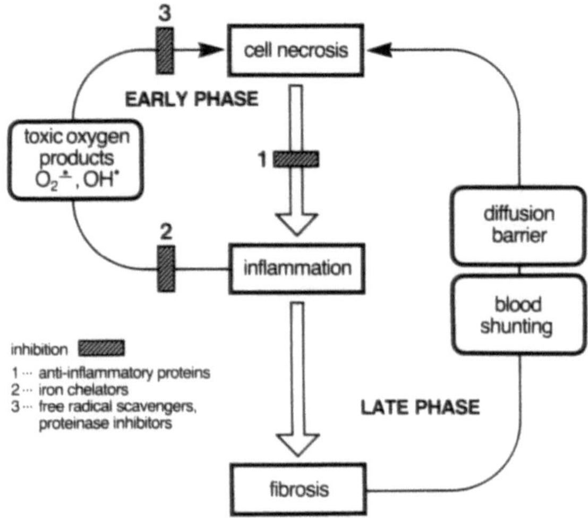

Fig. 4. Vicious circles in liver fibrogenesis and possible sites of inhibition. In the early phase, products of inflammatory cells, e.g., reactive oxygen species and proteinases, induce liver cell necrosis, the initiating event of fibrogenesis, followed by inflammation. In the late, dry phase, the increased deposition of extracellular matrix leads to blood shunting around the liver and increased diffusion barriers between the sinusoid and the hepatocyte resulting in parenchymal cell necrosis due to malnutrition

Table 1. Biological activities of tumor necrosis factor-α

Fibrogenic activities
   Mitogenic action on fibroblasts
   Increase number of EGF receptors on fibroblasts
   Stimulation of collagenase production
   Stimulation of hyaluronate production
   Decreased collagen gene transcription and collagen production
Inflammatory activities
   Stimulation of prostaglandin E_2 production
   Activation of granulocyte function
   Mediator of monocyte cytotoxicity
Miscellaneous activities
   Release of proteoglycans from cartilage
   Inhibition of proteoglycan synthesis in cartilage
   Suppression of lipoprotein lipase
   Mediation of endotoxin shock

mediator has been implicated in the lethality of the hepatotoxin galactosamine [11], and other data suggest that TNF might play an etiologic role in liver injury, e.g., in alcoholic hepatitis, in which increased production by monocytes was measured [12]. In addition, proteinases [13] and several other chemically not clearly defined hepatocytotoxic factors elaborated by activated macrophages might contribute in the early (inflammatory) phase to the persistence of hepatocyte injury and by this to ongoing fibrogenesis (Fig. 4). It

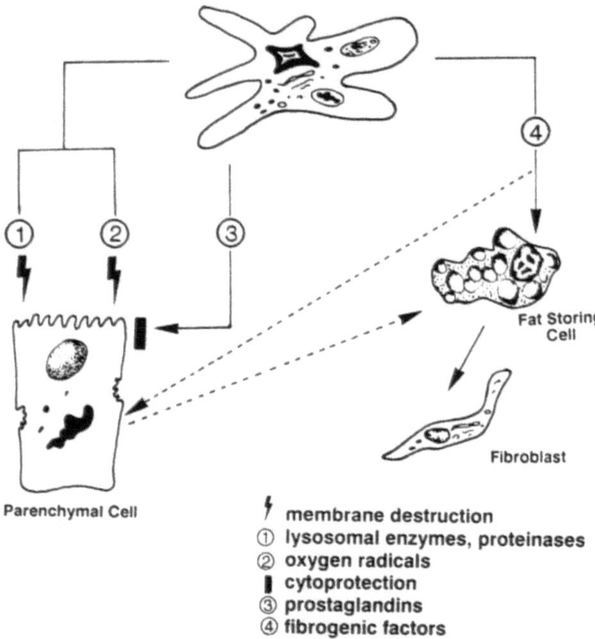

Fig. 5. Paracrine effects of activated liver macrophages and Kupffer cells on the hepatocyte and on the activation and transformation of fat storing cells to myofibroblast-like cells. Secreted proteinases (*1*) and oxygen radicals (*2*) exert injurious effects on parenchymal liver cells, whereas prostaglandins (*3*), synthesized by activated Kupffer cells, might be protective against liver cell necrosis. Fibrogenic mediators (*4*) elaborated by activated Kupffer cells include TGF-α, TGF-β, PDGF, and others which initiate proliferation, transformation, and enhanced connective tissue protein synthesis in fat storing cells, the principle extracellular matrix synthesizing cell type in liver

should be noted, however, that Kupffer cells produce also potentially protective agents, e.g., certain types of prostaglandins (PGI_2, PGE_2), which might counterbalance the deleterious effects of other mediators on liver cell integrity (Fig. 5).

Inflammation

Interactions between hepatocytes and stromal cells exist also in the inflammatory phase of fibrogenesis. As an example, rat [14] and human [15] hepatocytes metabolizing ethanol produce potent chemotactic activity for human polymorphonuclear leukocytes. Maximum effect is obtained with 10 mM ethanol; the activity was strongly reduced by 4-methylpyrazole and cyanamide, inhibitors of alcohol dehydrogenase and acetaldehyde dehydrogenase, respectively. The chemotactic factor which may be a polar lipid, might be relevant for the leukocytic infiltration observed in acute alcoholic hepatitis. Hepatocytes are also main targets in local (and general) inflammation. The most potent inducer of acute phase reaction, i.e.,

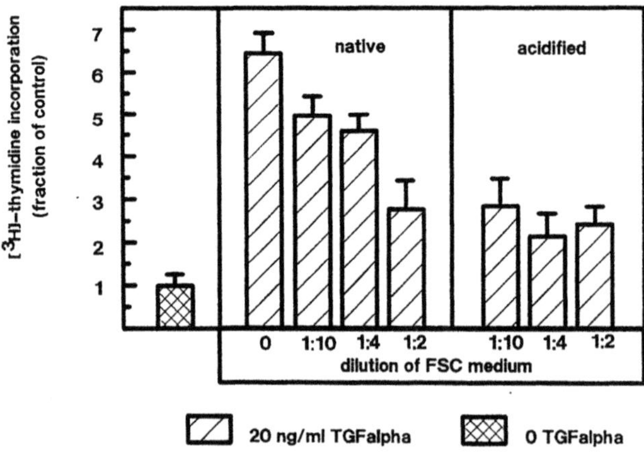

Fig. 6. Inhibition of TGF-α stimulated DNA synthesis in hepatocytes by native and acidified conditioned medium from secondary cultures of fat storing cells. TGF-α (20 ng/ml) was added 2 h and 20 h after plating, simultaneously with conditioned medium. Control represents DNA synthesis of parenchymal cells in the absence of TGF-α and fetal calf serum. Mean values ± S.D. of four experiments are shown

interleukin-6, is generated by macrophages and acts in a paracrine (local) and endocrine (systemic inflammation) way on the expression of acute phase protein genes [16–18]. Some of these proteins are potent scavengers of oxygen radicals and inhibitors of proteinases which contributes to suppression of the local inflammatory activity.

Parenchymal Cell Regeneration

Hepatocyte regeneration, a common sequel of necrosis, is strictly controlled by interactions with stromal cells, among which Kupffer cells, transformed fat storing cells (myofibroblast-like cells), and endothelial cells have been suggested to play prominent roles. Several growth factors, cytokines, and comitogenic factors have been implicated in the paracrine and autocrine regulation of liver cell multiplication [19], among which transforming growth factors (TGF)-α and β were identified as key regulators [20–23]. The expression of genes encoding TGF-α and TGF-β increases time dependently after partial liver resection [20–22]. TGF-α, which shares the same receptor with EGF (epidermal growth factor), is a potent mitogen for hepatocytes, whereas TGF-β negatively controls hepatocyte replication [20]. Therefore, TGF-β might provide an important stop signal for liver cell multiplication. TGF-α is expressed in hepatocytes and functions as a positive effector through an autocrine circuit which uses hepatocyte EGF receptor [21], but TGF-β is not synthesized in parenchymal liver cells [22]. This potent growth inhibitor is produced in Kupffer cells [24], endothelial cells [22], and transformed fat storing cells, i.e., the myofibroblast-like cells [25]. Using Northern blot hybridization, we identified in Kupffer cells and in myofibroblast-like cells

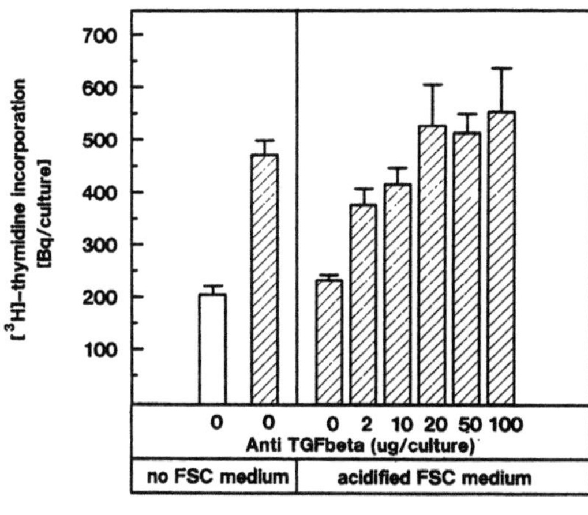

Fig. 7. Effect of anti-TGF-β antibodies on the inhibitory action of conditioned medium from fat storing cell (*FSC*) secondary cultures (myofibroblast-like cells) on hepatocellular [³H]thymidine incorporation. Transiently acidified FSC medium at a 1:4 dilution was incubated for 2 h with increasing amounts of antibody prior to the addition to hepatocyte cultures stimulated by TGF-α. Mean values ± S.D. of four experiments are shown

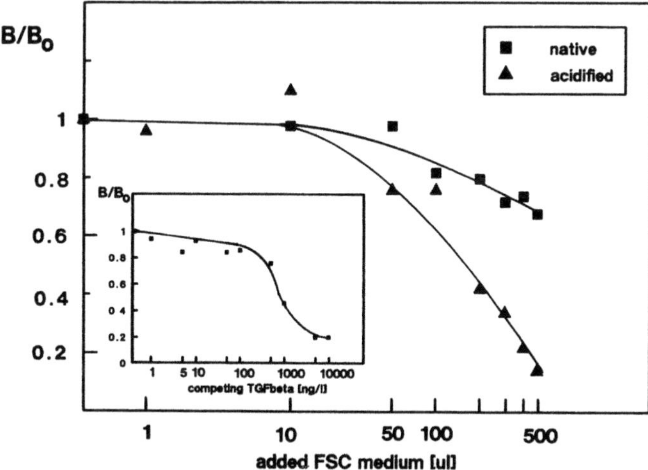

Fig. 8. Binding of ¹²⁵I-labeled TGF-β to hepatocytes at the first day of primary culture in the presence of increasing concentrations of native and transiently acidified conditioned medium from myofibroblast-like cell cultures. Control represents the binding of ¹²⁵I-labeled TGF-β in the absence of unlabeled TGF-β and conditioned medium. The *inset* shows binding in the presence of unlabeled TGF-β. Mean values of duplicate experiments are shown

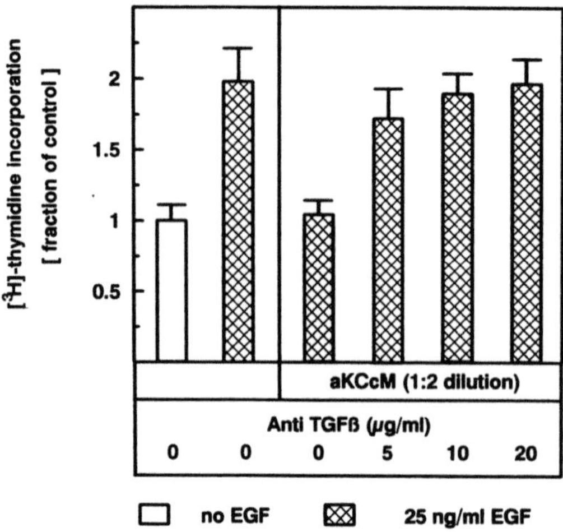

Fig. 9. Effect of anti-TGF-β antibodies on the inhibitory action of conditioned medium from Kupffer cell (*KC*) cultures on hepatocellular [³H]thymidine incorporation. Transiently acidified KC medium (*aKCcM*) at a 1:2 dilution was incubated for 2 h with increasing amounts of neutralizing anti-TGF-β prior to addition to hepatocytes stimulated by EGF. Mean values ± S.D. of four experiments are shown

transcripts of the genes of TGF-α and TGF-β and identified in the conditioned media of these cells both growth inhibitory (TGF-β) and stimulatory (TGF-α) activity [24]. DNA synthesis in cultured hepatocytes challenged with TGF-α was dose dependently reduced by conditioned media from transformed fat storing cells (Fig. 6). Transiently acidified conditioned media, in which latent inactive TGF-β is converted to the biologically active form, was far more potent than the native medium (Fig. 6). The antiproliferative activity was neutralized by incubation with anti-TGF-β antibodies (Fig. 7). In a radioligand assay the binding of ¹²⁵I-labeled TGF-β to hepatocytes is reduced in the presence of increasing concentrations of native and transiently acidified conditioned medium from transformed fat storing cells (Fig. 8). Kupffer cells also modulate the mitotic activity of hepatocytes. Data were reported which indicate that Kupffer cell conditioned media from intact liver and regenerating remnant liver significantly stimulate DNA synthesis in hepatocytes as compared with control media [26]. In our own experiments we found bidirectional, both inhibitory and stimulatory, effects of Kupffer cells on hepatocyte multiplication. The effects depend on the ratio of TGF-α and active TGF-β, since neutralization of one of these factors causes the opposite response in hepatocytes (Fig. 9). In conclusion, Kupffer cells and transformed fat storing cells control hepatocyte replication in both ways by secretion of TGF-α and -β. TGF-β is secreted mainly in an inactive precursor form which needs to be activated extracellularly to become growth inhibitory. The mechanism of activation, which is not yet known, may be a critical process in the control of hepatocyte multiplication.

Extracellular Matrix Production

Fibrosis is defined by: (1) a three- to sixfold increase of most of the extracellular matrix (ECM) molecules summarized in Fig. 1, (2) a disproportionate elevation of the various subspecies of individual ECM molecules (types of collagens, proteoglycans, and structural glycoproteins), (3) subtle changes of the microcomposition of specific types of ECM molecules, e.g., concerning the degree of hydroxylation of collagen α-chains, the number, length, and degree of sulfation (charge density) of glycosaminoglycans occupying the core protein of proteoglycans, and (4) the topographic redistribution of ECM in injured liver leading to an early and preponderant subendothelial deposition of connective tissue in the space of Disse (perisinusoidal fibrosis) and to other forms of local and diffuse fibrosis. Fibrosis plays a major role in the clinical consequences of liver cirrhosis since it hinders the systemic functions of hepatocytes and nonparenchymal cells by development of diffusion barriers and/or interferes with portal hemodynamics due to stenosis of intrasinusoidal blood flow. Furthermore, diffusion barriers between the sinusoid and hepatocytes contribute to progressive hepatocellular damage (necrosis) and thereby to persistence of the initiating event, which provides a pathogenetic vicious circle in the late phase of liver fibrosis (Fig. 4).

The excessive deposition of connective tissue in chronically injured liver is the result of an imbalance of synthesis and degradation. The most important mechanism concerns a stimulated synthesis, but changes in the degradation of the various components of ECM might be an important, presently not well understood, adjunct in the mechanism of fibrogenesis. Perisinusoidal lipocytes have been identified as the most important connective tissue producing cell type in liver [27,28]. This cell type, normally involved in the storage and metabolism of retinoids, has the capacity to transform into myofibroblast-like cells, to proliferate, and to synthesize a broad spectrum of those ECM components which accumulate during fibrogenesis [3,4]. These cells, which are localized in recessus between adjacent hepatocytes and, thus, have intimate contact with parenchymal liver cells, synthesize the major fractions of collagens [27], proteoglycans [29,30], hyaluronan [31,32], and structural glycoproteins [33,34]. A central question in the pathogenesis of liver fibrosis is related to the mechanism of fat storing cell activation leading to the transformed counterpart of these cells. Paracrine stimulation by activated liver macrophages, invaded monocytes, and degranulated thrombocytes leading to liberation of TGF-β, TGF-α, platelet-derived growth factor (PDGF), fibroblast growth factor (FGF), and others is probably of great importance. It is supposed that TGF-β is the most important fibrogenic mediator due to its multiple actions on the production of various connective tissue molecules in myofibroblast-like cells (Fig. 10). Furthermore, TGF-β suppresses the expression of collagenase and enhances the synthesis of TIMP (tissue inhibitor of metalloproteinases), which reduces the breakdown of newly synthesized and deposited matrix molecules. Although fat storing cells interact extensively with other adjacent

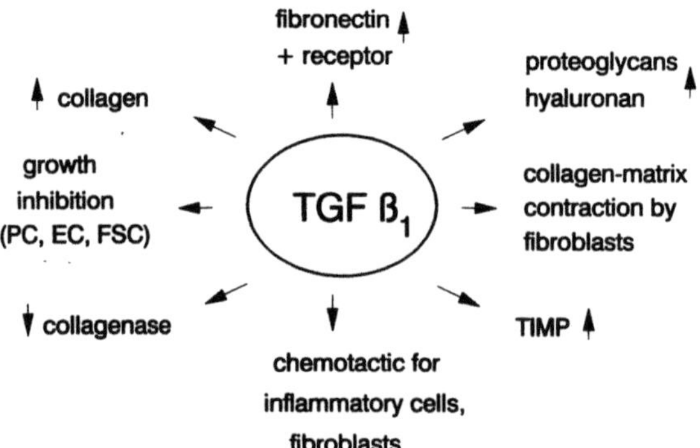

Fig. 10. Multiple functions of TGF-β in fibrogenesis. *PC*, parenchymal liver cells: *EC*, endothelial cells; *FSC*, fat storing cells; *TIMP*, tissue inhibitor of metalloproteinases

Table 2. Modes of hepatocyte-fat storing cell interactions

Soluble mediators
    Production of TGF-α by proliferating hepatocytes
    Scavenging of growth factors (PDGF, TGF-β) by secretion of α_2-macroglobulin
    Conversion of profibrogenic ethanol to fibrogenic acetaldehyde
    Ethanol-induced lipid peroxidation
    Secretion of an inhibitor of proliferation of transformed fat storing cells
Membrane contact
    Hepatocyte cell surface proteoheparan sulfate contact inhibition (?)
    Direct junctional transfer of substances

nonparenchymal cells, recent data also suggest important communications between hepatocytes and fat storing cells (Table 2). Conditioned media from monolayers of hepatocytes isolated from liver remnants 3 and 4 days after partial resection (Hep X) stimulated [³H]thymidine incorporation into DNA of fat storing cells kept in 0.5% fetal calf serum in a dose-dependent manner. Maximum stimulation of 87% was reached at a 1:2 dilution of conditioned medium from liver cells 4 days after Hep X. Similarly, the DNA content per well increased also (Fig. 11). Conditioned medium from normal liver cells and cells 1 day after Hep X did not significantly affect the DNA content and [³H]thymidine incorporation rate of fat storing cells. Medium from normal hepatocytes in 10% fetal calf serum added to proliferating fat storing cells in 10% fetal calf serum did not affect the DNA content or [³H]thymidine incorporation, ruling out any soluble proliferation inhibitor secreted by liver cells. The synthesis of medium proteoglycans by fat storing cells (kBq/mg DNA) was enhanced by a maximum of about 45% if conditioned media from regenerating and normal hepatocytes were added to fat storing cells in 0.5% fetal calf serum. This effect was mainly due to a strong increase of chondroitin

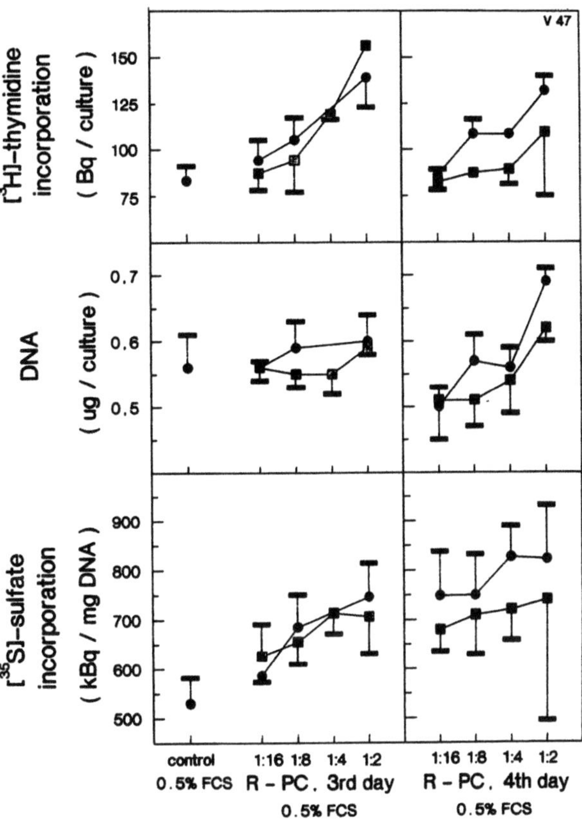

Fig. 11. Effect of various dilutions of conditioned media from regenerating hepatocytes (*R-PC*) isolated 3 and 4 days after partial liver resection on the proliferation ([³H]thymidine incorporation), DNA content per well, and glycosaminoglycan synthesis ([³⁵S] sulfate incorporation) of fat storing cells cultured under reduced fetal calf serum (*FCS*) conditions (0.5%). Control cultures received only 0.5% fetal calf serum

sulfate accompanied by a relative decrease of dermatan sulfate. Heparan sulfate remained essentially unchanged [35]. Qualitatively similar results were obtained with fat storing cells cocultured with normal and regenerating hepatocytes (not shown). The proliferation stimulatory effect of hepatocytes from regenerating liver might be at least partially due to TGF-α synthesized and secreted by proliferating parenchymal cells [21]. In a radioligand assay conditioned medium from regenerating hepatocytes competitively inhibited the binding of ^{125}I-labeled TGF-α to the TGF-α/EGF receptor of hepatocytes. It is concluded that conditioned medium from regenerating parenchymal cells (4 and 5 days after Hep X) but not from normal parenchymal cells stimulates the proliferation of fat storing cells due to TGF-α. Parenchymal cells do not secrete an inhibitor of fat storing cell proliferation. Both normal and regenerating parenchymal cells secrete a factor stimulating production and secretion of proteoglycans, in particular of chondroitin sulfate in fat storing cells [35]. Using a different experimental design, in which transformed fat storing cells which had first been cocultured with Kupffer cells were exposed in secondary culture to conditioned media from normal hepatocytes or were cocultured with hepatocytes, a strong inhibitory effect of liver cells on the multiplication of myofibroblast-like cells was demonstrated [36]. The effective factor has not yet been characterized but it might be a protein not identical with TGF-β. Preliminary studies in this laboratory have shown that fat storing cells cocultured with Kupffer cells render the former cells susceptible to proliferation inhibitory factor(s) secreted by parenchymal liver cells. Although the mechanism of inhibition is not yet known, we put forward the following hypothesis: Kupffer cells stimulate the expression of PDGF receptors on (transforming) fat storing cells [37]. Since it is known that the transformed (but not the original) fat storing cells are strongly stimulated by PDGF [38], α_2-macroglobulin secreted by parenchymal liver cells might act as a scavenger for PDGF [39] present in fetal calf serum and, thus, might inactivate this potent mitogenic stimulus. The hypothesis demonstrates a potential sequence of cellular interactions between stromal and epithelial liver cells which could be relevant for the pathogenesis of fibrosis. Injured parenchymal liver cells are unable to secrete α_2-macroglobulin and thus enhance passively the stimulatory potential of some Kupffer cell fibrogenic factors such as PDGF.

Another mode of potentially important epithelial-stromal cell interactions is realized by hepatocytes metabolizing some profibrogenic xenobiotics to fibrogenic substances, which activate the transformation of fat storing cells towards myofibroblast-like cells (Table 2). An example of this pathway is given by the metabolism of ethanol, which by itself is not fibrogenic [40–42]. Its oxidation product acetaldehyde (and lactate), however, generated in hepatocytes stimulates efficiently the synthesis of certain collagens and the proliferation of (transformed) fat storing cells (and fibroblasts) [41–45], although proteoglycan metabolism remains essentially unaffected [40]. Furthermore, ethanol-induced lipid peroxidation also stimulates collagen gene expression [46–48]. These observations made with cell culture studies suggest a specific fibrogenic effect of alcohol (metabolites) in the pathogenesis of alcohol-related liver diseases [49]. Recent comparative measurements of the serum levels of the NH_2-terminal propeptide of type III procollagen and laminin in patients with alcoholic and matched nonalcoholic liver cirrhosis support circumstantially this hypothesis [50]. Additional studies are required to see whether other xenobiotics might be activated also to fibrogenic factors.

Fat storing cells and hepatocytes might cooperate also via direct cell-cell contact (Table 2). Pericellular matrix components and other cell surface-associated binding sites on fat storing cells and parenchymal liver cells, e.g., fibronectin, laminin, type IV collagen, proteoheparan sulfate, and nidogen, are potential candidates which mediate intercellular communication between both cell types. In particular, cell surface-associated proteoheparan sulfate of hepatocytes might be important for regulating proliferation of fat storing cells, since heparin, synthetic heparin-oligosaccharides, and proteoheparan sulfate have been shown to inhibit proliferation of smooth muscle cells and other cell types (fibroblasts, some tumor cell lines). Thus, liver cell membrane associated proteoheparan sulfate might be an important physiologic regulator of the mitotic activity of fat storing cells in normal liver. Injured hepatocytes, which do not synthesize pericellular heparan sulfate, are unable to exert contact inhibition of fat storing cells, which then are susceptible to certain growth factors secreted by resident and invaded inflammatory cells. Following this concept, the interruption or abrogation of the membrane contact between hepatocytes and fat storing cells is the initiating event of the activation of fat storing cells, the central process of liver fibrogenesis. Experiments are underway to clarify this kind of communication between epithelial and stromal liver cells.

Matrix-Hepatocyte Interaction

Hepatocytes in vivo are surrounded by a framework of connective tissue to which the hepatocytes are probably anchored by specific receptors. Complex ECM and its individual components are used as culture substrata to improve the attachment and survival of cultured hepatocytes. Better maintenance of differentiated functions are known to be achieved by monolayer cells cultured on a defined matrix instead of pure plastic surfaces [51]. Sustained expression of liver-specific metabolic pathways by hepatocytes in culture is obtained when the cells are grown on a basement membrane-like matrix [52]. Individual components of the matrix cannot substitute for the complex. The induction of albumin gene transcription [53,54], albumin secretion [52,55], and replicative DNA synthesis [52] are strongly affected by collagen culture substrata. The finding that ECM affects the basal rate of DNA synthesis in hepatocytes raises the possibility that it may modulate also the response to mitogens, e.g., EGF and TGF-α, as is seen with mammary epithelial cells grown within collagen gel matrices [56] and with fibroblasts [57]. It is supposed that the mitogenic response of hepatocytes to EGF is strongly reduced if the cells are cultured on Matrigel, an Engelbreth-Holm-Swarm (EHS) tumor matrix [52]. Proteoglycans have significant effects in maintaining high albumin production of adult rat hepatocytes in vitro [58]. A number of ECM receptors or binding sites have been defined [59–62], but the signal transduction pathway between ECM components and gene activation is not clearly established. Hepatocyte-matrix interactions have potential clinical implications not only for the development of liver fibrosis but also for the control of liver regeneration and the perturbation of hepatocellular functions in fibrosis, in which the proximate matrix of the hepatocyte is greatly changed. Furthermore, epithelial-stromal interactions are also important in the pathobiology of primary hepatocellular carcinoma, known to be associated with qualitatively and quantitatively changed ECM [63]. Hepatocellular dysfunction in acute inflammation might be partially caused by disruption of this matrix and alteration of its interaction with the hepatocyte plasma membrane. Future studies on the effects of ECM (components) on hepatocytes (and other types of liver cells) are likely to be among the most important for understanding the regulation of differentiation in liver.

Summary and Conclusion

Recent data suggest strong cooperation between mesenchymal cell types and hepatocytes during the various phases of hepatic fibrogenesis (Fig. 12) [64]. A complex network of cytokines involving TGF-β, TGF-α/EGF, PDGF, FGF, and probably other cytokines regulates parenchymal cell replication, matrix biosynthesis, and the inflammatory response. Their is ample evidence that the response of a target cell to external factors is greatly influenced by the ECM surrounding the cell and by microenvironmental factors, e.g., local oxygen tension, hormone gradients and scavenger proteins neutralizing the effects of some bioactive molecules. Many of these interrelations concern fibrotic reactions in general, i.e., they are important in Dupuytren's disease, nonhepatic fibrotic lesions, and atherosclerosis. Experimental techniques have to be developed which allow study of in vitro communication of cells. Instead of monocultures, cocultures with two or even three cell types are needed which provide the possibility of a bidirectional interaction of the cell types under study. Conditioned media harvested from one cell type and exposed to another cell type allows only unidirectional signal transfer and, thus, are not optimum for studying cell interactions. A further problem concerns the ratio of cocultured cell types. It is known that in fibrotic reactions the pattern of cell types changes time dependently. For example, in liver the number of stromal cells increases steadily whereas that of parenchymal cells decreases. Consequently, the concentration of cytokines elaborated by the specific cell types will change strongly and induce different dose-dependent effects. Furthermore, expression of the receptors for specific growth factors are up- and down-regulated by other factors, changing the responsiveness of a certain target cell type (e.g., TGF-β stimulates the expression of TGF-β and PDGF receptors). Another type of interaction concerns the activation and inactivation of growth factors in the extracellular space. This process might be even more important for the pathogenesis of fibrosis than mere expression and secretion of biologically inactive/latent factors. Taken together, although valuable insights into the pathogenesis and uniformity of fibrotic tissue reactions were obtained in recent years, the highly complicated cascade of interacting cell types and molecular mediators requires innovative experimental designs which provide better models of the in situ interrelationship than conventional techniques used presently.

References

1. Peacock EE (ed) (1984) Wound repair, 3rd edn. Saunders, Philadelphia
2. Barbul A, Pines E, Caldwell M, Hunt TK (eds) Growth Factors and other aspects of wound healing. Prog Clin Biol Res 266

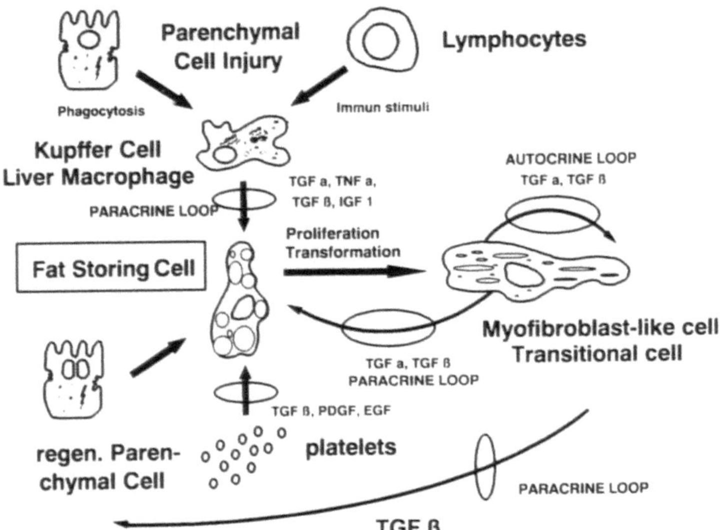

Fig. 12. Simplified model of the two-step activation process of fat storing cells in injured liver involving, first, paracrine activation by cytokines from activated macrophages/Kupffer cells, degranulated platelets, and regenerating hepatocytes and, second, autocrine stimulation by transformed fat storing cells (myofibroblast-like cells). The latter cell type exerts negative feedback control of parenchymal cell regeneration by secretion of TGF-β

3. Gressner AM, Bachem MG (1989) Mechanismen der Fibrogenese bei chronischer Leberentzündung. Z Klin Med 44:377–385
4. Gressner AM (1991) Liver fibrosis. Perspectives in pathobiochemical research and clinical outlook. Eur J Clin Chem Clin Biochem 29:293–311
5. Gressner AM, Bachem MG (1990) Cellular sources of noncollagenous matrix proteins: role of fat-storing cells in fibrogenesis. Semin Liver Dis 10:30–46
6. Nathan CF (1987) Secretory products of macrophages. J Clin Invest 79:319–326
7. Decker K (1990) Biologically active products of stimulated liver macrophages (Kupffer cells). Eur J Biochem 192:245–261
8. Shiratori Y, Kawase T, Shiina S, Okano K, Sugimoto T, Teraoka H, Matano S, Matsumoto K, Kamii K (1988) Modulation of hepatotoxicity by macrophages in the liver. Hepatology 8:815–821
9. Shiratori Y, Tanaka M, Umihara J, Kawase T, Shiina S, Sugimoto T (1990) Leukotriene inhibitors modulate hepatic injury induced by lipopolysaccharide-activated macrophages. J Hepatol 10:51–61
10. Gresser I, Woodrow D, Moss J et al. (1987) Toxic effects of recombinant tumor necrosis factor in suckling mice. Comparisons with interferon a/b. Am J Pathol 128:13–18
11. Lehmann V, Freudenberg MA, Galanos C (1987) Lethal toxicity of lipopolysaccharide and tumor necrosis factor in normal and D-galactosamine-treated mice. J Exp Med 165:657–663
12. McClain CJ, Cohen DA (1989) Increased tumor necrosis factor production by monocytes in alcoholic hepatitis. Hepatology 9:349–351
13. Tanner A, Keyhani A, Reiner R et al. (1981) Proteolytic enzymes released by liver macrophages may promote hepatic injury in a rat model of hepatic damage. Gastroenterology 80:647–654
14. Perez HD, Roll FJ, Bissell DM, Shak S, Goldstein IM (1984) Production of chemotactic activity for polymorphonuclear leukocytes by cultured rat hepatocytes exposed to ethanol. J Clin Invest 74:1350–1357

15. Roll FJ, Bissell DM, Perez HD (1986) Human hepatocytes metabolizing ethanol generate a non-polar chemotactic factor for human neutrophils. Biochem Biophys Res Commun 137:688–694

16. Le J, Vilcek J (1989) Interleukin 6: a multifunctional cytokine regulating immune reactions and the acute phase protein response. Lab Invest 61:588–602

17. Heinrich PC, Castell JV, Andus T (1990) Interleukin-6 and the acute phase response. Biochem J 265:621–636

18. van Snick J (1990) Interleukin-6: an overview. Annu Rev Immunol 8:253–278

19. Michalopoulos GK (1990) Liver regeneration: molecular mechanisms of growth control. FASEB J 4:176–187

20. Fausto N, Mead JE (1989) Biology of disease. Regulation of liver growth: protooncogenes and transforming growth factors. Lab Invest 60:4–13

21. Mead JE, Fausto N (1989) Transforming growth factor α may be a physiological regulator of liver regeneration by means of an autocrine mechanism. Proc Natl Acad Sci USA 86:1558–1562

22. Braun L, Mead JE, Panzica M, Mikumo R, Bell GI, Fausto N (1988) Transforming growth factor β mRNA increases during liver regeneration: a possible paracrine mechanism of growth regulation. Proc Natl Acad Sci USA 85:1539–1543

23. Gruppuso PA, Mead JE, Fausto N (1990) Transforming growth factor receptors in liver regeneration following partial hepatectomy in the rat. Cancer Res 50:1464–1469

24. Meyer DH, Bachem MG, Gressner AM (1990) Modulation of hepatic lipocyte proteoglycan synthesis and proliferation by Kupffer cell-derived transforming growth factors type β1 and type α. Bioochem Biophys Res Commun 171:1122–1129

25. Meyer DH, Bachem MG, Gressner AM (1990) Transformed fat storing cells inhibit the proliferation of cultured hepatocytes by secretion of transforming growth factor beta. J Hepatol 11:86–91

26. Katsumoto F, Miyazaki K, Nakayama F (1989) Stimulation of DNA synthesis in hepatocytes by Kupffer cells after partial hepatectomy. Hepatology 9:405–410

27. Friedman SL (1990) Cellular sources of collagen and regulation of collagen production in liver. Semin Liver Dis 10:20–29

28. Gressner AM, Schäfer S (1989) Comparison of sulphated glycosaminoglycans and hyaluronate synthesis and secretion in cultured hepatocytes, fat storing cells, and Kupffer cells. J Clin Chem Clin Biochem 27:141–149

29. Schäfer S, Zerbe O, Gressner AM (1987) The synthesis of proteoglycans in fat-storing cells of rat liver. Hepatology 7:680–687

30. Arenson DM, Friedman SL, Bissell DM (1988) Formation of extracellular matrix in normal rat liver: lipocytes as a major source of proteoglycan. Gastroenterology 95:441–447

31. Gressner AM, Haarmann R (1988) Hyaluronic acid synthesis and secretion by rat liver fat storing cells (perisinusoidal lipocytes) in culture. Biochem Biophys Res Commun 151:222–229

32. Gressner AM, Haarmann R (1988) Regulation of hyaluronate synthesis in rat liver fat storing cell cultures by Kupffer cells. J Hepatol 7:310–318

33. Ramadori G, Rieder H, Knittel T, Dienes HP, Meyer zum Büschenfelde KH (1987) Fat storing cells (FSC) of rat liver synthesize and secrete fibronectin.Comparison with hepatocytes. J Hepatol 4:190–197

34. Maher JJ, Friedman SL, Roll FJ, Bissell DM (1988) Immunolocalization of laminin in normal rat liver and biosynthesis of laminin by hepatic lipocytes in primary culture. Gastroenterology 94:1053–1062

35. Gressner AM (1989) Effects of conditioned media from normal and regenerating hepatocytes on proliferation and proteoglycan synthesis of rat liver fat storing cells in culture. Biol Chem Hoppe Seyler 370:902–903

36. Chen W, Steffan AM, Braunwald J, Nonnenmacher H, Kirn A, Gendrault JL (1990) Inhibition of fat-storing cell multiplication by a factor produced by normal cultured murine hepatocytes. J Hepatol 11:330–338

37. Friedman SL, Arthur MJP (1989) Activation of cultured rat hepatic lipocytes by Kupffer cell conditioned medium. J Clin Invest 84:1780–1785

38. Pinzani M, Gesualdo L, Sabbah GM, Abboud HE (1989) Effects of platelet-derived growth factor and other polypeptide mitogens on DNA synthesis and growth of cultured rat liver fat-storing cells. J Clin Invest 84:1786–1793

39. Ross R, Raines EW, Bowen-Pope DF (1986) The biology of platelet-derived growth factor. Cell 46:155–169

40. Gressner AM, Althaus M (1988) Effects of ethanol, acetaldehyde, and lactate on proteoglycan synthesis and proliferation of cultured rat liver fat-storing cells. Gastroenterology 94:797–807

41. Savolainen ER, Leo MA, Timpl R, Lieber CS (1984) Acetaldehyde and lactate stimulate collagen synthesis of cultured baboon liver myofibroblasts. Gastroenterology 87:777–787

42. Holt K, Bennett M, Chojkier M (1984) Acetaldehyde stimulates collagen and noncollagen protein production by human fibroblasts. Hepatology 4:843–848

43. Shiratori Y, Ichida T, Kawase T, Wisse E (1986) Effect of acetaldehyde on collagen synthesis by fat-storing cells isolated from rats treated with carbon tetrachloride. Liver 6:246–251

44. Moshage H, Casini A, Lieber CS (1990) Acetaldehyde selectively stimulates collagen production in cultured rat liver fat storing cells but not in hepatocytes. Hepatology 12:511–518

45. Brenner DA, Chojkier M (1987) Acetaldehyde increases collagen gene transcription in cultured human fibroblasts. J Biol Chem 262:17690–17695

46. Chojkier M, Solis-Herruzo JA, Brenner DA (1988) Lipid peroxidation stimulates collagen gene expression. A common pathway for fibrogenesis? (Abstr). Gastroenterology 94:A529

47. Yamada S, Yamada M, Murawaki Y, Hirayama C (1990) Increase in lipoperoxides and prolyl hydroxylase activity in rat liver following chronic ethanol feeding. Biochem Pharmacol 40:1015–1019

48. Neuschwander-Tetri BA (1990) Acetaldehyde mediates ethanol-induced lipid peroxidation in cultured rat hepatocytes (Abstr). Hepatology 12:933

49. Friedman SL (1990) Acetaldehyde and alcoholic fibrogenesis: fuel to the fire, but not the spark. Hepatology 12:609–612

50. Lotterer E, Gressner AM, Kropf J, Bircher J (1990) Alkoholtoxische Leberzirrhose: Gibt es einen spezifisch fibrogenetischen Effekt? (Abstr). Z. Gastroenterol 27:709–710

51. Reid LM, Narita M, Fujita M, Murray Z, Liverpool C, Rosenberg L (1986) Matrix and hormonal regulation of differentiation in liver cultures. In: Guillouzo A, Guguen-Guillouzo C (eds) Research in isolated and cultured hepatocytes. Libbey, London, INSERM, Paris, pp 225–258

52. Bissell DM, Choun MO (1988) The role of extracellular matrix in normal liver. Scand J Gastroenterol 23 Suppl 151:1–7

53. Bissell DM, Caron JM, Babiss LE, Friedman JM (1990) Transcriptional regulation of the albumin gene in cultured rat hepatocytes – role of basement membrane matrix. Mol Biol Med 7:187

54. Caron JM (1990) Induction of albumin gene transcription in hepatocytes by extracellular matrix proteins. Mol Cell Biol 10:1239–1243

55. Bissell DM, Arenson DM, Maher JJ, Roll FJ (1987) Support of cultured hepatocytes by a laminin-rich gel. J Clin Invest 79:801–812

56. Takahashi K, Suzuki K, Ono T (1990) Loss of growth inhibitory activity of TGFβ toward normal human mammary epithelial cells grown within collagen gel matrix. Biochem Biophys Res Commun 173:1239–1247

57. Colige A, Nusgens B, Lapiere CM (1990) Response to epidermal growth factor of skin fibroblasts from donors of varying age is modulated by the extracellular matrix. J Cell Physiol 145:450–457

58. Koide N, Shinji T, Tanabe T, Asano K, Kawaguchi M, Sakaguchi K, Koide Y, Mori M, Tsuji T (1989) Continued high albumin production by multicellular spheroids of adult rat hepatocytes formed in the presence of liver-derived proteoglycans. Biochem Biophys Res Commun 161:385–391

59. Bissell DM, Stamatoglou SC, Nermut MV, Hughes RC (1986) Interactions of rat hepatocytes with type IV collagen, fibronectin and laminin matrices. Distinct matrix-controlled modes of attachment and spreading. Eur J Cell Biol 40:72–78

60. Clement B, Yamada Y (1990) A M$_r$ 80K hepatocyte surface protein(s) interacts with basement membrane components. Exp Cell Res 187:320–323
61. Forsberg E, Paulsson M, Timpl R, Johansson S (1990) Characterization of a laminin receptor on rat hepatocytes. J Biol Chem 265:6376–6361
62. Clement B, Segui-Real B, Savagner P, Kleinman HK, Yamada Y (1990) Hepatocyte attachment of laminin is mediated through multiple receptors. J Cell Physiol 110:185–192
63. Donato MF, Colombo M, Matarazzo M, Paronetto F (1989) Distribution of basement membrane components in human hepatocellular carcinoma. Cancer 63:272–279
64. Gressner AM (1991) Major topics of fibrosis research: 1990 update. In: Wisse E, Knook DL, McCuskey RS (eds) Cells of the hepatic sinusoid, vol 3, pp 136–144

Proteoglycan – Collagen Fibril Interactions in Tissues

J.E. Scott

In the process of evolution, central physiological functions (neural, circulatory, etc.) have acquired defined anatomical locations, with the corollary that tissue/organ shape is maintained against internal and external stresses. The supporting framework, the connective tissues, are constructed of fibre-reinforced composite materials, in which the fibrils, mainly collagen, resist pulling forces and the interfibrillar spaces contain soluble polymers, characteristically proteoglycans (PGs), that keep the fibrils apart. Until recently there was little information on how the two components interacted together or if interactions were fundamentally similar in the enormous variety of connective tissues in all species. Answers to these questions are now possible as a result of ultrastructural work on tissues involving electron histochemistry accompanied by a new understanding of the secondary and tertiary structures in solution of the glycan side chains of the PGs.

Proteoglycan Binding Sites on Collagen Fibrils

It has long been thought that PGs interacted in different ways with different collagens in solution, and early attempts to localise PGs in tissues suggested that there might be specific association with collagen fibrils (reviewed by Scott 1988). However, unequivocal demonstrations of specific binding sites depended on the use of the dyes Cuprolinic or Cupromeronic blue (Scott 1980; Scott and Orford 1981), in "critical electrolyte concentration" (CEC) methods, to stain PGs. After counterstaining with UO_2^{2+} to show the collagen fibril banding pattern (a–e), it was established that sulphated PGs were present at the d and e bands in all the soft mammalian connective tissues so far examined (skin, sclera, corneal stroma, etc.) (Scott 1991). These interactions were also present in very abnormal tissue (dermatosparactic calf skin; Scott et al. 1989) and in liver fibrosis (J.E. Scott, T.G. Bosworth, A.M. Cribb, and A. Gressner, unpublished). Wherever a clear banding pattern (a–e) was observable, PG binding at the d or e bands was seen.

Biochemical analysis and specific enzyme digestions proved these PGs to be the small PGs, containing dermatan sulphate (DS) as the glycan chain(s). Intervertebral disc showed similar interactions at the d band, where the PG

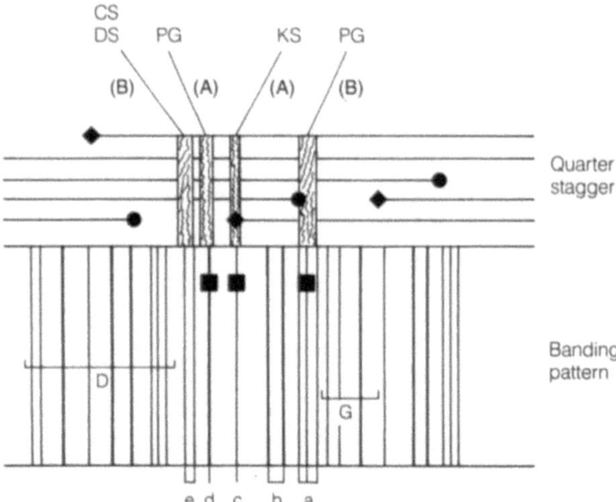

Fig. 1. Map embodying the hypothesis of one proteoglycan (*PG*): one binding site. Binding sites of chondroitin sulphate (*CS*), *dermatan sulphate* (*DS*) and *keratan sulphate* (*KS*) small PGs are shown against the quarter-staggered array of collagen molecules (*upper half*) and a–e banding pattern of stained collagen fibrils (*lower half*). ◆, NH$_2$-terminal; ●, COOH-terminal; *D*, D period (about 65 nm); *G*, gap zone; ■, major sites of glycosylation, which are also sites of cross linking in the a and c bands. (From Scott 1991)

glycan is chondroitin sulphate (CS). These PGs have a globular protein head, with a DS tail, giving rise to the name "tadpole" PGs (Scott 1988). Other members of this PG class, containing keratan sulphate (KS), are found in quantity in corneal stroma but almost nowhere else. These PGs also associate with collagen fibrils at specific binding sites, in this case at the a and c bands. Only in corneal stroma are these bands seen to be occupied. The frequency of occupation varies dramatically from species to species, being almost zero in very small animals (mouse, frog) to over 50% in large animals (cow, human etc). By contrast, DS PGs were present in large amounts at the d and e bands in all corneas so far examined.

There are thus tissue and species specificities in the incidence and frequency of these interactions. CEC techniques using Cupromeronic blue established that the PGs at the different bands were different, giving rise to the hypothesis of one binding site, one PG (Scott and Haigh 1988) (Fig. 1).

Available evidence suggests that binding is via the PG protein core to the collagen fibril (Scott 1988), but there is little hard chemical evidence on the primary structures of the binding sites, either on the PG or the collagen. However, the situation is unique in that there are two binding sites per fibril D period for both the DS PGs and KS PGs. Since the structures of the pair of KS PG protein cores must be very similar, it was assumed that the two KS PG binding sites on the collagen fibril would also be similar. A search for homologous amino acid sequences, one in the a and the other in the c band, revealed that a nine amino acid stretch (Hyl-Gly-His-Arg-Gly-Phe-Ser-Gly-

Leu) in the two α1 chains, at residues 87–96 in the a band, was indeed repeated in the right place (residues 930–938 in the c band) and nowhere else. The match in the α2 chains was almost as good, and out of 27 relevant amino acids on the three adjacent chains, 26 were identical. The less than perfect homology is important, since if both homologies were identical, it would be expected that a/c band occupancies should also be identical, and this is not the case (Scott and Haigh 1988). It is particularly interesting that this region is the cross-linking zone, and the presence of PG at this point may help to control chemical stabilisation of the fibril.

Similar logic applied to the DS PGs produced an 11 amino acid sequence (Gly-Asp-Arg-Gly-Glu-Thr-Gly-Pro-Ala-Gly-Pro) in the two α1 chains in the d band (residues 886–896) that repeated in the e band in several closely similar variants (e.g., residues 856–866).

These sequences were absent from all proteins that were not fibril-forming collagens (J.E. Scott and R.W. Glanville 1992). Although these findings do not prove that the sequences are binding sites, it would be a striking coincidence if they were not.

These interactions are with the surface of the fibril. In some tissues, particularly those with thick fibrils, and in the mutable connective tissues of echinoderms, there are *intra*-fibrillar PGs, with the glycan chains oriented along the axis of the fibril. It was suggested that these PGs were associated with subfibrillar modules (the protofibrils), which were seen in dissociating or frayed collagen fibrils (Scott 1991).

The regular specific binding of PGs to fibril surfaces endows the interfibrillar space with a degree of order that was previously unsuspected. The "amorphous ground substance" is clearly not amorphous. It now appears that there are further levels of sophistication involving the glycan chains.

Ordered Structures of the Glycosaminoglycans in Solution

The consensus attributed random coil structures to the solution form of hyaluronan (HA) (Laurent 1989), and only X-ray fibre diffraction indicated *possible* solid phase (but not solution) secondary and tertiary structures. The first unequivocal evidence for secondary structures in solution came from periodate oxidation kinetics, which produced a model (Scott and Tigwell 1978) that was later confirmed by computer simulation. Subsequent nuclear magnetic resonance (NMR) studies established the full secondary structures of HA and chondroitin-4-sulphate (CS4) in solution (reviewed in Scott 1989). In HA, each tetrasaccharide unit in the polymer may have four H-bonds and a water bridge in the form of a twofold helix.

The space filling mdoel of this secondary structure showed a remarkably large hydrophobic patch, of about eight C–H groups spread over three sugar units, repeated on both sides of the flat tape-like polymer. Each face of the tape was identical, giving rise to the term "ambidexteran," i.e., able to perform equally well with both hands (Scott 1992a). So large a hydrophobic patch suggested that HA might self-aggregate, driven by hydrophobic bonding. Rotary shadowing and electron microscopy showed that HA indeed formed essentially infinite meshworks, even in dilute solution, and computer dynamics gave insight into possible mechanisms of aggregation (Scott et al. 1991). Hydrogen bonds and hydrophobic bonding stabilise duplexes and higher aggregates, and electrostatic repulsion hinders aggregation.

Applying this analysis to the other glycosaminoglycans (GAGs) revealed that aggregation was possible, particularly chondroitin-6-sulphate (CS6) and undersulphated KS. Electrostatic repulsion increases with the addition of sulphate ester to the twofold helix, but this effect is much greater in CS4, where the anionic sulphate esters are in the polymer midline, than in CS6, where they are at the edges of the polymer, as far apart as possible (Scott 1992a). Not only was homoaggregation possible, but so was heteroaggregation between, e.g., HA and CS, or undersulphated CS and KS (Scott et al. 1992).

It has been known for some time that DS chains could aggregate in aqueous solutions, with the glucuronic:iduronic ratio playing an important role in deciding the strength of the interactions (Fransson et al. 1979).

Given that GAGs can participate in secondary, tertiary and quaternary structures in solution, is this of ultrastructural significance in the tissue?

Glycosaminoglycans as Tissue Organisers

Most techniques that diagnose secondary and higher order structures in solution (NMR, etc.) are not yet usable on tissues. It follows, however, that tertiary structures must be of a larger size than single molecules. Isolated and purified PGs stained with Cupromeronic blue appeared only slightly longer than expected from rotary shadowing or biophysical measurements on the unstained molecules. However, PGs stained in corneal stroma were sometimes over twice as long as stained isolated PGs, and this was interpreted to mean that aggregated forms were present in tissues (Scott 1992a). It was clear from electron micrographs that PG glycans were bridging two or more collagen fibrils, tangentially. The interfibrillar distance is constant at about 66 nm in the corneal stroma of many species, and this is also the length of a DS chain of the corneal DS PG (Scott 1992a). Assuming that PG protein cores were attached to collagen fibrils, a scheme was produced incorporating these observations (Fig. 2), in which the DS chains duplexed (or formed higher aggregates) in antiparallel arrays, joining the collagen fibrils from d/e band to d/e band, i.e., in register. It was proposed that the interfibrillar distance was determined by the GAG length, which acted as a yardstick, being shorter in those tissues in which collagen fibrils were closer together (Scott 1992a). The yardstick function keeps the fibrils in corneal stroma in a highly ordered array, which is essential for transparency.

Direct evidence that the dumbbell forms postulated in Fig. 2 actually occur and are stable came from rotary shadowing electron microscopy of DS PG solutions (Ward et al. 1987).

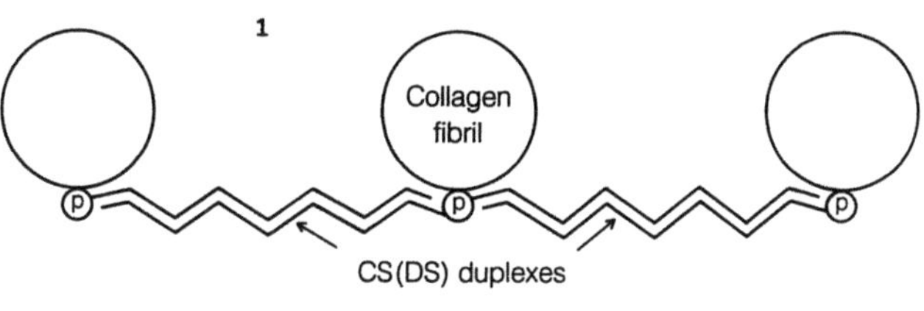

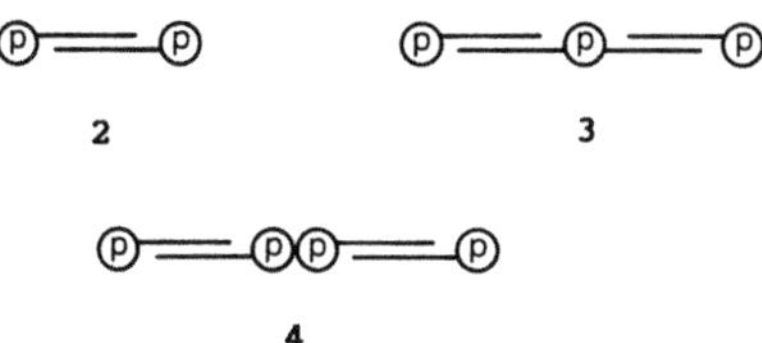

Fig. 2. Scheme (*1*) of DS (CS) proteoglycan (PG): collagen interactions in connective tissues, incorporating glycan duplexes or aggregates. *P*, protein core of PG. Structures like these have been seen in Cupromeronic blue-stained tissues (Scott 1992a). Small PGs have one or two glycan chains that could aggregate in ways shown in *2–4*. Some of these structures have been observed in electron micrographs of rotary shadowed DS PG solution. (Ward et al. 1987)

The bridge and tie motifs observed in corneal stroma have been seen in many other connective tissues and must be regarded as one of the most common PG:collagen interactions, in which pairs of PGs and collagen fibrils associate together in a quaternary structure.

The significance of the design of the tadpole PGs thus emerges. They are bifunctional cross-linking molecules, PG protein associating with collagen protein and glycans with glycans.

A similar structure, in which type II collagen fibrils in vitreous humor are tied together in regular bundles by GAGs (probably CS6 and/or undersulphated CS4) at regular intervals of about 60 nm along the fibrils, like the rungs in a ladder, may make use of type IX collagen instead of a tadpole PG. This collagen has an attached GAG chain which is of a kind able to duplex and bridge the gaps between fibrils in a regular way but at concentrations of collagen and GAG about 50 times lower than those in the otherwise analogous quaternary structures in the corneal stroma (Scott 1992b). The principles are the same, a protein-protein (i.e., collagen type II-collagen type IX) interaction anchors the associated GAG, which then aggregates to a similarly anchored GAG on a neighbouring fibril forming a bridge and a tie.

Glycosaminoglycans as Shock Absorbers

In the corneal stroma CS and KS were shown to swell, keeping the fibrils apart (Hedbys 1961). This is the postulated function of the three-dimensional arrays of GAG bridges and ties, in which swelling pressure derives from their osmotic pressure and that of their counterions. Intervertebral disc showed another type of GAG structure, consisting of rings resembling motor car tyres, encircling the fibril (Scott and Haigh 1986). These rings were independent of each other but were at the d band, separated by a D period. Following the car tyre analogy, it seemed that these structures might keep the fibrils apart by physically intervening rather than by spacing the fibrils, as the bridges and ties are postulated to do.

Proteoglycans as Regulators of Collagen Fibril Diameter

Collagen fibrils are of very different diameters in different tissues and at different ages. The mechanisms that control these diameters have been the subject of much controversy in the past few decades. One factor, which correlates well with observations in developing tissues, may be the presence of interfibrillar PG glycans, which hold the fibrils apart and prevent them from fusing (Scott and Parry 1992).

Conclusion

The polymers of connective tissues are characteristically very large, with thousands of amino acids and hundreds or thousands of sugars. There are almost infinite possibilities for interactions between them. It would speculate that there are already more interactions postulated in the literature than actually exist in the tissues, and that the tissues rely on certain simple structures, held together by the interactions described above, which appear in the majority of connective tissues.

References

Fransson L-A, Nieduszynski I, Phelps C, Sheehan JK (1979) Interactions between dermatan sulphate chains. III. Light-scattering and viscometry studies of self-association. Biochim Biophys Acta 586:179–188

Hedbys BO (1961) The role of polysaccharides in corneal swelling. Exp Eye Res 1:81–91

Laurent TC (1989) Ciba Found Symp 143:1–5

Scott JE (1980) Localisation of proteoglycans in tendon by electron microscopy. Biochem J 187:887–891

Scott JE (1988) Proteoglycan-fibrillar collagen interactions. Biochem J 252:313–323

Scott JE (1989) Secondary structures in hyaluronan solutions: chemical and biological implications. Ciba Found Symp 143:6–20

Scott JE (1991) Proteoglycan:collagen interactions in connective tissues. Ultrastructural, biochemical, functional and evolutionary aspects. Int J Biol Macromol 13:157–161

Scott JE (1992a) Supramolecular organisation of extracellular matrix glycosaminoglycans, in vitro and in the tissues. FASEB J 6:2639–2645

Scott JE (1992b) The chemical morphology of the vitreous. Eye 6:553–555

Scott JE, Glanville RW (1993) Homologous sequences in fibrillar collagens may be proteoglycan binding sites. Biochem Soc Trans 21:123S

Scott JE, Haigh M (1986) Proteoglycan- collagen interactions in intervertebral disc. Chondroitin sulphate proteoglycan associates with collagen fibrils in rabbit annulus fibrosus at the d–e bands. Biosci Rep 6:879–888

Scott JE, Haigh M (1988) Identification of specific binding sites for keratan sulphate proteoglycans and chondroitin-dermatan sulphate proteoglycans on collagen fibrils in cornea by the use of cupromeronic blue in "critical electrolyte concentration" techniques. Biochem J 253:607–610

Scott JE, Orford CR (1981) Dermatan sulphate-rich proteoglycan associates with rat tail-tendon collagen at the d band in the gap region. Biochem J 197:213–216

Scott JE, Parry DAD (1993) Control of collagen fibril diameters in tissues. Int J Macromol 14:292–293

Scott JE, Tigwell MJ (1978) Periodate oxidation and the shapes of glycosaminoglycuronans in solution. Biochem J 173:103–114

Scott JE, Haigh M, Nusgens B, Lapierre CM (1989) Proteoglycan:collagen interactions in dermatosparactic skin and tendon. An electron histochemical study using cupromeronic blue in a critical electrolyte concentration method. Matrix 9:437–442

Scott JE, Cummings C, Chen Y, Brass A (1991) Secondary and tertiary structures of hyaluronan in aqueous solution, investigated by rotary shadowing-electron microscopy and computer simulation. Hyaluronan is a very efficient meshwork-forming polymer. Biochem J 274:699–705

Scott JE, Chen Y, Brass A (1992) Secondary and tertiary structures involving chondroitin and chondroitin sulphates in solution, investigated by rotary shadowing/electron microscopy and computer simulation. Eur J Biochem 209:675–680

Ward NP, Scott JE, Coster L (1987) Dermatan sulphate proteoglycans from sclera examined by rotary shadowing and electron microscopy. Biochem J 242:761–766

Changes in the Biochemical Properties of Diseased Tissue as Pathogenetic Factors in Dupuytren's Contracture

H. Millesi, R. Reihsner, J. Menzel, G. Hamilton, and R. Mallinger

The purpose of this study was to investigate the biomechanical properties of Dupuytren's disease (DD) tissue with special reference to viscoelasticity and to set the result in relation to (a) normal palmar aponeurosis (NPA) and (b) different stages of the disease.

Viscoelastic Properties of Dense Connective Tissue

Ideally, elastic material reacts immediately to any deforming force with a corresponding change of shape and reassumes the original shape as soon as the deforming force stops acting. In reality, however, an elastic material that behaves in this theoretical way does not exist. Especially in living tissues, deformation is always accompanied by a dislocation of internal structures, which occurs against a certain amount of friction and takes some time. Accommodation to a final shape takes place slowly and requires energy. From our preliminary studies, which examined the parameters listed below, we knew that the viscous fraction is low in NPA but significantly increased in tissues obtained from patients with DD. We were not interested in extreme values such as tensile strength, because these values may be influenced strongly by individual factors. We wanted to determine the changes in parameters as expressed in physiological values. We therefore selected strain levels of 2.5%, 5%, 7.5%, and 10%.

Residual Elongation. After the specimens had been elongated to the strain levels mentioned above, they were deloaded, i.e., the strain was reduced. The location where the zero point had again been reached and the length of the residual elongation were then measured. A high residual elongation does not mean that in situ the tissue becomes longer and longer. First, it is quite possible that the residual elongation might spontaneously disappear if one waits long enough. In our study, however, we did not wait. The residual elongation therefore refers to this waiting time. Secondly, before being taken, the specimen is incorporated in the whole tissue complex in situ, where it is exposed not only to longitudinal stress like the isolated specimen after it has been obtained but also to transverse forces which are elicited by longitudinal strain. If the longitudinal strain is removed, these forces pull in a transverse direction and help restore the original situation. Since these forces are moreover subject to the laws of viscoelasticity, the fiber bundles elongated by the longitudinal strain may become shorter than they had originally been if the transverse forces continue to act in a retardant manner (see below).

Hysteresis. In an ideal elastic tissue, the loading and unloading graphs coincide. If the unloading curve differs from the loading graph, a hysteresis loop is formed. The area within the normalized hysteresis loop is a measure of the energy loss during the load cycle.

Relaxation. The specimens are elongated to the strain levels mentioned above. The elongation is kept constant. The stress that is necessary to achieve this elongation decreases as a result of internal structural dislocations. This decrease can be measured as a function of time (time constant tau) or by the normalized difference between the initial and final values of stress (kappa), respectively.

Retardation. In contrast to the relaxation test, the stress is kept constant in the retardation test if the selected strain level is reached. Since structural dislocations induced by stress are slow to develop against friction, elongation continues to progress, even if the stress remains constant. Retardation can also be measured by a time constant (tau) and the normalized difference between the initial and final value of strain (kappa).

Inverse Relaxation. The specimen is loaded to a selected strain level, e.g., 5%; it is then deloaded to a lower level, e.g., 2.5%. The stress required to maintain this strain level increases.

Inverse Retardation. The specimen is loaded to a selected strain level, e.g., 5%; it is then deloaded to a lower level, e.g., 2.5%. If the stress is kept constant at this level, the specimen becomes shorter. In our opinion, this is an important observation, since it demonstrates that under certain conditions, a connective tissue sample can become shorter without interference by external or cellular forces.

Recovery Time. If a first loading and unloading test is followed immediately by a second one, the second test differs significantly from the first because of the lasting effect of the first test. For the second test to result in exactly the same graph as the first, it must be performed after a certain time interval. This interval must elapse in order to allow the dislocated structures resulting from the first test to return to the original configuration. This is the recovery time, which is measured in minutes.

Morphology

We distinguished the following morphologic classes:

Normal Palmar Aponeurosis. In NPA, the individual fiber bundles are well defined and the loose tissue between the bundles is transparent. When illuminated from an oblique angle, fiber bundles in a state of relaxation show a cross striation as an expression of the wavy course. With delicate longitudinal stress, the cross striation disappears because the fiber bundles elongate. The cross striation reappears if the stress is removed.

Apparently Normal Palmar Aponeurosis. In patients with DD, some areas of palmar aponeurosis still present normally, especially at the radial side. Under the light microscope, this tissue does not appear different from NPA tissue; the only actual difference is that ANPA tissue is derived from patients with DD.

Thickend Fiber Bundles. Patients with DD display thickened fiber bundles (THFB) still showing the original bundle structure; the cross striation, however, has disappeared. Apparently, the fiber bundles are already in a relaxed state when the finger is exposed to a certain stress. The light microscope reveals THFB due to increased collagen synthesis. This is the result of the activity of the *local* fibroblasts, because at this stage there is no fibroblast proliferation whatsoever. THFB do not contain elastic fibers (EF). In the loose connective tissue (LCT) between fiber bundles, however, there are accumulations of thick and fragmented EF. Due to the thickening of individual fiber bundles (FB), the epi- or peritenonal tissue is compressed and disappears, and the THFB fuse to larger units.

Contracture Bands. These bands consist of thickend and fused FB. At some locations there are fusiform enlargements. The original structure of the FB has disappeared except for traces, and at this stage the tissue shrinks and contractures develop. Microscopically, there are nodules of cellular proliferation consisting mainly of fibroblasts, which originate from perivascular spaces. These cells break down the preexisting collagen framework and produce new collagen in patterns resembling vascular structures rather than corresponding to functional requirements. CB tissue contains a higher percentage of type III collagen, which is produced during wound healing and scar formation. In some areas, the cells are similar to secretory fibroblasts and continue to produce collagen; other fibroblasts resemble myofibroblasts. In later stages, the collagen content increases and the number of cells is reduced to a few irregularly distributed accumulations with a scar-like appearance. CB do not contain EF.

Material and Methods

The study was performed in two phases. In the first phase we studied specimens obtained from patients operated upon for carpal tunnel syndrome ($n = 23$) as NPA (classified as group 1). Group 2 ($n = 13$) consisted of specimens from patients with DD matching the definition of ANPA. In group 3 ($n = 11$) we examined specimens with THFB. Group 4 ($n = 13$) consisted of specimens of CB not showing the scar-like residual stage. In group 5 ($n = 5$) there were specimens of CB showing the scar-like residual stage. The number of specimens in the second study are given in each table.

Mechanical Tests

Uniaxial strain-controlled tensile tests were performed at a rate of 1% per minute. Strain was defined as the alteration of length per original length of specimens. Displacements were measured with a potentiometer, at an open length of 100 mm and a resolution of 10 µm. Loads were recorded with a load cell, at a maximum load of 100 N and a resolution of 10 mN.

In the case of hysteresis tests, the unloading phase immediately follows the loading procedure. From the load cycle we obtained the residual strain, i.e., the strain remaining after complete removal of the load, and the normalized hysteresis loop, i.e., the ratio of the area between the loading and unloading graph to the area below the loading graph, which represents the strain energy. The normalized hysteresis loop is a measure of the energy loss during the load cycle.

Stress relaxation was conducted at constant strain levels of 2.5%, 5.0%, and 7.5%. During relaxation the stress required to keep strain constant decreases as a function of time. The resulting relaxation graph can be described in terms of the time constant (tau) and the normalized difference between the initial and final stress values. The time constant is defined as the inverse of the initial slope. The normalized difference between the initial and final stress values represents the viscous stress component. On the other hand, if strain is kept constant after partial deloading of a sample, stress increases as a function of time. This phenomenon is called inverse relaxation.

Retardation or creep tests were performed starting from the following initial strain values: 2.5%, 5.0%, and 7.5%. After achieving these strain levels, the load was kept constant, and the strain was plotted as a function of time. Analogous to the relaxation graph, the retardation graph can be characterized by a time constant. The viscous component of stress is defined according to the increase of strain during retardation as the normalized difference between the initial and final strain values. If stress is kept constant after partial deloading of a sample, strain decreases as a function of time. This experimental procedure is called inverse retardation. If load cycles are repeated several times, the loading and unloading graphs of a cycle generally do not coincide with the previous ones. After a certain time interval between load cycles has elapsed, the original biomechanical properties of the specimens can be restored. This time interval is called recovery time.

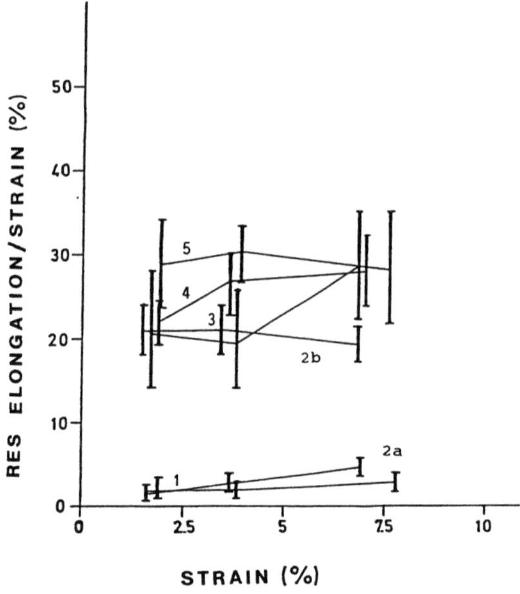

Fig. 1. Normalized residual elongation for three strain levels

Results

First Study

Residual Elongation. Figure 1 illustrates normalized residual elongation for strain levels 2.5%, 5.9%, and 7.5%. It is evident that residual elongation in group 1 was very low (1 in Fig. 1). The residual elongations in groups 3, 4, and 5 (3, 4, 5 in Fig. 1) consisted of 20% to 30%. The 13 patients in group 2 (presenting with ANPA) fell into two different groups. Group 2a was not only normal from the morphologic point of view, it also behaved like NPA patients with respect to residual elongation. Even though they were morphologically normal, however, the tissue obtained from patients in group 2b displayed biomechanical behavior that was similar to that of the tissue obtained from the pathologic groups.

Mechanical Relaxation. Figure 2a presents the initial slope of the relaxation curve for different strain levels (2.5%, 5.0%, and 7.5%). With a 2.5% strain level, there was a significant difference between group 1 (NPA) and groups 3, 4, and 5. Group 2 was in the middle between the two extremes. With a 5% strain level, the values for groups 1 and 2 came closer to those for the pathologic tissue; at a 7.5% strain level, the difference was minimal. If one analyzes the patients in group 2, two characteristic subgroups can be distinguished (Fig. 2b). Some of them behaved more like the NPA specimens (2a in Fig. 2b), and others were more similar to the pathologic tissue (2b in Fig. 2b). The same was true of the viscous fraction (kappa) in the relaxation

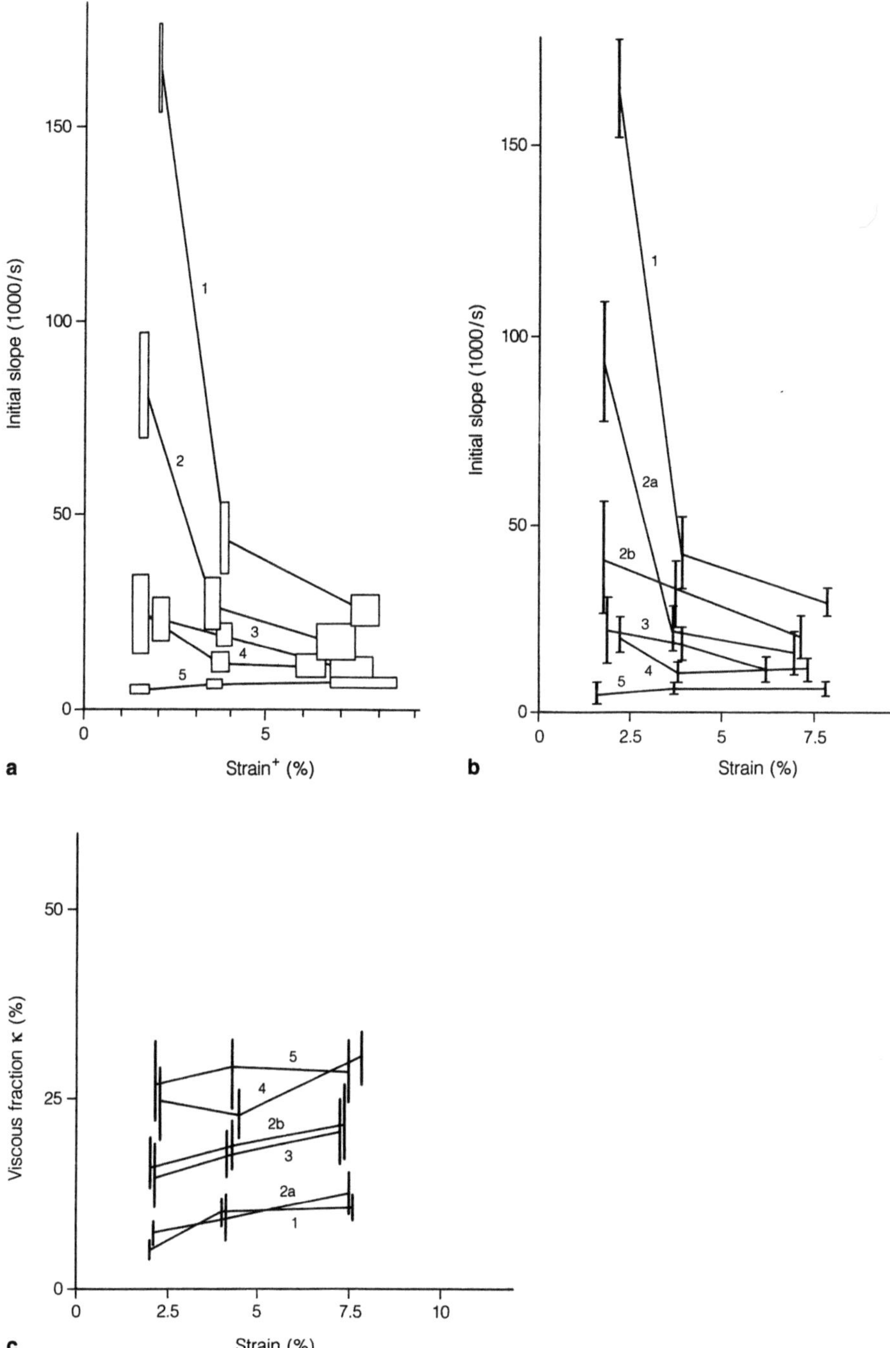

Fig. 2. **a** Initial slopes of relaxation curves for three strain levels for the five groups of patients. **b**, **c** Values for group 2 for initial slope and for viscous fraction divided into two subgroups

Table 1a,b. Residual strain

a Strain levels for unloading phase

Tissue	(n)	2.5%	5.0%	10.0%
NPA	23	0.22 +/− 0.13	0.18 +/− 0.07	0.89 +/− 0.08
ANPA	13	0.30 +/− 0.15	0.50 +/− 0.20	0.80 +/− 0.20
THFB	16	0.50 +/− 0.08	1.50 +/− 0.30	3.00 +/− 0.70
CB	13	0.70 +/− 0.20	1.50 +/− 0.20	3.10 +/− 0.50

b Levels of significance

p	NPA	ANPA	THFB	CB
NPA	−	ns	0.05	0.05
ANPA	ns	−	ns	0.05
THFB	0.05	ns	−	ns
CB	0.05	0.05	ns	−

Table 2a,b. Hysteresis loop

a Strain levels for unloading phase

Tissue	(n)	2.5%	5.0%	10.0%
NPA	23	5.0 +/− 0.8	5.0 +/− 1.0	8.2 +/− 1.3
ANPA	13	7.0 +/− 2.0	10.0 +/− 3.0	15.0 +/− 5.0
THFB	16	16.0 +/− 2.0	16.0 +/− 1.0	21.0 +/− 2.0
CB	13	19.0 +/− 3.0	21.0 +/− 4.0	30.0 +/− 2.0

b Levels of significance

p	NPA	ANPA	THFB	CB
NPA	−	ns	0.01	0.01
ANPA	ns	−	0.01	0.01
THFB	0.01	0.01	−	ns
CB	0.01	0.01	ns	−

test (Fig. 2c). It is interesting to note that changes in biomechanical properties preceded morphologic changes in light microscopic studies.

Second Study

Residual Elongation. Table 1 represents the strain level for the unloading phase of NPA, ANPA, THFB, and CB. The numbers of the specimens are given under n. The values are proportional to strain levels of 2.5%, 5.0%, and 10.0%. Table 1b presents the levels of significance. As in the first study, there was a difference between NPA and ANPA; in this series, however, the difference is not significant. The values for THFB differed significantly from those for NPA. While they were much higher than the values for ANPA, this

Table 3a,b. Relaxation time

a Strain levels for relaxation phase

Tissue	(n)	2.5%	5.0%	10.0%
NPA	19	6.1 +/− 0.4	22.6 +/− 4.8	39.4 +/− 6.2
ANPA	11	12.0 +/− 2.0	36.8 +/− 7.3	57.8 +/− 15
THFB	11	40.0 +/− 15	82.0 +/− 20	95.0 +/− 32
CB	5	196 +/− 39	156 +/− 26	154 +/− 38

b Levels of significance

p	NPA	ANPA	THFB	CB
NPA	–	0.05	0.01	0.01
ANPA	0.05	–	ns	0.01
THFB	0.01	ns	–	0.01
CB	0.01	0.01	0.01	–

Table 4a,b. Retardation time

a Initial strain levels

Tissue	(n)	2.5%	5.0%	10.0%
NPA	20	7.9 +/− 0.9	44.0 +/− 8.7	47.0 +/− 3.8
ANPA	13	11.0 +/− 1.2	43.0 +/− 7.9	80.0 +/− 6.9
THFB	5	15.0 +/− 1.3	53.0 +/− 9.2	80.0 +/− 5.4
CB	8	45.0 +/− 8.2	77.0 +/− 14	77.0 +/− 8.3

b Levels of significance

p	NPA	ANPA	THFB	CB
NPA	–	0.05	0.01	0.01
ANPA	0.05	–	0.05	0.01
THFB	0.01	0.05	–	ns
CB	0.01	0.01	ns	–

difference was not statistically significant, however. The values for CB differed from those for NPA and ANPA, but not from those for THFB.

Hysteresis. NPA and ANPA do not differ significantly with respect to hysteresis. There is a clear significant difference between the two groups and THFB and CB specimens, however (Tables 2a and 2b).

Relaxation Time. The values for NPA and CB specimens at various strain levels are shown in Tables 3a and 3b. There is a strong difference between NPA and ANPA at 2.5% strain. The results of this test confirm the results of the first study with respect to the difference between NPA and ANPA.

Retardation Time. Values for retardation time are presented in Table 4a, and levels of significance for a strain level of 2.5% are provided by Table 4b. There

Table 5a,b. Inverse relaxation

a Values obtained

Tissue	(n)	tau	kappa
NT	7	4.2 +/− 1.0	0.03 +/− 0.02
NPA	9	6.3 +/− 1.7	0.62 +/− 0.40
ANPA	8	12.0 +/− 2.6	2.40 +/− 0.80
THFB	5	7.1 +/− 1.4	6.20 +/− 2.90
CB	8	18.8 +/− 5.0	11.80 +/− 4.20

b Levels of significance

p (tau)	NT	NPA	ANPA	THFB	CB
NT	−	ns	0.01	ns	0.005
NPA	ns	−	ns	ns	0.005
ANPA	0.01	ns	−	ns	ns
THFB	ns	ns	ns	−	0.005
CB	0.005	0.005	ns	0.005	−

p (kappa)	NT	NPA	ANPA	THFB	CB
NT	−	ns	ns	0.005	0.001
NPA	ns	−	ns	0.005	0.001
ANPA	ns	ns	−	0.005	0.001
THFB	0.005	0.005	0.005	−	ns
CB	0.001	0.001	0.001	ns	−

was a significant difference between NPA and ANPA as well as between these and other groups. CB and THFB were the only groups that did not differ significantly. This again confirms the results of the first study.

Inverse Relaxation. Table 5a provides the values for inverse relaxation time (tau) and the viscous fraction obtained by the inverse relaxation test (kappa). Table 5b shows the difference in levels of significance between the groups for both tau and kappa for loading to 5% and deloading to 2.5% strain. There was no significant difference between NPA and ANPA; both groups differed significantly from CB for tau and THFB for kappa, however.

Inverse Retardation. Table 6a demonstrates inverse retardation time (tau) and the viscous fraction obtained by the inverse retardation test (kappa). There was no significant difference between NPA and ANPA specimens; THFB and CB specimens clearly differed, however.

Mechanical Recovery. Figure 3 shows the recovery time with a load strain test investigating a specimen of NPA. After ten minutes the loading curve once again resembled the original one. Figure 4 represents a typical test of a CB specimen. Even after 420 min, the loading curve still differed from the original one. Mechanical recovery values in minutes for the different groups, including specimens with normal tendons, are given in Fig. 5. There was already a

Table 6a,b. Inverse retardation

a Values obtained

Tissue	(n)	tau	kappa
NT	9	217 +/− 45	6.4 +/− 1.3
NPA	9	143 +/− 27	3.3 +/− 0.6
ANPA	3	222 +/− 17	9.2 +/− 0.4
THFB	4	489 +/− 59	23.8 +/− 2.8
CB	9	1050 +/− 234	43.2 +/− 3.9

b Levels of significance

p (tau)	NT	NPA	ANPA	THFB	CB
NT	–	ns	ns	0.01	0.005
NPA	ns	–	ns	0.005	0.005
ANPA	ns	ns	–	0.005	0.005
THFB	0.01	0.005	0.005	–	ns
CB	0.005	0.005	0.005	ns	–

p (kappa)	NT	NPA	ANPA	THFB	CB
NT	–	ns	ns	0.001	0.001
NPA	ns	–	ns	0.001	0.001
ANPA	ns	ns	–	0.001	0.001
THFB	0.001	0.001	0.001	–	ns
CB	0.001	0.001	0.001	ns	–

Table 7a,b. Mechanical recovery

a Values

Tissue	(n)	Interval (min)
NPA	9	12.2 +/− 1.2
ANPA	8	21.3 +/− 1.3
THFB	5	45.0 +/− 8.7
CB	8	210 +/− 45

b Levels of significance

p (interval)	NPA	ANPA	THFB	CB
NPA	–	ns	0.005	0.005
ANPA	ns	–	0.01	0.01
THFB	0.005	0.01	–	0.05
CB	0.005	0.01	0.05	–

difference in recovery time between NPA (12.2 +/− 1.2) versus ANPA (21.3 +/− 1.3), but this is not significant. There was a much bigger difference compared to THFB. The striking increase in recovery time is shown by the difference between CB and the other groups (Fig. 5), however.

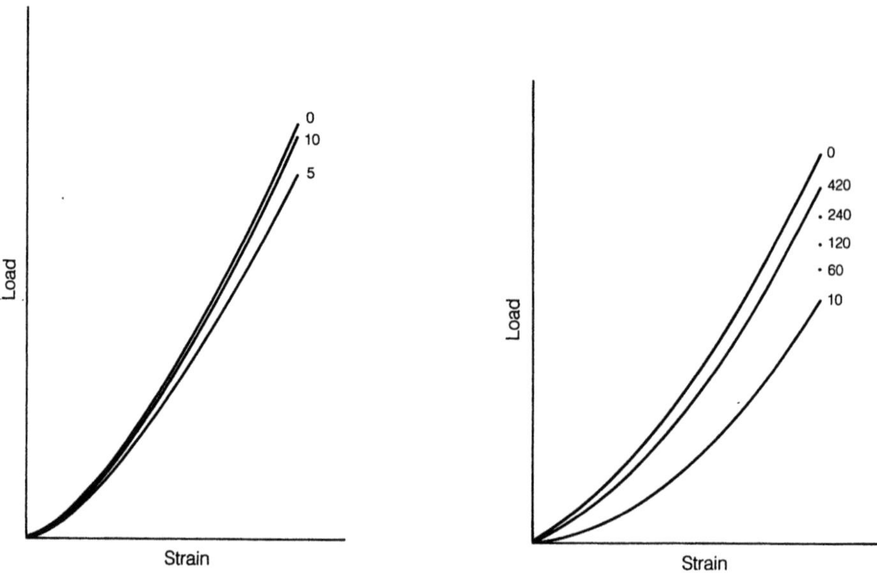

Fig. 3 *(left)*. Recovery time with load strain test for normal palmar aponeurosis

Fig. 4 *(right)*. Loading curves for contracture band recovery after different periods of time

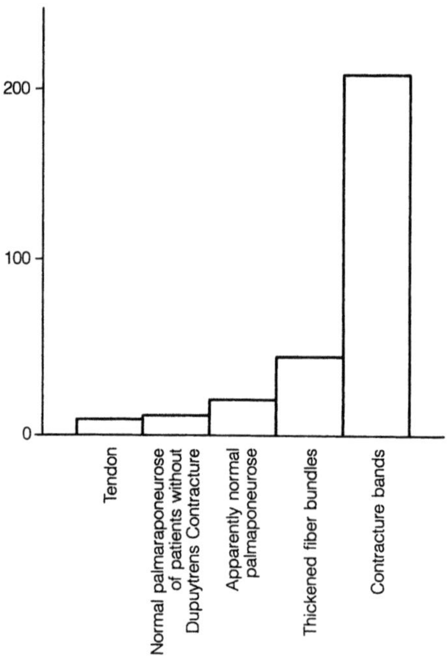

Fig. 5. Recovery period (in min) for the different groups

188   H. Millesi et al.

Discussion

In NPA specimens, the residual strain was rather uniformly small. It increased in some of the ANPA and significantly increased in THFB and CB specimens. The return to zero after loading with elongation was certainly supported by EF. We may therefore assume that EF functioning was less than optimal in these patients. A quantitative study would be necessary to prove this observation. It is very difficult to explain differences in relaxation times between these groups. Inverse relaxation arises in the transient zone between ANPA and THFB. Thickening of the fiber bundles accompanied by fusion and loss of the peri- and epitenonal structures may be the morphologic background for this change in mechanical properties. Prolonged mechanical recovery times are linked to specimens which are in the process of developing contracture. It will be our next task to analyze these results in the light of our clinical data.

Summary

The mechanical properties of different specimens obtained from patients with DD and of palmar aponeurosis specimens obtained from patients without DD who are suffering from carpal tunnel syndrome have been studied. The residual elongation after loading and unloading to 2.5% strain increased in some cases of ANPA in patients with DD. The same was true for the relaxation time. This means that these particular mechanical changes precede the typical morphology. Inverse relaxation and inverse retardation increase if the structure of the fiber bundle changes. The mechanical recovery time is strongly linked to the process of contracture.

Fibromatoses

Localization and Morphology of Different Fibromatoses

W. Mohr and D. Wessinghage

Fibromatoses can be regarded as tumorous proliferations "intermediate in their biological behavior between benign fibrous lesions (e.g. nodular fasciitis) and fibrosarcoma" (Enzinger and Weiss 1988) (Fig. 1). They are usually divided into superficial (Dupuytren-type) and deeply located groups. Since they do not metastasize they should not be called low-grade fibrosarcomas (Allen 1977). Below, some of the more common types of fibromatoses with the exception of Dupuytren's disease, will be briefly summarized. The different fibrous proliferations of infancy and childhood will not be discussed.

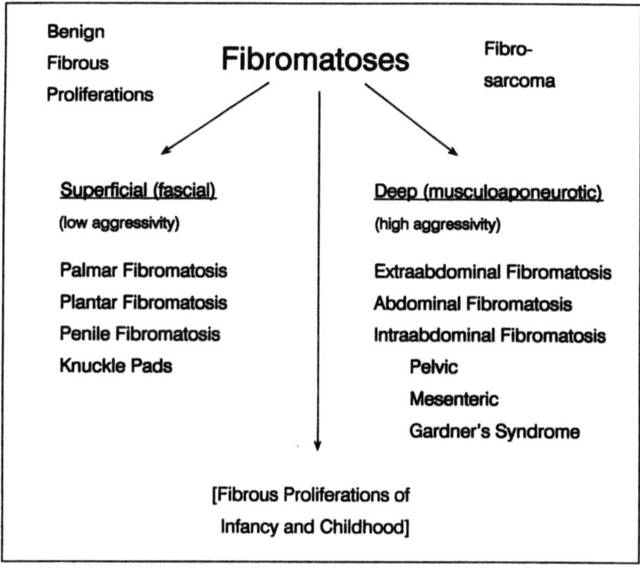

Fig. 1. Classification of fibromatoses

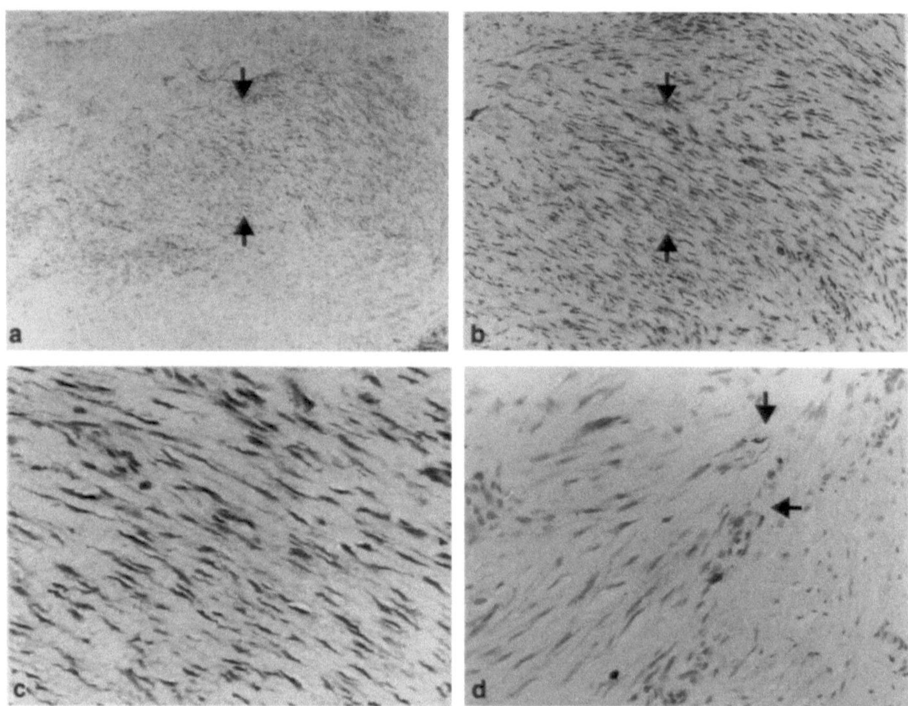

Fig. 2a–d. Fibromatosis of plantar aponeurosis (Ledderhose's disease) of a 36 year old male patient. **a** Aponeurosis with a hypercellular nodule (*arrows*). H and E; ×35. **b** Higher magnification of the area marked in **a**: hypercellular nodule. H and E; ×85. **c** Higher magnification of the area marked in **b**. Spindle-shaped fibroblasts surrounded by collagenous fibrils. H and E; ×220. **d** Iron deposits (*arrows*) in some of the spindle-shaped cells. Prussian blue, nuclear fast red; ×220

Superficial Fibromatoses

Plantar Fibromatosis

Ledderhose (1897) recognized the nodules in the plantar aponeurosis as an equivalent of Dupuytren's disease and characterized the disease as a proliferation of cells and blood vessels with a tendency for the lesion to shrink. According to Pirie (1987) and Rao and Luthra (1988) contractures rarely occur.

The prevalence of the disease is unknown; Yost et al. (1955) observed one case in 430 patients whose feet were examined. The disease often develops in younger individuals (Allen 1977). According to Enzinger and Weiss (1988) 55% of the affected persons are younger than 30 years. This is in accordance with the observations of Albers et al. (1985), who described a mean age of 38 years, and Wilson (1987), who found two thirds of the patients to be under 40 years of age. While Enzinger and Weiss (1988) stated that males were twice as often affected as females, Kirby et al. (1989) observed six women among their

11 patients. The association of this disorder with Dupuytren's disease is of interest: Fibromatoses of the palmar aponeurosis are simultaneously present in 5%–20% of patients with Dupuytren's disease. Weckesser (1964) observed plantar nodules in 7% of these patients. The etiology of the disease is unknown; Ledderhose (1897) assumed traumas to be the inducing event.

Morphologically, the disease does not differ from Dupuytren's contracture (Pirie 1987). Hypercellular foci of fibroblast-like cells are present in the plantar aponeurosis (Fig. 2a–c), and mitoses can often be observed (Aviles et al. 1971). Iron deposits may be found (Fig. 2d), but mast cells are rarely encountered. Involvement of the overlying skin may occur (Rao and Luthra 1988).

Penile Fibromatosis

This condition, also known as Peyronie's disease, is characterized as a "fibrous thickening or mass in the shaft of the penis" (Enzinger and Weiss 1988).

Neither incidence nor prevalence of the disease are known. According to McRoberts (1969) about 1500 cases have been reported. Based on 100 routine autopsy specimens, Smith (1969) concluded that subclinical disease with early inflammation and subsequent development of fibrosis is a rather common condition in American males for it was observed in 23%. As in Dupuytren's disease, patients between 55 and 75 years are affected; the disease is more common in patients with palmar and plantar fibromatosis than in the general population (Enzinger and Weiss 1988). Weckesser (1964) observed Peyronie's disease in 5% of patients with Dupuytren's disease. The etiology is unknown (McRoberts 1969). Smith (1966) suggested that the process is initiated by an inflammation leading to a fibrous replacement of the corpus cavernosum.

Histologically the disease is characterized by fibrosis of the corpus cavernosum mainly beneath the tunica albuginea; ossification may also occur (Smith 1966; Allen 1977).

Knuckle Pads

Knuckle pads are "fibrous thickenings on the dorsal aspect of the proximal interphalangeal joints and the paratenon of the extensor tendon" (Enzinger and Weiss 1988).

The incidence and prevalence are unknown. The disease occurs, predominantly in males, in the fourth to sixth decade of life (Enzinger and Weiss 1988). Also in this disorder has an association with Dupuytren's disease been documented. According to Mikkelson (1977), patients with Dupuytren's disease suffer four times more often than the general population. Weckesser (1964) observed knuckle pads in 6% and Skoog (1948) in 44% of patients with Dupuytren's contracture. Histologically the disease is not different from Dupuytren's contracture.

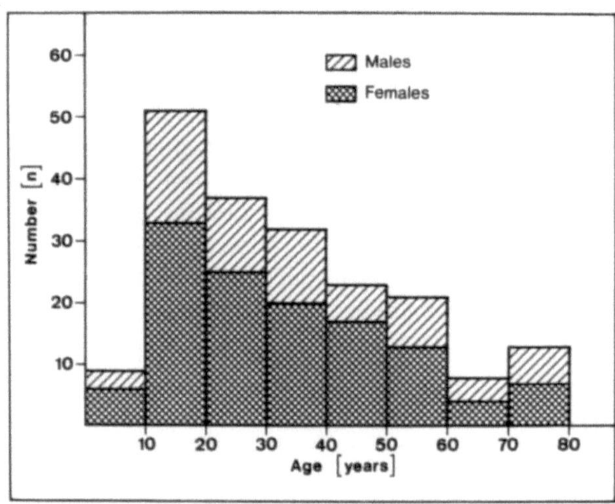

Fig. 3. Age and sex destribution of extraabdominal fibromatosis. (From Rock et al. 1984)

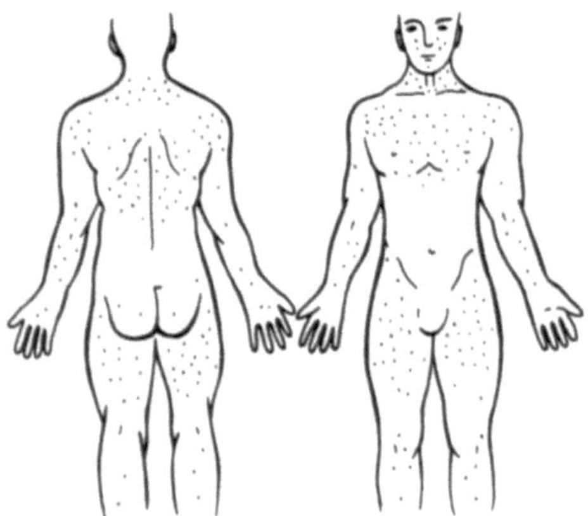

Fig. 4. Localization of extraabdominal fibromatosis. (From Reitamo et al. 1982 and Enzinger and Weiss 1988)

Deep Fibromatoses

Extraabdominal Fibromatosis (Extraabdominal Desmoid)

Clinically these desmoid tumors appear as poorly circumscribed, deep-seated masses that may be mistaken for sarcoma.

Reitamo et al. (1982) calculated an incidence for extra- and abdominal fibromatosis of 2.4–4.3/1 000 000. Individuals of all ages can be affected; however, younger patients more commonly suffer from this disease (Fig. 3). While Enzinger and Weiss (1988) noted that males and females are equally affected, Rock et al. (1984) found a predominance of females (Fig. 3). The localizations of this condition are summarized in Fig. 4: shoulder (22.1%), chest wall and back (17.2%), and thigh (12.5%) predominate (Enzinger and

196   W. Mohr and D. Wessinghage

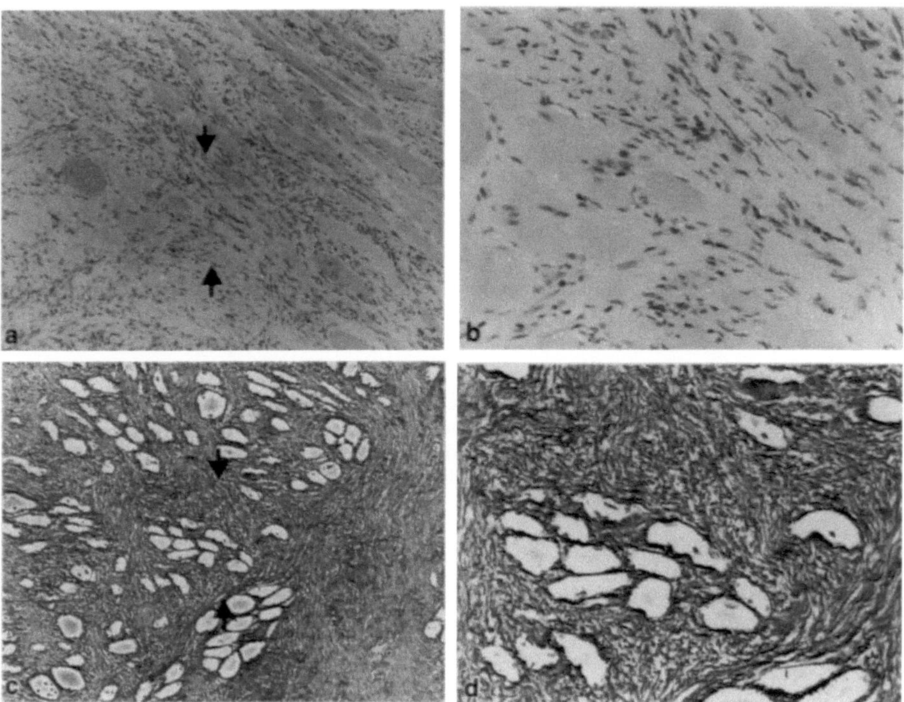

Fig. 5a–d. Fibromatosis of the vocal cord of a 17 year old female patient. **a** Hypercellular fibrous tissues between muscle bundles. H and E; ×85. **b** Higher magnification of the area marked in **a**. Between the muscle bundles spindle-shaped fibroblasts are surrounded by collagenous fibers. H and E; ×220. **c** Replacement of the muscle-cells by fibrous tissue rich in argyrophilic fibers. Gomori's silver stain impregnation; ×85. **d** Higher magnification of the area marked in **c**. Remnants of muscle-cells are surrounded by argyrophilic fibers. Gomori's silver stain impregnation; ×220

Weiss 1988). Mammary fibromatosis is a very rare finding (Rosen and Ernsberger 1989). Pathologists need to be familiar with this condition, which may be misdiagnosed as fibrosarcoma. Spontaneous regression of this lesion has been documented (Jenkins et al. 1986). The etiology and pathogenesis are unknown.

The macroscopic gray-white tumor consists histologically of spindle-shaped fibroblasts surrounded by collagenous fibers. No atypical cells are present. Invasion of the striated musculature occurs even in such rare localizations as the vocal cords (Fig. 5). Electron microscopy exhibits the presence of myofibroblasts (Stiller and Katenkamp 1975).

Abdominal Fibromatosis (Abdominal Desmoid)

This kind of tumor usually develops in the abdominal wall (Fig. 6) in females during gravidity or the first year following childbirth; however, nullipara, and

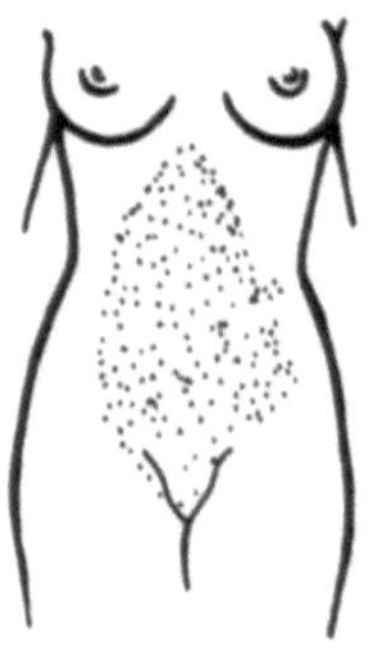

Fig. 6. Localization of abdominal fibromatosis. (From Reitamo et al. 1982)

Fig. 7a–c. Abdominal fibromatosis of a 27 year old male patient. **a** Macroscopically fibrous ▷ tissue invades the skeletal musculature. *Bar*, 1 cm. **b** Histology of the tumorous tissue exhibiting fibrous tissue poor in cells. H and E; ×85. **c** Higher magnification of the area marked in **a**. Between collagenous fibers spindle-shaped fibrocytes are found. H and E; ×220

in rare instances males, are affected (Caldwell 1976). The prevalence and incidence of this fibromatosis have not been well documented. Reitamo et al. (1982) reported an incidence of extra- and abdominal fibromatosis in about 2.4–4.3 cases/1 000 000. At the Memorial Hospital 17 cases were seen in 50 316 and at Johns Hopkins five in 21 000 surgical specimens (Caldwell 1976). The etiology and pathogenesis are unknown, but hormonal factors may be involved. Spontaneous regression of this desmoid has also been documented (Caldwell 1976).

The gross and microscopic appearance of these tumors is identical to that of extraabdominal fibromatosis. A firm gray-white tissue may be found that invades the musculature (Fig. 7a). Histologically, spindle-shaped cells surrounded by collagenous fibers are present (Fig. 7b,c). Older tumors may exhibit calcifications (Fig. 8).

Intraabdominal Fibromatoses

The different types of these tumors are summarized in Table 1. Morphologically, they are indistinguishable from fibromatoses at other sites. Even multinodular tumors exhibit a fibrous tissue of spindle-shaped fibroblasts surrounded by collagenous fibers (Roscher et al. 1988). Psammomatous calcification may be present (Lee and Sen 1985; Roscher et al. 1988). Mitoses and occasionally myxoid areas can also be observed (Yannopoulos and Stout 1963).

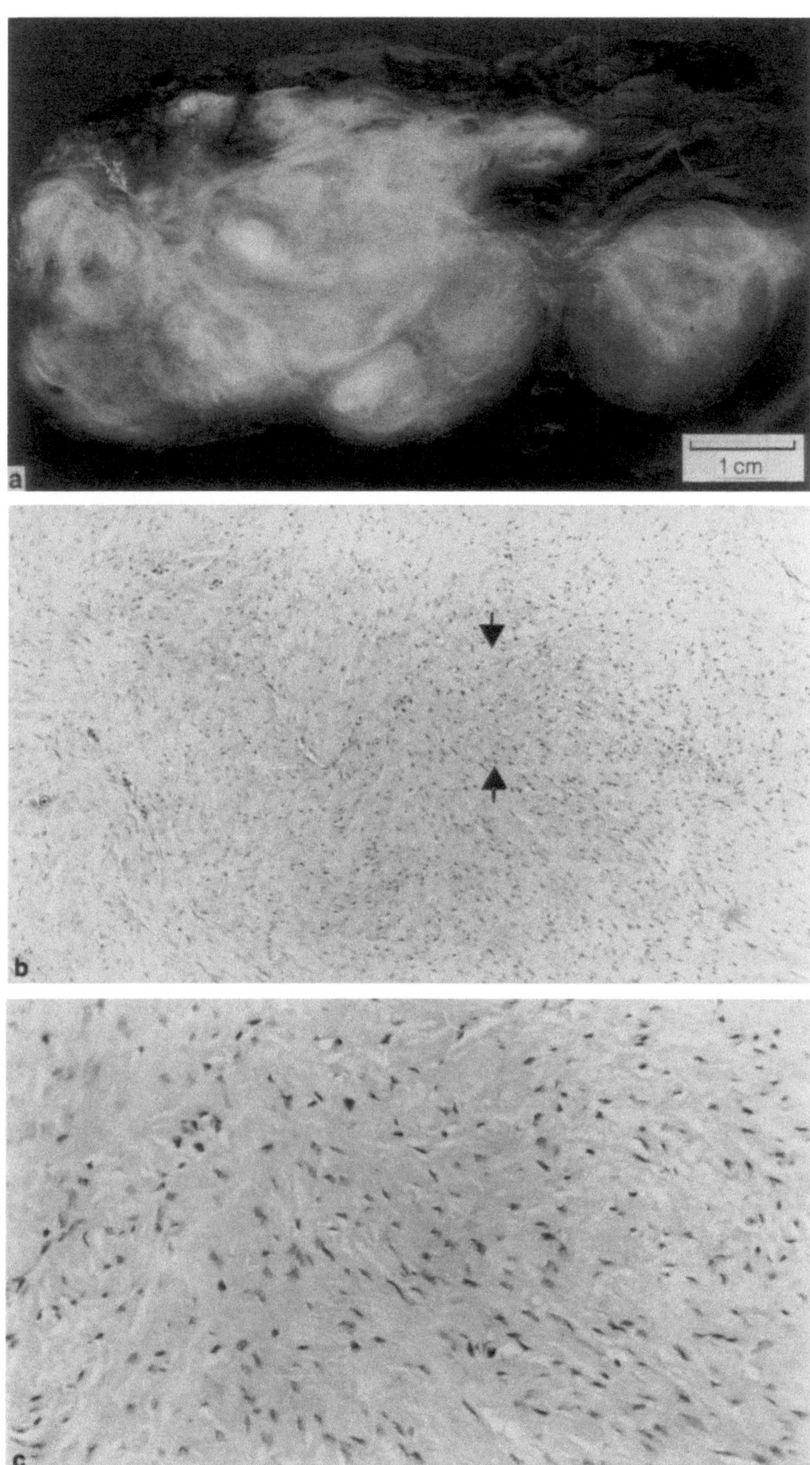

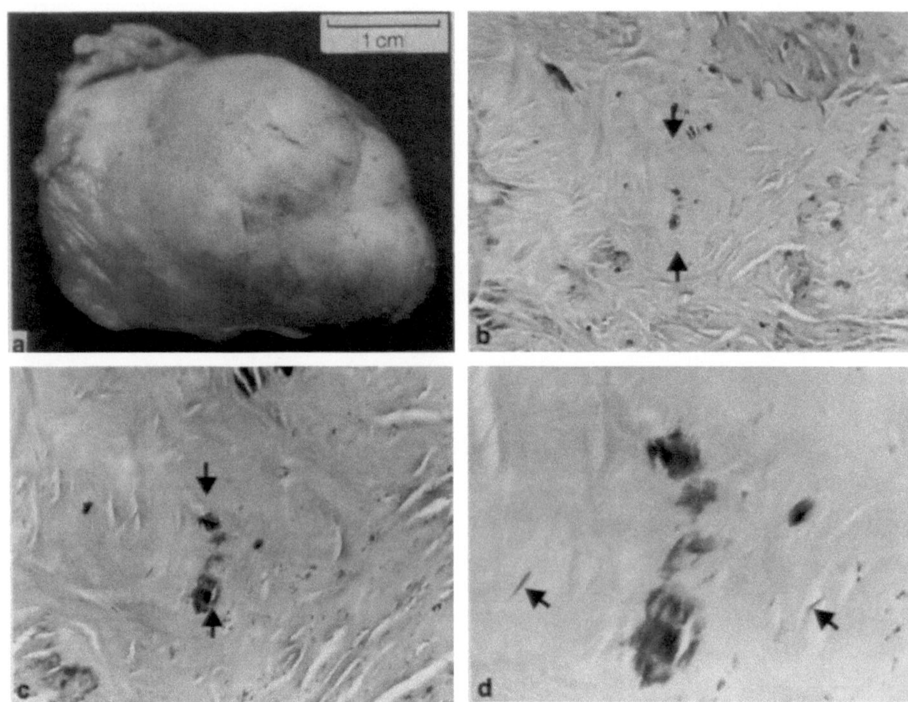

Fig. 8a–d. Structure of a well demarcated abdominal desmoid of a 54 year old female patient. **a** Nodule; *bar*, 1 cm. **b** Fibrous tissue with calcification. H and E; ×35. **c** Higher magnification of area marked in **b**. Dense fibrous tissue with some calcification is shown. H and E; ×85. **d** Higher magnification of the area marked in **c**. Between the broad collagenous fibers only some spindle-shaped fibrocytes (*arrows*) beneath a calcified focus are found. H and E; ×220

Table 1. Classification of intraabdominal fibromatoses

Pelvic fibromatosis	Mesenteric fibromatosis	Gardner's syndrome (Intestinal polyposis, osteomata, cutaneous cysts)
Preferentially females	Females and males equally affected	Females affected more than males
20–35 years[a]	10 months–60 years[b]	Diagnosis at 25–35 years[a]

[a] Enzinger and Weiss 1988.
[b] Yannopoulus and Stout 1963.

References

Albers W, Sühler H, Blümlein H (1985) M. Ledderhose. Die Fibromatose des Fußes, Klinik und Therapie. Chir Prax 34:293–296

Allen PW (1977) The fibromatoses: a clinicopathologic classification based on 140 cases. Am J Surg Pathol 1:255–270

Aviles E, Arlen M, Miller T (1971) Plantar fibromatosis. Surgery 69:117–120

Caldwell EH (1976) Desmoid tumor: musculoaponeurotic fibrosis of the abdominal wall. Surgery 79:104–106

Enzinger FM, Weiss SW (1988) Soft tissue tumors, 2nd edn. Mosby, St Louis

Jenkins NH, Freedman LS, McKibbin B (1986) Spontaneous regression of a desmoid tumour. J Bone Joint Surg [Br] 68:780–781

Kirby EJ, Shereff MJ, Lewis MM (1989) Soft-tissue tumors and tumor-like lesions of the foot. An analysis of eighty-three cases. J Bone Joint Surg [Am] 71:621–626

Ledderhose (1897) Zur Pathologie der Aponeurose des Fußes und der Hand. Langenbecks Arch Klin Chir 55:694–712

Lee Y-S, Sen BK (1985) Dystrophic and psammomatous calcifications in a desmoid tumor. A light microscopic and ultrastructural study. Cancer 55:84–90

McRoberts JW (1969) Peyronie's disease. Surg Gynecol Obstet 129:1291–1294

Mikkelson OA (1977) Knuckle pads in Dupuytren's disease. Hand 9:301–305

Pirie L (1987) Pathology of plantar fibromatosis (Abstr). J Bone Joint Surg [Br] 69:679

Rao GS, Luthra PK (1988) Dupuytren's disease of the foot in children: a report of three cases. Br J Plast Surg 41:313–315

Reitamo JJ, Häyry P, Nykyri E, Saxén E (1982) The desmoid tumor. I. Incidence, sex-, age- and anatomical distribution of the Finnish population. Am J Clin Pathol 77:665–673

Rock MG, Pritchard DJ, Reiman HM, Soule EH, Brewster RC (1984) Extra-abdominal desmoid tumors. J Bone Joint Surg [Am] 66:1369–1374

Roscher R, Gaedicke G, Mohr W (1988) Mesenteriale Fibromatose im Kindesalter. Monatsschr Kinderheilkd 136:393–396

Rosen PP, Ernsberger D (1989) Mammary fibromatosis. A benign spindle-cell tumor with significant risk for local recurrence. Cancer 63:1363–1369

Skoog T (1948) Dupuytren's contraction with special reference to aetiology and improved surgical treatment, its occurrence in epileptics, note on knuckle-pads. Acta Chir Scand 96 Suppl 139:1–190

Smith BH (1966) Peyronie's disease. Am J Clin Pathol 45:670–678

Smith BH (1969) Subclinical Peyronie's disease. Am J Clin Pathol 52:385–390

Stiller D, Katenkamp D (1975) Cellular features in desmoid fibromatosis and well-differentiated fibrosarcomas. An electron microscopic study. Virchows Arch [Pathol Anat] 369:155–164

Weckesser EC (1964) Results of wide excision of the palmar fascia for Dupuytren's contracture: special reference to factors which adversely affect prognosis. Ann Surg 160:1007–1013

Wilson DW (1987) Clinical aspects of plantar fibromatosis (Abstr). J Bone Joint Surg [Br] 69:679

Yannopoulos K, Stout AP (1963) Primary solid tumors of the mesentery. Cancer 16:914–927

Yost J, Winters T, Fett HC (1955) Dupuytren's contracture. A statistical study. Am J Surg 90:568–571

Thermal Stability and Fibrillogenesis of Collagen from Tissue of Patients with Dupuytren's Disease

H. Notbohm, S. Mosler, and J. Hoch

Introduction

Dupuytren's disease (DD) is a spontaneously occurring tissue rearrangement with a number of biochemical and cellular variations compared to normal fibroblast activity (McFarlaine 1983; Gabbiani and Majno 1972). Fibroblasts are influenced by a number of environmental factors, e.g., cytokines, drugs, or biomechanical stress, which modulate gene expression and therefore the rate of collagen production and extracellular matrix formation. The extracellular matrix of connective tissue is basically constructed of collagen fibrils and various noncollagenous extracellular matrix proteins (Piez 1984). Specific collagen types and proteoglycans modulate the biomechanical character of tissues including skin, bone, cornea, or palmar aponeurosis (Romanic et al. 1991; Birk et al. 1990; Scott 1988; Lapiere et al. 1977). In pathological situations such as fibrosis, the pattern of collagen expression is changed (Bailey et al. 1977).

In Dupuytren's contracture, mainly quantitative changes in the amount of extracellular matrix components are observed. In addition, beyond the formation of nodules and bands, the ultrastructure of the collagen fibers is altered. Areas of active proliferation are characterized by their cellularity and by a meshwork of fibrils (polymeric collagen) which only focally coalesce into discrete fibers but which then separate again. An important feature is that both the constituent fibrils and the fibers themselves tend to be oriented in one direction in contrast to what occurs in mature tissue (Hunter et al. 1975).

The events leading to altered production of collagen fibrils and contraction of the tissue are presently not clear. It has been suggested that contraction is due to the transformation of fibroblasts into myofibroblasts, since myofibroblasts have been found in diseased palmar aponeurosis (Gabbiani and Majno 1972). Hereditary factors, sex, metabolic diseases, and drugs such as alcohol may be initiating factors in DD. (Hueston 1990).

The biochemical changes of DD tissue include the following:

1. A change in the relative content of the different collagen types, especially an increase in collagen III (Bailey et al. 1977)
2. Increased proteoglycan content relative to collagen (Tunn et al. 1988)
3. A lysyl overmodification of collagen I (Bailey et al. 1977)

4. Increase fibronectin content in the tissue (Brokaw et al. 1985; Menzel 1984)
5. Fewer cross-links in the tissue than found in normal aponeurosis (Bailey, this volume)

Organization of the extracellular matrix is a self-regulated process involving the various collagen types and proteoglycans. Posttranslational modifications of collagen, such as hydroxylation of prolyl and lysyl residues and glycosylation of hydroxylysine, may also have a regulatory effect on extracellular matrix formation.

It was our aim to acquire biochemical data, with respect to the changes listed above, from collagen obtained from Dupuytren's nodules. These data were compared to the special ultrastructural features found in DD tissue and to the unbalanced biochemical turnover which leads to a net overproduction of collagen.

Materials and Methods

Biochemical Analysis of Skin, Palmar Aponeurosis, and Tissue from DD Patients

Tissue samples were manually homogenized under liquid nitrogen using a stainless steel homogenizer followed by dialysis against 0.05% acetic acid for 3 days. All dialysis steps were carried out in the presence of phenylmethansulfonylfluoride (3 mg/l) to inhibit proteases. After centrifugation at $100\,000 \times g$ (1 h, 4°C), an aliquot (5 ml) of the supernatant was lyophilized and analyzed on SDS-PAGE (Bätge et al. 1990). The remainder was used for the extraction procedures described below. Skin, palmar aponeurosis, and tissue from DD patients was defatted and then homogenized prior to extraction.

Extraction of Collagens

Limited pepsin digestion was used to solubilize bulk collagen. Samples (2–10 g dry weight) were stirred in a pepsin (0.1 mg/ml) (Boehringer Mannheim, FRG) solution at 4°C for 24 h. After centrifugation at $65\,000 \times g$ (1 h, 4°C), supernatants were neutralized and stored at $-20°C$. This digestion procedure was repeated six times; for determination of the total collagen composition all neutralized supernatants were pooled.

Sequential Salt Precipitations

In order to separate collagen I from the other collagen types, sequential neutral salt precipitations were performed by consecutive dialysis against 1.0, 1.8, and 2.5 M NaCl solutions (0.05 M Tris, pH 7.4) (Miller and Rhodes 1982). The 2.5 M precipitate consisted of highly purified collagen I. After centrifugation (65 000 × g, 1 h, 4°C), the pellet was redissolved in 0.05% acetic acid and dialyzed against the same solvent to remove residual salt. For all further studies only the fraction precipitating at 2.5 M NaCl was used.

Electrophoretic Separation

Small aliquots of each tissue sample were lyophilized and redissolved in SDS sample buffer at a concentration of 1 mg/ml. Each sample was heated to 95°C for 2 min and quenched on ice prior to sample loading (Laemli 1970). After separation of collagen the polyacrylamide gels were stained with Coomassie blue and the relative amounts of the different components were measured by densitometric scanning using a video scanner (Computer and Vision, Lübeck, FRG). Relative amounts of collagen types were determined by measuring the integrated absorption of the bands in a lane.

Amino Acid Analysis

Lyophilized collagen I was hydrolyzed with 6 M HCl and 0.1% mercaptoethanol under nitrogen. Analysis was performed on a Beckman 6300 amino acid analyzer (Beckman, Munich, FRG). The relative content of hydroxylysine and hydroxyproline per mole of fractionated collagen was expressed as Hyl/(Hyl + Lys) and Hypro/(Pro + Hypro), respectively.

In Vitro Fibril Formation and Fibril Melting

Fibrillogenesis. Self-assembly conditions followed a modification of the method described by Williams et al. (1978): 100 µg/ml collagen I, 30 mM Tris, 30 mM K_2HPO_4, 150 mM NaCl. In order to reach 90% saturation of fibril formation within 2 h for all samples, the incubation was performed at 37.0°C and pH 7.4 in a thermocontrolled Gilford quartz cuvette, unless otherwise stated.

Fibril Melting. After 18 h the sample was exposed to a linear temperature gradient of 0.5°C/min. Assembly and disassembly was monitored by continuous recording of the absorbance at 313 nm in a Gilford spectrophotometer.

Definition of the Characteristic Values

Fibrillogenesis and fibril melting is a process which can be described with an unsymmetric sigmoid function. We have differentiated this curve and determined the following parameters, which mainly characterize the process of collagen assembly: (1) turning point (maximum of the differentiated curve), (2) maximal slope (height of the differentiated curve), and (3) maximal turbidity

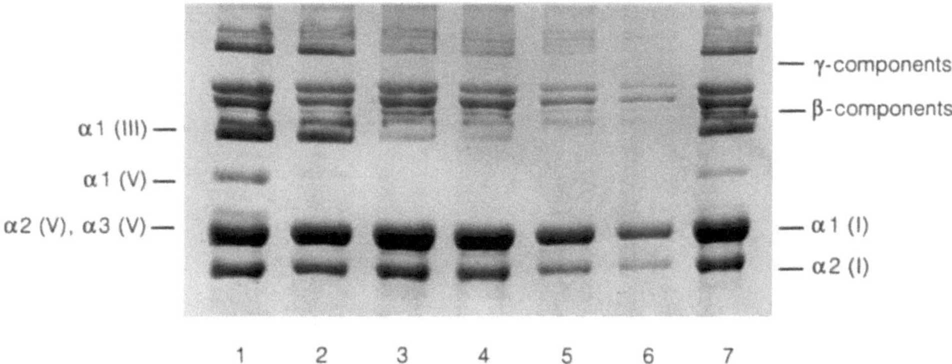

Fig. 1. SDS gel electrophoresis of pepsin extracts of Dupuytren's nodules. *Lanes 1–6* are successively extracted collagens; *lane 7* displays the overall composition of collagens

(area under the differentiated curve). For the melting curve, the value of the maximal transition rate (the maximum of the differentiated curve) is defined here as the fibril melting temperature, T_m.

Results

Unaffected tissue from palmar aponeurosis was taken during hand surgery from patients suffering from carpal tunnel syndrome. Tissue from five DD patients came from nodules of the midhand.

Composition of Collagens

The tissue material from the DD patients was totally digested after five rounds of pepsin digestion. Densitometric evaluation of the electrophoretically separated proteins of the digests showed only collagen types, I, III, and V. Samples taken from every digest and from the collagen composition of the total pool were analyzed by gel electrophoresis (Fig. 1).

Amino Acid Composition

The collagen I α-chains are lysyl-overhydroxylated in Dupuytren's nodules. The value of the relative content of hydroxylysine (Hyl/Hyl + Lys) is 0.25 compared to 0.17 in normal aponeurosis. The relative hydroxyproline content (Hyp/Hyp + Pro), 0.44, is unchanged (Table 1).

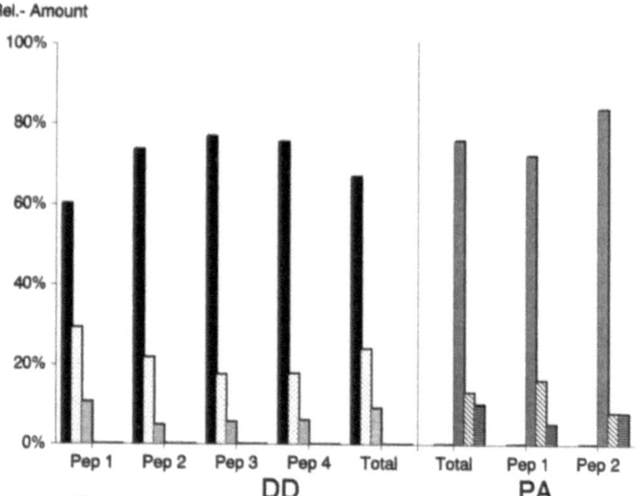

Fig. 2. Histograms of the densitometrically determined relative collagen concentrations of the α-bands of collagen types I, III and V (from left to right; see Fig. 1). *Pep*, successive pepsin digests (also shown is the total pool of pepsin-soluble collagen); *DD*, Dupuytren's disease; *PA*, palmar aponeurosis

Table 1. Biochemical and biophysical data regarding collagen type I

Human tissue	Fibril T_m (°C)	Triple helix T_m (°C)	Hyl/Hyl + Lys	Hyp/Hyp + Pro
Skin	49.9	41.5	0.12	0.41
Palmar aponeurosis	n.d.	42.2	0.17	0.46
Dupuytren's disease nodules	50.2	42.8	0.25	0.46

T_m, fibril melting temperature; Hyl, hydroxylysine; Lys, lysine; Hyp, hydroxyproline; Pro, proline.

Composition of Collagen Types

Electrophoretic separation and subsequent determination of the relative content of collagen types in the individual pepsin digests and in the total tissue are shown in Fig. 2. Most of the collagen III is present in the first digest and collagen V is nearly absent in the last digests. The overall content of collagen III is higher in tissues derived from DD patients.

Thermal Stability of Collagen

Collagen I (2.5 M NaCl sediment) from DD patients has as higher melting temperature than collagen from normal aponeurosis. The T_m value of collagen

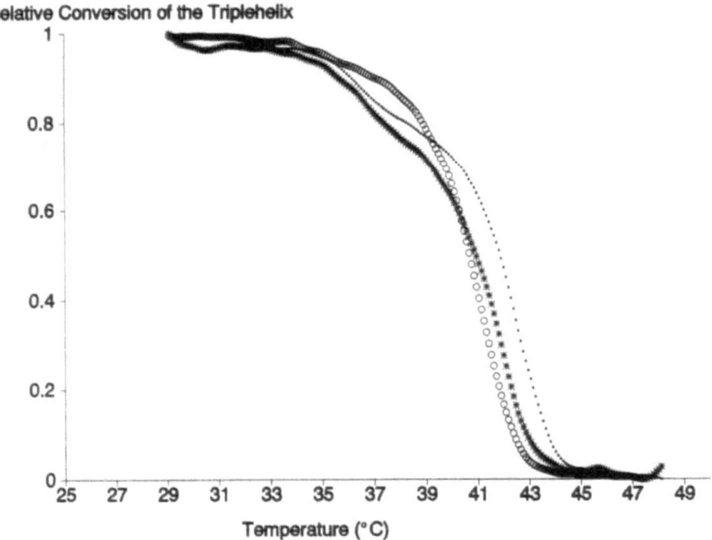

Fig. 3. Melting curve of solute collagen molecules in 0.05% acetic acid. Ellipticity at 221 nm is normalized in terms of triple helix to random coil conversion. □, collagen I from Dupuytren's disease patients; *, collagen I from normal aponeurosis; ○, collagen I from control skin

from DD patients is 42.8°C. For the unaffected aponeurosis we measured 42.2°C. Denaturation curves of skin, DD collagen and palmar aponeurosis collagen obtained from circular dichroism (CD) measurements are shown in Fig. 3.

Fibrillogenesis of Heterotypic Collagen

Various mixtures of the collagen precipitated at $1.8\,M$ NaCl (collagen I + collagen III) and at $2.5\,M$ NaCl (pure collagen I) were incubated together in order to determine the effect of minor collagen types on fibril formation.

In Fig. 4 the maximum turbidity values, which are proportional to the mass per unit length of the collagen fibrils, are summarized. The mass per unit length of collagen fibrils decreases by a factor of five with increasing amounts of collagen III. Also, as shown in Fig. 4, the amount of collagen which is not assembled into fibrils represents only 20% of the total amount of collagen. Free collagen concentration is increased by 5% if the collagen III concentration is raised. The structure of the in vitro formed collagen fibrils was demonstrated to be the same as native collagen by negatively stained electron micrographs (not shown).

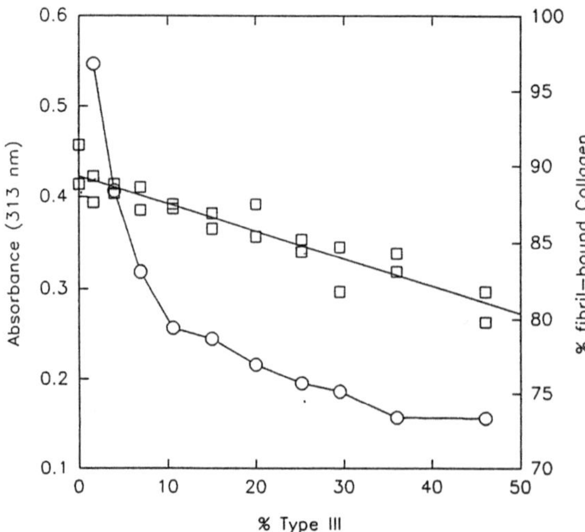

Fig. 4. Influence of collagen III on fibril structure. Amount of collagen III in a solution with collagen I (always 100 µg/ml) is plotted against maximum turbidity (O) and against relative amount of collagen in the supernatant after sedimentation of the fibrils (□)

Fibrillogenesis and Fibril Stability of Collagen I from Palmar Aponeurosis and from Dupuytren's Disease Patients

In Fig. 5a overhydroxylated collagen of DD patients is compared with normal skin collagen (highly purified collagen from normal palmar aponeurosis cannot be obtain in sufficient quantity). Lysyl-overhydroxylated collagen from DD patients did not show different dynamic patterns of fibrillogenesis as compared to collagen I from control skin, but the mass per unit length was nearly twice as high for the overhydroxylated collagen. The thermal stability of fibrils formed in vitro from these isolated collagens was also not significantly different (Fig. 5b). The melting temperature was about 50°C for both control skin collagen I and collagen I from DD patients. Presumably, because of the thicker fibrils of DD patients, melting is slightly shifted to higher temperatures.

Discussion

In comparing the collagenous extracellular matrix components of normal palmar aponeurosis and palmar aponeurosis altered by the typical symptoms of DD contracture, two changes, the results of an as yet unknown initiating biochemical mechanism, can be found: (1) quantitative changes in the collagen composition and (2) posttranslational collagen modification. Posttranslational modification of collagen stabilizes the collagen triple helix, which is a structural prerequisite for the molecule to withstand proteolytic degradation. Therefore, the degree of posttranslational modification indirectly influences the net collagen production rate. Additionally, collagen fibril structure and fibril

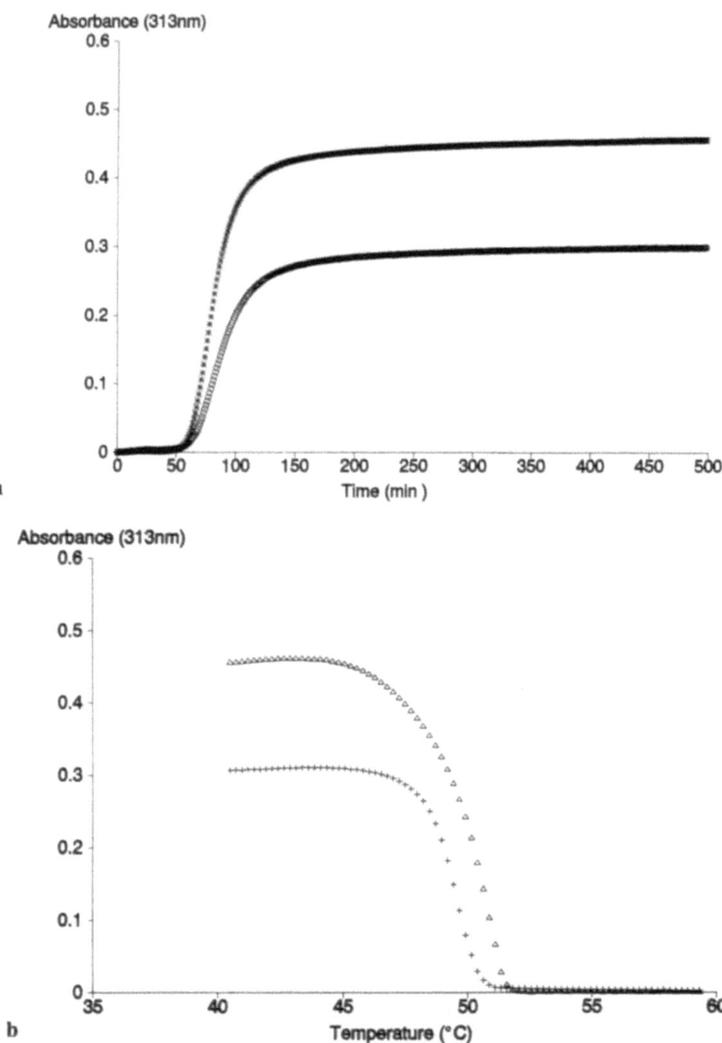

Fig. 5. a Turbidity-time curve of neutralized collagen at 37°C monitored at 313 nm; *, skin collagen I; ○, overhydroxylated collagen I from Dupuytren's disease patients. b Turbidity-temperature curve of fibrils to determine the melting temperature of fibrils; +, skin collagen I; △, collagen from Dupuytren's disease patients

stability is influenced by collagen type composition and posttranslational modification (Notbohm et al. 1992). It is well known that prolyl overhydroxylation can affect triple helix stability. The influence of lysyl overhydroxylation and underhydroxylation have been demonstrated recently for collagen from pathologically altered bone and skin (Fig. 6, Notbohm et al. 1992). A decrease of the melting temperature of about 1°C was observed when the hydroxylysine content increased by a factor of three. Collagen I from DD patients is lysyl- but not prolyl-overhydroxylated, as compared to collagen I

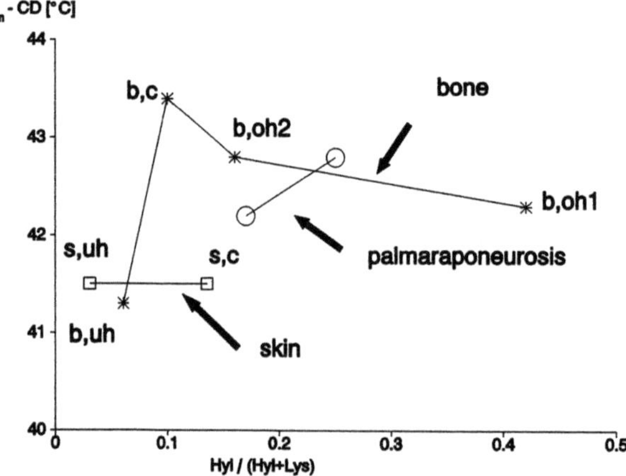

Fig. 6. Melting temperatures of collagen I from normal palmar aponeurosis and collagen I from Dupuytren's disease patients in relation to the relative hydroxylysine content (O) (*Hyl/Hyl* + *Lys*); *CD*, circular dichroism. The data from bone (*) and skin (□) are taken from Notbohm et al. (1992)

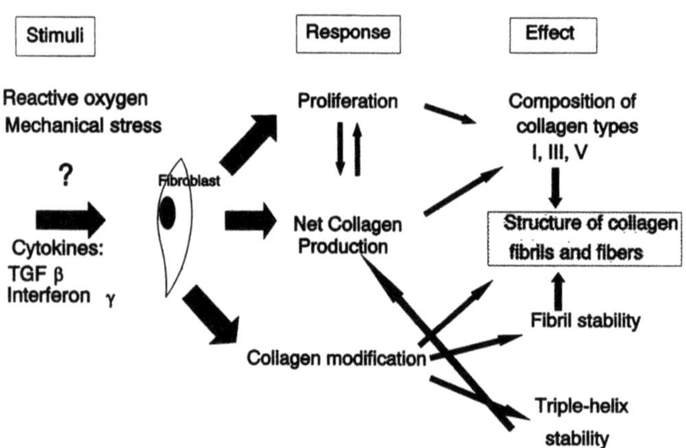

Fig. 7. Interactions initiated by heterotypic collagens and posttranslational modifications of collagen molecules

from normal palmar aponeurosis, and had a higher melting temperature. One can expect that collagen from a tissue with a deficient collagen mass (e.g., osteogenesis imperfecta; Brenner et al. 1989) would melt at a lower temperatures than collagen from tissue with a surplus of extracellular matrix (fibrosis).

Fibrils of tissue from DD patients were investigated by electron microscopy (Hunter and Ogdnon 1975). Most frequently, the tissue was described as consisting of more irregularly arranged fibrils which were also smaller in diameter. From our in vitro studies, we can conclude that overhydroxylated collagen I from DD nodules does not produce fibrils of smaller diameter. Therefore, changes in collagen type composition may play a dominant role in the formation of smaller fibrils. Furthermore, in agreement with in vivo observations that formation of thick bundles of fibers is impaired in DD nodules, the in vitro experiments demonstrated that fibrils did not tend to form bundles when greater amounts of collagen III were present in solution. The interdependencies of collagen metabolism and extracellular matrix formation are summarized in Fig. 7.

In conclusion, our observations provide preliminary evidence that changes in extracellular matrix biochemistry and structure do not initiate Dupuytren's contracture. The characteristics of these alterations strongly argue for a mechanism which induces an acceleration of fibrogenesis.

Acknowledgements. The authors thank C. Sesselmann and G. Buchholz for technical assistance.

References

Bätge B, Notbohm H, Diebold J, Lehmann H, Bodo M, Deutzmann R, Müller PK (1990) A critical crosslink region in human bone derived collagen type I. Eur J Biochem 192:153–159

Bailey AJ, Sims TJ, Gabbiani G, Bazin S, Le Lous M (1977) Collagen of Dupuytren's disease. Clinical Sci Molec Med 53:499–502

Birk D, Fitch JM, Babiarz JP, Doanne KJ, Linsenmayer TF (1990) Collagen fibrillogenesis in vitro: interaction of types I and V collagen regulates fibril diameter. J Cell Sci 95:649–657

Brenner RE, Vetter U, Nerlich A, Wörsdorfer O, Teller WM, Müller PK (1989) Biochemical analysis of callus tissue in osteogenesis imperfecta type IV. J Clin Invest 20:8–14

Brokaw JL, Doillon CJ, Hahn R, Birk DE, Berg RA, Silver FH (1985) Turbimetric and morphological studies of type I collagen fibre self assembly anf the influence of fibronectin. Int J Biol Macromol 7:135–140

Gabiani G, Majno G (1972) Dupuytren's contracture: fibroblast contraction? An ultrastructural study. Am J Pathol 66:131–146

Hueston JT (1990) Cell-controlling factors in Dupuytren's contracture. Ann Chir Main Memb Super 9(2):135–137

Hunter JAA, Ogdnon C (1975) Dupuytren's contracture II: scanning electron microscopic observations. Br J Plastic Surg 28:19–25

Laemli UK (1970) Cleavage of structural proteins during the assembly of the head of bacteriophage T4. Nature 227:680–685

Lapiere CM, Nusgens B, Pierard GE (1977) Interaction between collagen type I and III in conditioning bundles organisation. Connective Tiss Res 5:21–29

Menzel EJ (1984) Fibronectin in der Dupuytren'schen Kontraktur. Handchirurgie 16:164–167

Miller EJ, Rhodes RK (1982) Preparation and characterisation of the different types of collagen. Meth Enzymol 82:33–64

Notbohm H, Mosler S, Bodo M, Lehmann HW, Müller PK (1992) Comperative study on the thermostability of collagen I of skin and bone: Influence of posttranslational hydroxylation of prolyl and lysyl residues. J Protein Chem 11:635–643

Piez K (1984) Molecular and aggregate structures of the collagens. In: Piez KA, Redy AH (eds) Extracellular matrix biochemistry Elsevier, New York, pp 1–13

Romanic AM, Adachi E, Kadler KE, Hojima Y, Prockop DJ (1991) Copolymerisation of pNcollagen III and collagen I-pNcollagen -III. J Biol Chem 266:12703–12709

Scott JE (1988) Proteoglycan- fibrillar collagen interactions. Biochem J 252:313–323
Tomasek JJ, Schultz RJU, Haaksma (1987) Extracellular matrix-cytoskeletal connections at the surface of the specialized contractile fibroblast (myofibroblast) in Dupuytren's disease. J Bone Joint Surg 69(9):1400–1407
Tunn S, Gurr E, Pallasch Delbrück A, Buhr T, Flory J (1985) The distribution of unsulfated and sulfated glycosaminoglycans in Palmar Fascia from patients with Dupuytren's disease and healthy subjects. J Clin Chem Clin Biochem 23:77–87
Williams BR, Gelman RA, Poppke DC, Piez KAJ (1978) Collagen fibril formation. Biol Chem 253:6578–6585

Macrophage Activity, Fibronectin, and SPARC Protein in Experimentally Induced Granuloma

S. Shoshan, I. Babayof, I. Peleg, F. Grinnell, N. Ron, S. Funk, and E.H. Sage

Introduction

Repair of injured tissue is a sequence of events in which cells with distinct functions are attached to the wound, proliferate, and secrete extracellular matrix material to finally restore structure and function.

It has now become clear that migration to the site of injury, proliferation, and metabolic activity of fibroblasts are regulated by factors originating from platelets, monocytes/macrophages, lymphocytes, and connective tissue cells themselves [1–3].

The role of macrophage activity is of particular importance in view of the multiple involvement of these cells in the tissue repair process [4]. It is now well established that activated macrophages synthesize and secrete proteolytic enzymes, phagocytose cell and tissue debris, and bring about chemotactic migration of fibroblasts to the site of injury, owing to growth factors secreted by them; macrophages also play a key role, albeit indirectly, during the reparative phase of healing, i.e., during formation of the fibrous scar and its remodeling [5,6]. It has also been demonstrated that the prolonged presence of activated macrophages in experimentally induced granulation tissue results in a conspicuously increased deposition of collagen leading to fibrosis (S. Shoshan and L.M. Wahl, unpublished). Macrophage activity may thus affect the ultimate outcome either of a healing process following injury or during repair following various insults.

The ability of macrophages to phagocytose particulate matter is largely dependent on nonspecific opsonin found in plasma [7]. This opsonin, $\alpha2$-globulin, is known as fibronectin, a glycoprotein consisting of two similar but not identical subunits of about 230 kDa. Fibronectin is also a component of extracellular matrices and it also resides on cell surfaces. It is secreted into cell culture medium and is assembled into insoluble matrix under and/or around cultured cells such as fibroblasts, epithelial cells, and macrophages [8]. Fibronectins play an important role in tissue repair and wound healing by (a) affecting cell adhesion, (b) stimulating cell spreading, cell attachment and cell migration, and (c) taking part in formation of the initial deposition of connective tissue (granulation tissue) at the site of injury [9–11]. Thus, it has been shown that fibronectin depletion, due to its binding to gelatin following thermal injuries, brought about impairment of healing, while its supplementation improved the healing process [12–14].

Experimental studies on cultured cells and fibronectin-coated latex beads have shown that fibronectin acts as an opsonizing agent and, as such, enhanced phagocytic activity of macrophages, fibroblasts, and epithelial cells [15,16].

Another protein has been recently shown at sites of high cellular activity – turnover and remodeling – in a variety of tissues [17]. It was termed SPARC, because it is a secreted protein, acidic and rich in cysteine [18]. This is a calcium binding protein also known as osteonectin [19] and BM-40 [20]. The exact role of SPARC in developmental processes and cellular activities is not completely understood as yet. Most recent findings indicate the involvement of SPARC in inhibiting cell cycle progression in bovine aortic endothelial cells, resulting in the inhibition of cell proliferation. This finding led to the assumption that this function of SPARC may have a regulatory purpose: by inhibiting further proliferation of already proliferating cells, SPARC promotes other cellular events, such as migration [21].

The present study was initiated to examine whether the opsonizing effect of fibronectin could be demonstrated on macrophage activity in vivo using fibronectin-coated latex beads and whether SPARC is present in granulation tissue, which represents an environment in which cell and matrix turnover is markedly increased.

Material and Methods

Polyvinyl alcohol sponges (PVSs) were implanted subcutaneously on the back of 60 ether-anaesthesized guinea pigs, two sponges at each side of and along the vertebral column at an equidistance of 1 cm. In another series of 60 ether-anaesthesized guinea pigs, full-thickness dermal excision wounds, 7 mm in diameter, were inflicted on the back of the animals using a biopsy punch. The animals were divided into three groups as follows:

Group A: Untreated control group. Animals with wounds and PVSs received no treatment.

Group B: Uncoated latex beads. A suspension of latex beads was put onto the wound and into the PVS.

Group C: Fibronectin-coated latex beads [16]. A suspension of latex beads which were precoated with fibronectin were put onto the wounds and into the PVS.

After 5 days, 30 animals were killed with an overdose of pentobarbital; the other 30 animals were killed after 10 days. The granulation tissues from both the wounds and the PVSs were examined as follows: (1) histologically following fixation with Boin's fixative, parafin embedding, sectioning and staining with hematoxylin and eosin; (2) immunocytochemically using polyclonal antibodies to SPARC [17]. A few PVS samples were processed for scanning electron microscopic examination.

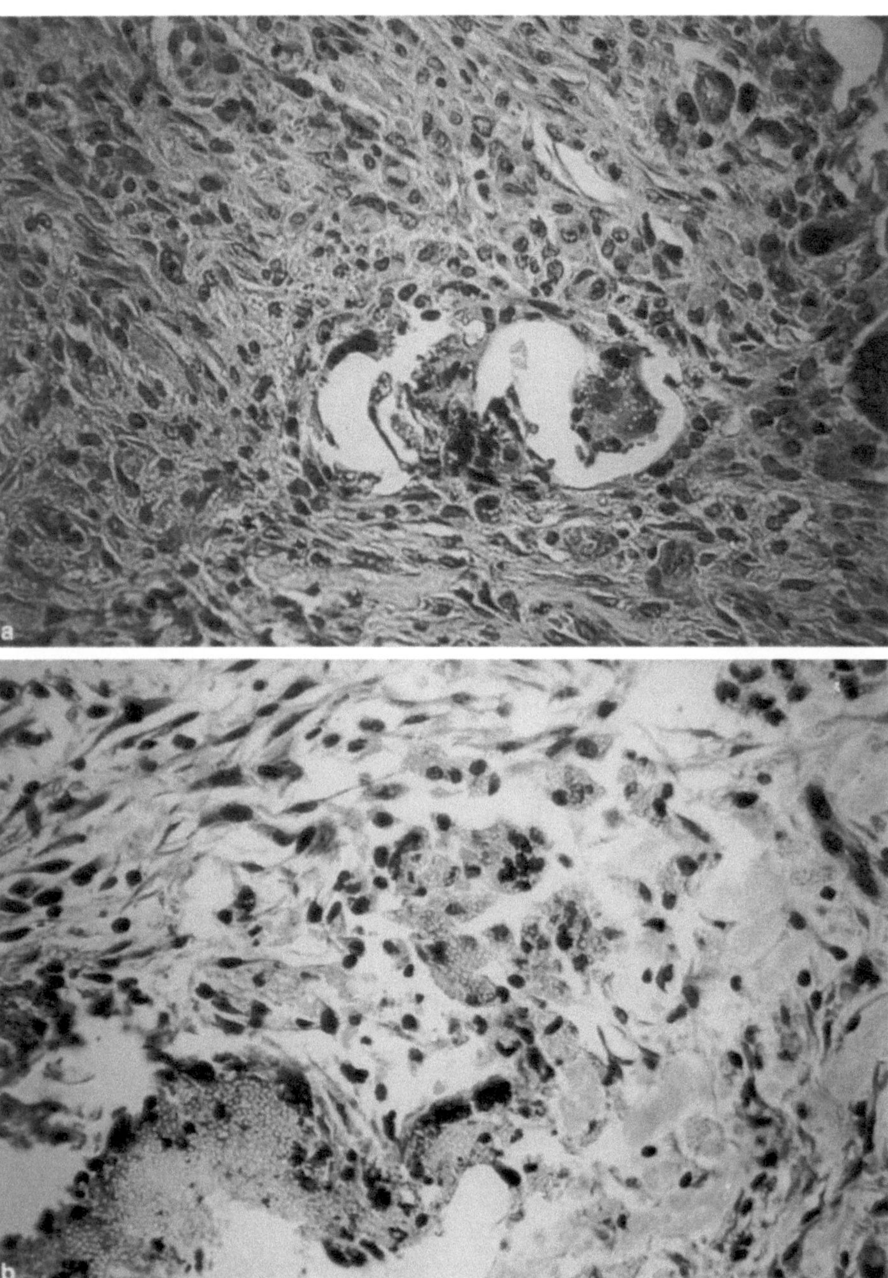

Fig. 1a,b. Photomicrographs of **a** 5 day wound granulation tissue with fibronectin-coated latex beads. Note engulfed beads by many cells, some of which have an extended cytoplasm and are multinucleated. **b** 5 day wound granulation tissue with uncoated latex beads. Note both the less densely arranged fibroblasts and the clusters of beads. Relatively few cells are seen with phagocytosed latex beads. H and E, ×500

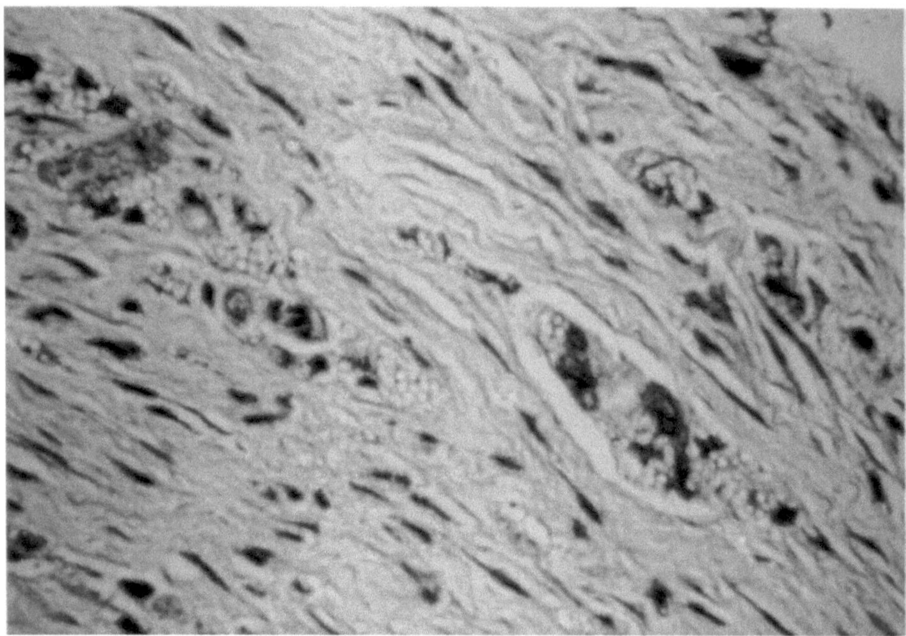

Fig. 2. Photomicrograph of a 10 day wound at a site away from the granulation tissue, in the hypodermis, to show residual macrophages with engulfed fibronectin-coated latex beads. H and E, ×500

Results

Excision Wounds

The granulation tissue at 5 days postwounding showed an abundance of macrophages with ingested fibronectin-coated beads, whereas the uncoated beads were seen in clusters in the interstitium and only a few were seen to be phagocytosed (Fig. 1).

At 10 days postwounding, uncoated latex beads were still seen in granulation tissue which showed typical features of the proliferative phase of healing, namely, a tissue rich in budding new capillaries directed towards the wound surface, invading fibroblasts, and a residual presence of components of the late inflammatory phase, including a few macrophages. This picture was very similar to that seen in the untreated controls.

The granulation tissue of wounds onto which fibronectin-coated latex beads were applied showed an entirely different histologic picture after 10 days: It was a dense fibroblast-rich tissue and, surprisingly, with almost complete disappearance of latex-loaded macrophages from the wound site. Only in a few instances were cells with engulfed latex beads in their cytoplasm detected somewhere away from the wound site, mostly in the hypodermis (Fig. 2). The granulation tissues from all the wounds were rich in SPARC, which was

216   S. Shoshan et al.

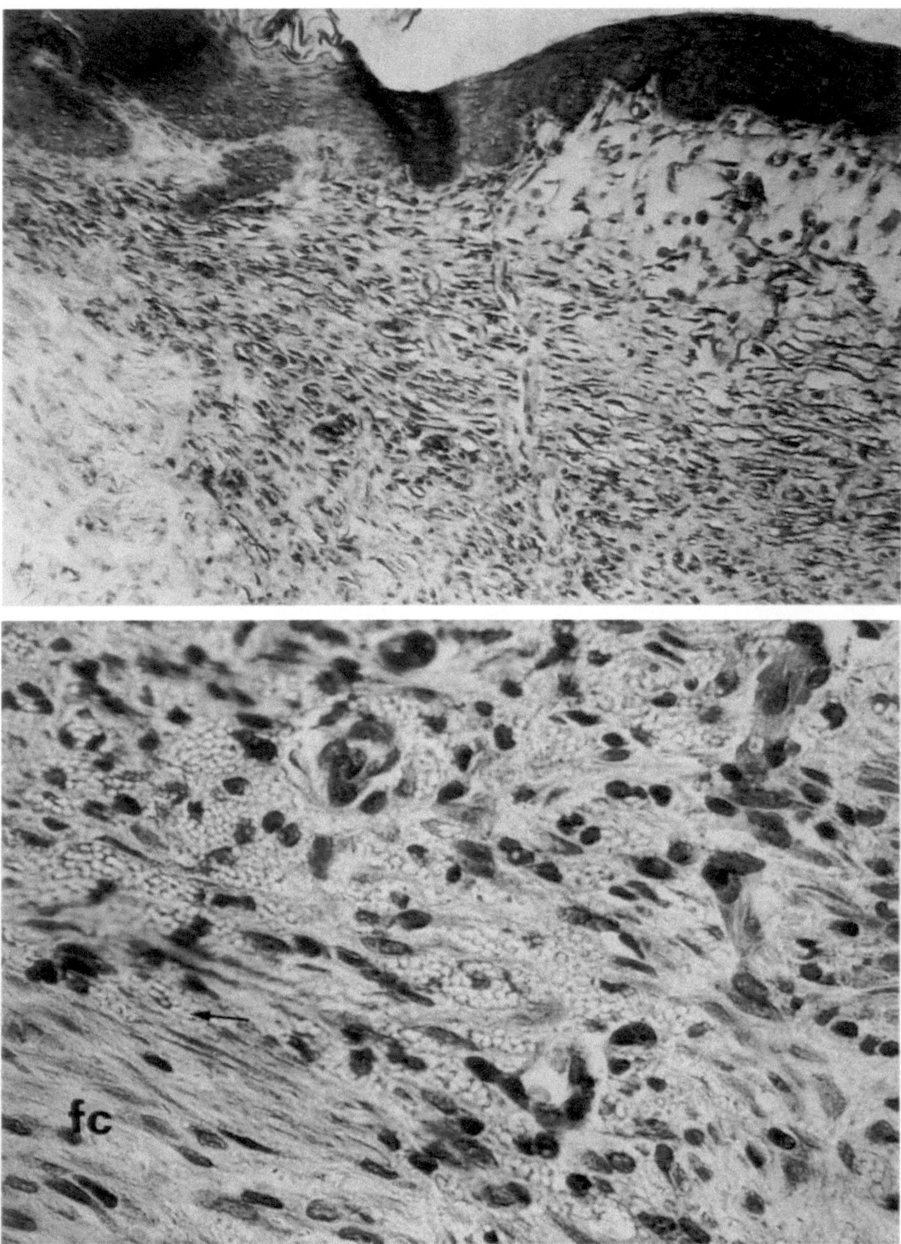

Fig. 3 *(above)*. Photomicrograph of a 10 day, wound to show SPARC in the granulation tissue in blood vessel walls and macrophages. No latex beads are present. H and E, ×125

Fig. 4 *(below)*. Photomicrograph of a section of polyvinyl alcohol sponge (PVS) to show fibronectin-coated latex beads engulfed by many cells including a fibroblast *(arrow)* 10 days after implantation. Note the thick dense fibrous capsule at the *lower left (fc)*. H and E, ×800

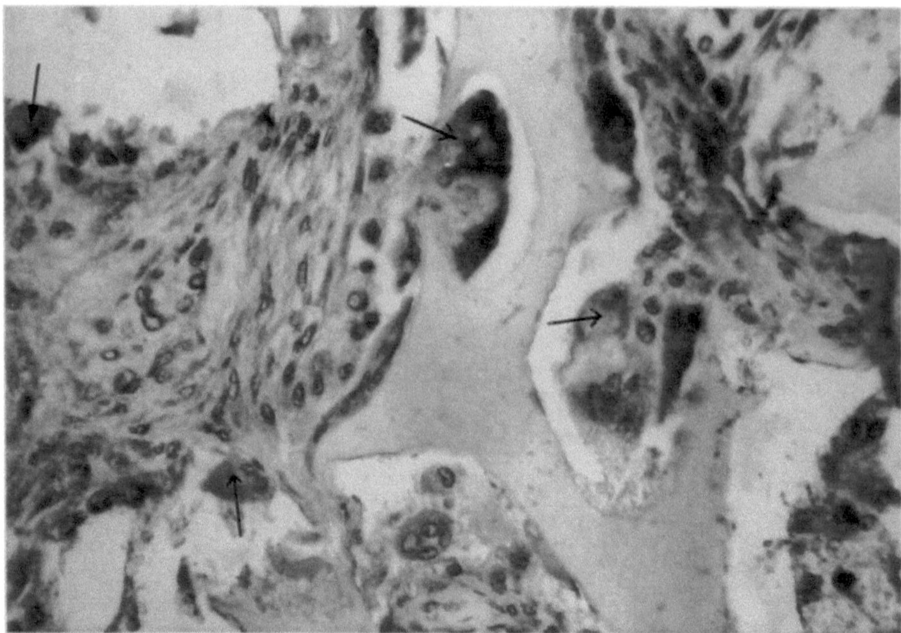

Fig. 5. Photomicrograph of a section of polyvinyl alcohol sponge (PVS) to show positive SPARC reactivity with anti-SPARC antibodies. Note positive reactions within multinucleated giant cells (*arrows*). Counterstained with H and E, ×500

Fig. 6a,b. Scanning electron micrograph of a polyvinyl alcohol sponge (PVS) 10 days after ▷ implantation. **a** Note the cluster of uncoated nonphagocytosed latex beads. × 1500. **b** Note phagocytosed and engulfed fibronectin-coated latex beads. ×3000

especially abundant in and near the cells of the newly sprouting blood vessels and in macrophages both with and without ingested latex beads (Fig. 3).

Polyvinyl Alcohol Sponges

The histologic picture of the granulation tissue that grew into the PVS which had been infiltrated with fibronectin-coated latex beads differed largely from that found in the PVS with uncoated latex beads after 5 days. The former showed macrophages with extended cytoplasm loaded with engulfed latex beads (Fig. 4), while the latter was distinguished by clusters of beads outside the cells.

A positive reactivity with anti-SPARC antibodies was found in cells in all PVSs after 5 and 10 days. However, unlike in the wounds, macrophages, multinucleated giant cells, and fibroblasts were seen laden with phagocytosed fibronectin-coated latex beads after 10 days (Fig. 5). Scanning electron microscopy demonstrates this phenomenon within the PVS (Fig. 6).

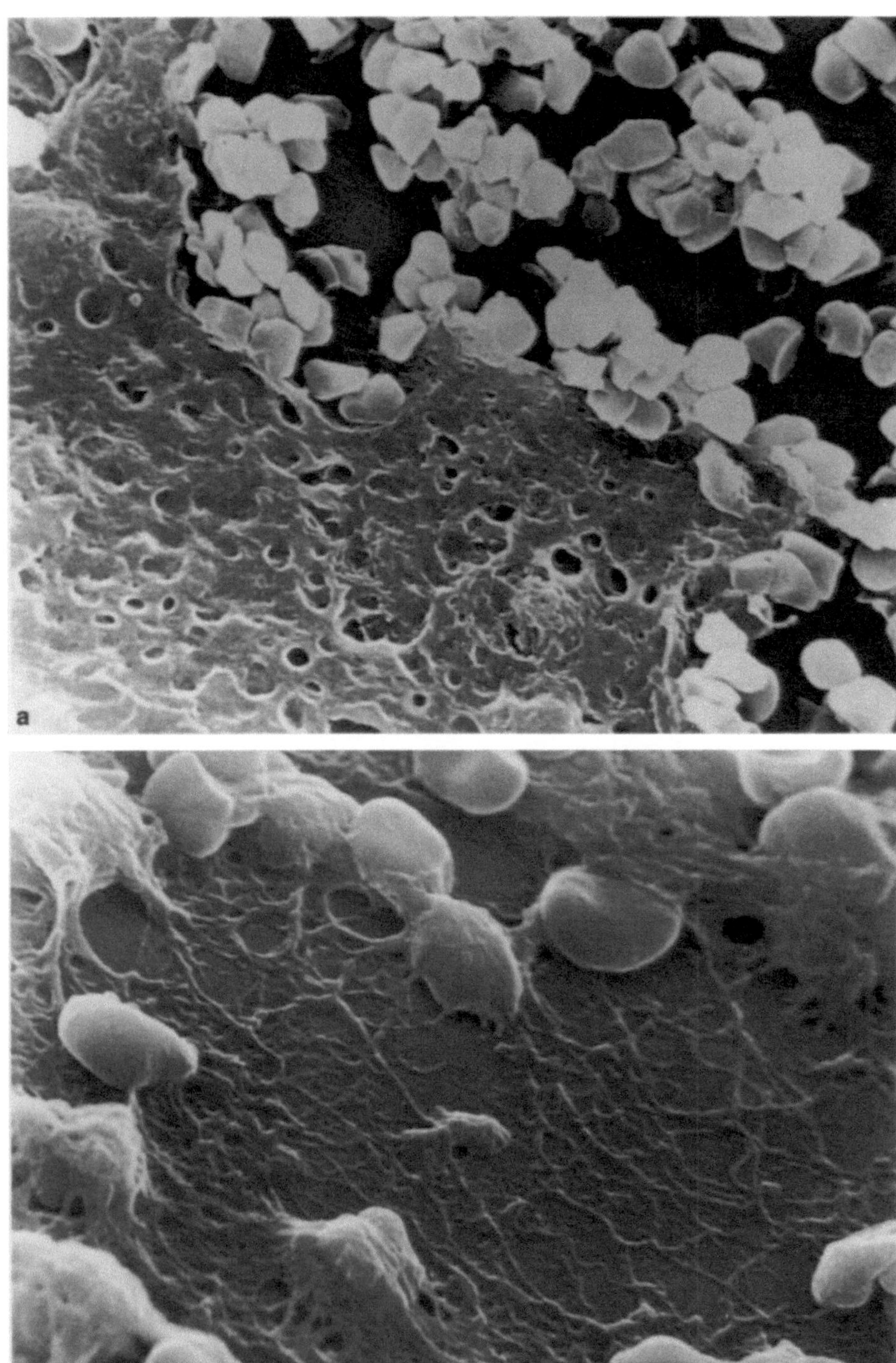

Discussion

The results obtained from these in vivo studies indicate the importance of fibronectin as an opsonizing agent which is instrumental in activating macrophage phagocytosing abilities in both wound granulation tissues and in a foreign body (PVS)-induced granuloma, as already shown in previous studies [9,10]. We found, however, an unexpected phenomenon in the healing excision wound, namely the relatively early and almost complete disappearance of macrophages from the granulation tissue together with the engulfed fibronectin-coated latex beads. The fact that the few macrophages which were detected were found at sites away from the wound, at the periphery or deep in the hypodermis, indicates an intensive removal mechanism which, we feel, deserves further investigation. The presence of SPARC protein in granulation tissue was not surprising in view of the active metabolic nature of that tissue and of the cells that populate it. Moreover, the finding of dense fibrous granulation tissue in the 10 day old wounds which were treated with fibronectin-coated latex beads corroborates the recently expressed idea [21] that SPARC may play a role in setting the stage for cell activities, such as migration, following prior proliferation. This seems to be of particular interest in association with the presence of fibronectin-activated macrophages and the observed increased fibroblast migration.

The histologic picture found in 10 day old granulomata in the PVS animals injected with fibronectin-coated latex beads was entirely different from that seen in the "open" excision wounds, namely, there were multiple, foreign body, multinucleated giant cells and singly nucleated macrophages laden with engulfed latex beads. This may be explained by the encapsulation of the granulomata with a rather thick fibrous capsule, thus preventing the "escape" of the laden macrophages. Thus, we suggest that both macrophages and fibronectin may play a role in the development of fibrotic lesions when the affected tissue is persistently activated by some factors. The activated tissue becomes rich in SPARC which in turn brings about migration of cells leading to fibrosis.

References

1. Shoshan S (1981) Wound healing. Int Rev Connect Tissue Res 9:1–26
2. Clark RA, Henson PM (eds) (1988) Molecular and cellular biology of wound repair. Plenum, New York
3. Wahl SM, Wahl LM (1981) Modulation of fibroblast growth and function by monokines and lymphokines. Lymphokines, vol 2: A forum for immunoregulatory cell products, p 179
4. Riches DWH (1988) The multiple roles of macrophages in wound-healing. In: Clark RA, Henson PM (eds) Molecular and cellular biology of wound repair. Plenum, New York, p 213
5. Werb Z, Gordon S (1975) Elastase secretion by stimulated macrophages. Characterization and regulation. J Exp Med 142:361–377
6. Leibovich SJ, Ross R (1976) A macrophage-dependent factor that stimulates the proliferation of fibroblasts in vitro. Am J Pathol 84:501–504

7. Blumenstock F, Saba TM, Weber P, Cho E (1976) Purification and biochemical characterization of a macrophage stimulating alpha-2-globulin opsonic protein. J Reticuloendothel Soc 19:157–172

8. McDonald JA (1988) Fibronectin – a primitive matrix. In: Clark RA, Henson PM (eds) Molecular and cellular biology of wound repair. Plenum, New York, p 405

9. Grinnell F (1984) Fibronectin and wound healing. J Cell Biochem 26:107–116

10. Grinnell F, Billingham RE, Burgess L (1986) Distribution of fibronectin during wound healing in vivo. J Invest Dermatol 76:181–189

11. Mosher DF (1984) Physiology of fibronectin. Annu Rev Med 35:561–575

12. Deno DC, McCafferty MH, Saba TM, Blumenstock FA (1984) Mechanism of acute depletion of plasma fibronectin following thermal injury in rats. Appearance of a gelatin like ligand in plasma. J Clin Invest 73:20–34

13. Nagelschmidt M, Becker D, Bonninghoff N, Engelhardt GH (1987) The effect of fibronectin therapy and fibronectin deficiency on healing of rat burns and excision wounds. Res Exp Med (Berl) 187:217–223

14. Nagelschmidt M, Becker D, Bonninghoff N, Engelhardt GH (1987) Effect of fibronectin therapy and fibronectin deficiency on wound healing: a study in rats. J Trauma 27:1267–1271

15. Takashima A, Grinnell F (1984) Human keratinocyte adhesion and phagocytosis promoted by fibronectin. J Invest Dermatol 83:352–358

16. Grinnell F, Geiger B (1986) Interaction of fibronectin-coated beads with attached and spread fibroblasts. Binding, phagocytosis, and cytoskeletal reorganization. Exp Cell Res 162:449–461

17. Sage EH, Vernon RB, Decker J, Funk S, Iruela-Arispe ML (1989) Distribution of the calcium-binding protein SPARC in tissues of embryonic and adult mice. J Histochem Cytochem 37:819–829

18. Mason IJ, Taylor A, Williams JG, Sage EH, Hogan BL (1986) Evidence from molecular cloning that SPARC, a major product of mouse embryo parietal endoderm, is related to an endothelial cell 'culture shock' glycoprotein of Mr 43 000. EMBO J 5:1465–1472

19. Termine JD, Kleinman HK, Whitson SW, Conn KM, McGarvey ML, Martin GR (1981) Osteonectin, a bone-specific protein linking mineral to collagen. Cell 26:99–105

20. Dziadek M, Paulsson M, Aumailley M, Timpl R (1986) Purification and tissue distribution of a small protein (BM-40) extracted from a basement membrane tumor. Eur J Biochem 161:455–464

21. Funk SE, Sage EH (1991) The Ca2(+)-binding glycoprotein SPARC modulates cell cycle progression in bovine aortic endothelial cells. Proc Natl Acad Sci USA 88:2648–2652

Modulation of Fibroblastic Cytoskeletal Features During Dupuytren's Disease

G. Gabbiani

The mechanisms leading to retraction of the palmar fascia during Dupuytren's disease have not, at present, been fully elucidated (for review see [1]). Several years ago, our laboratory described the presence within the nodule of fibroblasts having several ultrastructural features of smooth muscle cells, including microfilament bundles with dense bodies scattered within [2]. These cells, called myofibroblasts, have been proposed to play a retractile role in several conditions such as granulation tissue contraction, parenchymal organ retraction, fibromatosis, and the stromal reaction to epithelial tumors (for review see [3]). The coincidence of the presence of myofibroblasts with retractile phenomena has supported this hypothesis. However, direct proof of the presence and activity of contractile elements in myofibroblasts was possible only after suitable techniques were developed to localize and quantify cytoskeletal and contractile proteins within the affected organs. For this purpose, advances in our understanding of cytoskeletal and contractile element morphology and biochemistry in different cells have been of great help (for review see [4]). Presently, we know that the cytoskeleton of mesenchymal cells is composed of intermediate filaments which consist of a single protein, vimentin. In muscle cells, however, most of the intermediate filaments have been shown to contain another related, but not identical, protein, desmin. Nonetheless, vascular smooth muscle cells always express vimentin and only a portion of them additionally contain desmin. Desmin has been increasingly found in a number of nonmuscle mesenchymal cells such as endothelial cells [5, 6], podocytes [7], and stromal cells from various locations [7–10]. Vimentin and desmin thus serve as markers of tissue origin. Another such marker is the presence of a specific actin isoform, since the six actin isoforms expressed in mammalian tissue show a tissue-specific distribution [4]. For example, α-smooth muscle actin is present in all smooth muscle cells. Finally, isoforms of myosin heavy and light chains can also be typical of smooth muscle (particularly under normal conditions) and hence help in the identification of cells involved in different pathological changes [11]. Using different markers, we have defined four cytoskeletal phenotypes among myofibroblasts: (1) phenotype V represented by myofibroblasts positive for vimentin only; (2) phenotype VA represented by myofibroblasts positive for vimentin and α-smooth muscle actin; (3) phenotype VAD represented by myofibroblasts

Table 1. Cytoskeletal features of normal soft tissue and of nonmalignant soft tissue proliferative lesions

Tissue type	Total number of cases	Number of cases containing V cells	Number of cases containing VA cells	Number of cases containing VAD cells	Number of cases containing VD cells
Normal soft tissue	10	10	0	0	0
Normally healing granulation tissue	8	8	0	0	0
Eschar	2	2	0	0	0
Normally healed scar	18	18	0	0	0
Hypertrophic scar	15	15	15	4	0
Superficial (fascial) fibromatosis[a]					
Palmar	25	25	25	22	0
Plantar	2	2	2	2	0
Deep (musculoaponeurotic) fibromatosis					
Extraabdominal	8	8	8	6	1
Abdominal	5	5	5	4	1
Intraabdominal fibromatosis (Gardner's syndrome)	1	1	0	0	1
Stromal reaction to mammary carcinoma	10	10	10	3	0

V cells, myofibroblasts positive for vimentin only; VA cells, myofibroblasts positive for vimentin and α-smooth muscle actin; VAD cells, myofibroblasts positive for vimentin, α-smooth muscle actin, and desmin; VD cells, myofibroblasts positive for vimentin and desmin.
[a] Results presented are from proliferative nodules.

positive for vimentin, α-smooth muscle actin, and desmin; and (4) phenotype VD represented by myofibroblasts positive for vimentin and desmin. When we studied normally healing granulation tissue with these criteria, we found that during granulation tissue contraction a large proportion of myofibroblasts develop expression of α-smooth muscle actin but not desmin and smooth muscle myosin [12], and hence acquire, at least in part, smooth muscle features. When contraction stops and the wound is fully epithelialized, myofibroblastic cells containing α-smooth muscle actin disappear, probably by apoptosis. The scar becomes classically less cellular and composed of typical fibroblasts with well developed rough endoplasmic reticulum; there are no microfilaments or α-smooth muscle actin. In more permanent retractile conditions, and in particular in Dupuytren's Disease, myofibroblasts expressing α-smooth muscle actin are constantly present, and furthermore some of them also express desmin [13] (Table 1). However, at present, myofibroblasts expressing smooth muscle myosin have not been described [11,14]. This is typical of Dupuytren's nodule, whereas in cordae tendineae fibroblasts do not express any smooth muscle cytoskeletal features, thus more closely resembling scar fibroblasts than nodular fibroblasts [1]. On the basis of these results, we propose that, during the development of Dupuytren's Disease, fibroblasts acquire contractile features and produce the centripetal force leading to palmar retraction. For this purpose, myofibroblasts have the capacity of developing connections to the surrounding extracellular matrix and hence to act on the whole tissue [3]. Traction, rather than contraction, forces have been shown to be responsible for the retractile activity of cultured fibroblasts on their substratum [15]. In analogy with these observations, we suggest that the retractile activity of myofibroblasts during Dupuytren's disease is more dependent on isometric than on isotonic contraction.

The mechanisms leading to the development of cytoskeletal features similar to those of smooth muscle cells in fibroblasts, including the factors which regulate the appearance of α-smooth muscle actin and desmin in vivo and in vitro are as yet unknown. The more likely candidates are cytokines, which can be locally liberated by vascular cells, inflammatory cells and fibroblastic cells themselves, and extracellular matrix components, which have been shown to influence the shape, replication, and development of cytoskeletal features in fibroblastic and smooth muscle cells (for review see [3]). Working along these lines, we have observed that γ-interferon, a cytokine mainly produced by T helper lymphocytes, is capable of inhibiting the expression of α-smooth muscle actin in both smooth muscle [16] and fibroblastic [17] cells. When γ-interferon is applied to Dupuytren's nodules, it produces an improvement of the retractile condition. In hypertrophic scars, in addition to reduction of the size of the lesion, γ-interferon elicits the disappearance of α-smooth muscle actin in myofibroblasts (unpublished observation). Although further studies are needed to confirm these preliminary results, we feel that work in these directions can help not only in understanding the pathogenesis of Dupuytren's disease, but also suggest future directions for treatment. In this respect, we have observed, in an experimental model in the rat in vivo, that application of granulocyte/ macrophage-colony stimulating factor (GM-CSF) to rat subcutaneous tissue induces not only the proliferation of fibroblasts and the formation of ultrastructurally typical myofibroblasts, but also the expression of α-smooth muscle actin in a significant proportion of these cells [18]. GM-CSF is mainly known for its hematopoietic effect [19], but some extrahematopoietic activity has been attributed to this factor. Thus, GM-CSF stimulates migration of human endothelial cells [19] and in vitro proliferation of different nonhematopoietic cells of mesenchymal origin, such as endothelial cells [20], bone marrow fibroblast precursors, and several transformed cell lines [21]. Moreover, in transgenic mice expressing GM-CSF, fibrotic nodules developed in areas where macrophages accumulate [22]. These lesions have been interpreted as occurring following chronic macrophage activation induced by GM-CSF. However, another study did not detect any side effects in response to long-term GM-CSF treatment in mice [23]. Clearly, these results need further study in order to be confirmed, but they indicate that progress in understanding cytokine influence on fibroblastic cells may furnish explanations of the mechanisms leading to the development of a contractile phenotype in fibroblasts. It is well known that heparin and heparan sulfates inhibit smooth muscle cell replication and increase the expression of α-smooth muscle actin in these cells [24]. We have also observed that heparin and heparan sulfates exert a similar action on fibroblastic cells, and hence they could also participate in the regulation of the fibroblastic phenotype during wound healing and different retractile diseases [25].

In conclusion, the early observation that fibroblasts modify their phenotype during wound healing and fibrocontractive diseases has been supported by several biochemical and functional studies which support the idea that myofibroblasts are a key cell in understanding retractile phenomena. Further studies on the factors regulating the phenotype of myofibroblasts will probably be useful for understanding their behavior in vivo and possibly modifying this behavior in different clinical settings.

Acknowledgements. This work has been supported in part by the Swiss National Science Foundation, grant number 3.108-0.88. We thank Mrs. M.-M. Rossire for typing the manuscript.

References

1. Schürch W, Skalli O, Gabbiani G (1990) Cellular biology. In: McFarlane RM, McGrouther DA, Flint MH (eds) Dupuytren's disease: biology and treatment. Churchill Livingstone, Edinburgh, pp 31–47 (The hand and upper limb, vol 5)
2. Gabbiani G, Majno G (1972) Dupuytren's contracture: fibroblast contraction? Am J Pathol 66:131–146
3. Sappino AP, Schürch W, Gabbiani G (1990) Differentiation repertoire of fibroblastic cells: expression of cytoskeletal proteins as marker of phenotypic modulations. Lab Invest 63:144–161
4. Skalli O, Gabbiani G (1990) The biology of the myofibroblast and its relation to the development of soft tissue and epithelial tumours. In: Fletcher CDM, McKee PH (eds) Pathobiology of soft tissue tumours. Churchill Livingstone, Edinburgh, pp 83–103
5. Fujimoto T, Singer SJ (1986) Immunocytochemical studies of endothelial cells in vivo. I. The presence of desmin only, or of desmin plus vimentin, or vimentin only, in the endothelial cells of different capillaries of the adult chicken. J Cell Biol 103:2775–2786
6. Toccanier-Pelte MF, Skalli O, Kapanci Y, Gabbiani G (1987) Characterization of stromal cells with myoid features in lymph nodes and spleen in normal and pathologic conditions. Am J Pathol 129:109–118
7. Stamenkovic I, Skalli O, Gabbiani G (1986) Distribution of intermediate filament proteins in normal and diseased human glomeruli. Am J Pathol 125:465–475
8. Glasser SR, Julian J (1986) Intermediate filament protein as a marker of uterine stromal cell decidualization. Biol Reprod 35:436–474
9. Skalli O, Ropraz P, Trzeciak A, Benzonana G, Gillessen D, Gabbiani G (1986) A monoclonal antibody against α-smooth muscle actin: a new probe for smooth muscle differentiation. J Cell Biol 103:2787–2796
10. Franke WW, Moll R (1987) Cytoskeletal components of lymphoid organs. I. Synthesis of cytokeratins 8 and 18 and desmin in subpopulations of extrafollicular reticulum cells of human lymph nodes, tonsils and spleen. Differentiation 36:145–163
11. Benzonana G, Skalli O, Gabbiani G (1988) Correlation between the distribution of smooth muscle or non muscle myosins and α-smooth muscle actin in normal and pathological soft tissues. Cell Motil Cytoskeleton 11:260–274
12. Darby I, Skalli O, Gabbiani G (1990) α-smooth muscle actin is transiently expressed by myofibroblasts during experimental wound healing. Lab Invest 63:21–29
13. Skalli O, Schürch W, Seemayer T, Lagacé R, Montandon D, Pittet B, Gabbiani G (1989) Myofibroblasts from diverse pathologic settings are heterogeneous in their content of actin isoforms and intermediate filament proteins. Lab Invest 60:275–285

14. Eddy RJ, Petro JA, Tomasek JJ (1988) Evidence for the nonmuscle nature of the "myofibroblast" of granulation tissue and hypertrophic scar. An immunofluorescence study. Am J Pathol 130:252–260
15. Harris AK, Stopak D, Wild P (1981) Fibroblast traction as a mechanism for collagen morphogenesis. Nature 290:249
16. Hansson GK, Hellstrand M, Rymo L, Rubbia L, Gabbiani G (1989) Interferon γ inhibits both proliferation and expression of differentiation-specific α-smooth muscle actin in arterial smooth muscle cells. J Exp Med 170:1595–1608
17. Desmoulière A, Rubbia-Brandt L, Abdiu A, Walz T, Macieira-Coelho A, Gabbiani G (1992) α-Smooth muscle actin is expressed in a subpopulation of cultured and cloned fibroblasts and is modulated by γ-interferon. Exp Cell Res 201:64–73
18. Rubbia-Brandt L, Sappino AP, Gabbiani G (1991) Locally applied GM-CSF induces the accumulation of α-smooth muscle actin containing myofibroblasts. Virchows Arch [B] 60:73–82
19. Clark SC, Kamen R (1987) The human hematopoietic colony-stimulating factors. Science 236:1229–1237
20. Bussolino F, Wang JM, Defilippi P, Turrini F, Sanavio F, Edgell CJS, Aglietta M, Arese P, Mantovani A (1989) Granulocyte- and granulocyte-macrophage-colony stimulating factors induce human endothelial cells to migrate and proliferate. Nature 337:471–473
21. Dedhar S, Gaboury L, Galloway P, Eaves C (1988) Human granulocyte-macrophage colony-stimulating factor is a growth factor active on a variety of cell types of nonhemopoietic origin. Proc Natl Acad Sci USA 85:9253–9257
22. Lang RA, Metcalf D, Cuthbertson RA, Lyons I, Stanley E, Kelso A, Kannourakis G, Williamson DJ, Klintworth GK, Gonda TJ, Dunn AR (1987) Transgenic mice expressing a hemopoietic growth factor gene (GM-CSF) develop accumulations of macrophages, blindness, and a fatal syndrome of tissue damage. Cell 51:675–686
23. Pojda Z, Molineux G, Dexter TM (1989) Effects of long-term in vivo treatment of mice with purified murine recombinant GM-CSF. Exp Hematol 17:1100–1104
24. Clowes AW, Clowes M, Kocher O, Ropraz P, Chaponnier C, Gabbiani G (1988) Arterial smooth muscle cells in vivo: relationship between actin isoform expression and mitogenesis and their modulation by heparin. J Cell Biol 107:1939–1945
25. Desmoulière A, Rubbia-Brandt L, Grau G, Gabbiani G (1992) Heparin induces α-smooth muscle actin expression in cultured fibroblasts and in granulation tissue myofibroblasts. Lab Invest 67:716–726

Oxygen Free Radicals and Dupuytren's Disease

G.A.C. Murrell and M.J.O. Francis

Introduction

Dupuytren's contracture is associated with increasing age [1], sex (M > F) [1], diabetes mellitus [2,3], heavy alcohol consumptior [4], HIV infection [5], cigarette smoking [6], epilepsy [7] and Colles' fractures [8], but rarely with rheumatoid arthritis [9]. Two important features of the palmar fascia of Dupuytren's contracture are an increase in the number of fibroblasts [10], and an increase in the relative amounts of type III collagen [11]. It is likely that these phenomena are associated, as fibroblasts cultured at high density decrease type I collagen production and thus increase the relative amounts of type III collagen [12]. Changes in the glycosaminoglycan content can also be explained by high cell density [13].

The question remains: what are the stimuli for fibroblast proliferation? Evidence for localized ischemia [14] (van Lacken and Gropper, in preparation) and preliminary clinical results indicating that allopurinol may improve Dupuytren's contracture [15,16] suggest that xanthine oxidase-catalyzed free radical release may be important in the pathogenesis of Dupuytren's contracture.

What Is a Free Radical?

A free radical is any group of atoms capable of independent existence that contain one or more unpaired electrons (an unpaired electron is one that occupies an atomic or molecular orbital by itself). The presence of one or more unpaired electrons causes the species to be attracted slightly to a magnetic field and sometimes makes the species highly reactive.

Consideration of the above broad definition shows that there are many free radicals in chemistry and biology. Free radicals may be formed by radiolysis (decomposition of a chemical compound by the action of ionizing radiation), photolysis (decomposition of a chemical compound by the action of radiant energy from light), homolysis (splitting of a group of atoms into one or more groups of atoms), and during oxygen reduction reactions. They have half lives in the order of milliseconds. An important principle of free radical chemistry is that the reaction of a free radical with a nonradical species produces a different free radical, which may be more or less reactive than the original radical. Reactivity depends on availability of reaction pathways as well as the "intrinsic" reactivity of the free radical species.

Oxygen Free Radicals

Oxygen as it occurs naturally has two unpaired electrons and hence qualifies as a radical. Oxygen is a good oxidizing agent, i.e., good at absorbing electrons from the molecule it oxidizes. If a single electron is added to the ground state O_2 molecule the product is the superoxide radical (O_2^-). Addition of a further electron will given O_2^{2-}, the peroxide anion (with no unpaired electrons), which readily becomes hydrogen peroxide (H_2O_2). Although H_2O_2 is not a free radical, it is an integral part of the free radical cascade and for this reason is often classified with free radical species. Traces of the transition metal ions Fe^{2+} and Cu^{2+} can catalyze the reaction of O_2^- with H_2O_2 to form the hydroxyl radical (OH·) (via the Haber-Weiss reaction).

Free Radicals in Medicine

Oxygen free radicals are becoming recognized as being important in more and more physiological and pathological processes. The roles for oxygen free radicals in the bactericidal activities of phagocytic cells and in mediating tissue damage after acute ischemia are now well established [17,18]. During ischemia the purine bases xanthine and hypoxanthine accumulate and endothelial xanthine dehydrogenase is converted to xanthine oxidase (Fig. 1). The purine base-xanthine oxidase reaction releases superoxide (O_2^-) and hydrogen peroxide (H_2O_2), which in high concentrations are toxic to tissues and cultured cells.

To determine if free radicals could be important in the pathogenesis of Dupuytren's contracture we measured the concentration of substrates able to react with exogenous xanthine oxidase to produce O_2^- in Dupuytren's and control palmar fascia. These substrates are most likely to be hypoxanthine and xanthine; for clarity they are expressed as hypoxanthine concentrations. A sixfold increase in hypoxanthine was found in Dupuytren's palmar fascia compared with control palmar fascia (Fig. 2). In a single large piece of Dupuytren's tissue examined and sectioned, the hypoxanthine concentration increased with cell density and was two times greater in tissue classified as "nodule" 0.32 (SE 0.03) than in "cord" 0.14 (SE 0.03) µmol hypoxanthine/g wet weight; ($p < 0.005$). The mean xanthine oxidase activity in Dupuytren's contracture tissue from six patients was 13 (SE 6.1); range (1–41) mU/g wet weight. Samples of normal palmar fascia from control patients were too small for the xanthine oxidase activity assay [19].

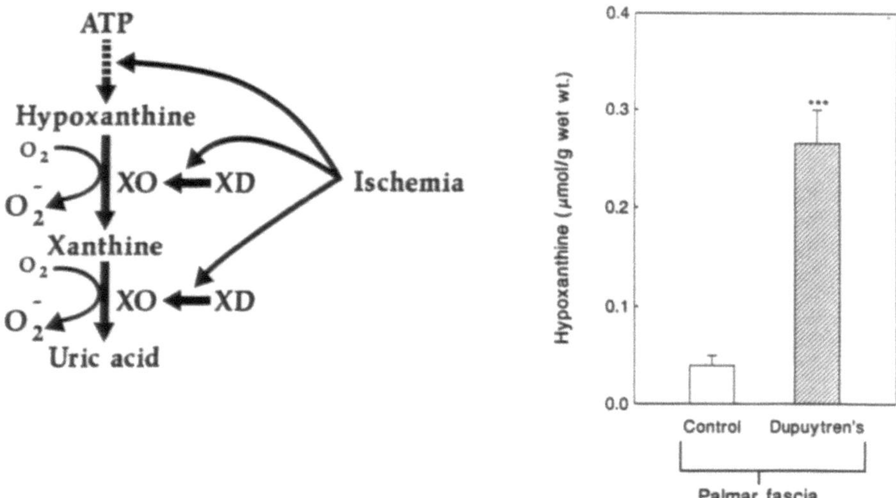

Fig. 1 *(left)*. The mechanism for ischemia-induced free radical damage. *ATP*, adenosine triphosphate; *XO*, xanthine oxidase, *XD*, xanthine dehydrogenase

Fig. 2 *(right)*. Hypoxanthine concentrations in control and Dupuytren's palmar fascia. $n = 10$ for both groups; mean (SEM), ***$p < 0.001$

Oxygen Free Radicals Stimulate Fibroblast Proliferation

The effects of oxygen free radicals on cultured human fibroblasts were then examined. Passage 3–5 fibroblasts from skin biopsies or operative Dupuytren's contracture palmar fascia specimens were cultured in Dulbecco's modification of Eagle's medium (DMEM) supplemented with 10% (v/v) fetal calf serum. Each well of a 1.6 cm 24 multiwell tissue culture plate was seeded with 4×10^4 fibroblasts and cultured for 48 h (near confluence). The medium was then replaced with 1.0 ml of media containing the agents to be tested. In thymidine incorporation experiments, this media also contained 1.0 µCi [^{3}H]thymidine and carrier thymidine to a final concentration of 5.0 µM thymidine. After 4 h of incubation at 37°C the cell layer was harvested, processed, and the radioactive, acid insoluble fraction measured by liquid scintillation spectrometry to give an estimation of the rate of cell proliferation. Cell density was determined using a 1 mm^2 eyepiece graticule at 6 and 24 h. Cell morphology parameters were calculated at 4 h using a Zeiss modulator system for quantitative digital image analysis (MOP AM02) [20].

Oxygen free radicals were generated by three systems (xanthine oxidase and hypoxanthine, glyceraldehyde in phosphate buffered saline and H_2O_2). Oxygen free radicals in high concentrations ($>10^{-3}$ U/ml xanthine oxidase with $10^{-3} M$ hypoxanthine; $>10^{-4} M$ H_2O_2; $>10^{-3} M$ glyceraldehyde) visibly damaged cultured human fibroblasts, reduced cell density and inhibited thymidine incorporation. In contrast, lower concentrations of free radicals (10^{-4}–10^{-7} U/ml xanthine oxidase; 10^{-4}–$10^{-6} M$ glyceraldehyde; $10^{-6} M$ H_2O_2) stimulated

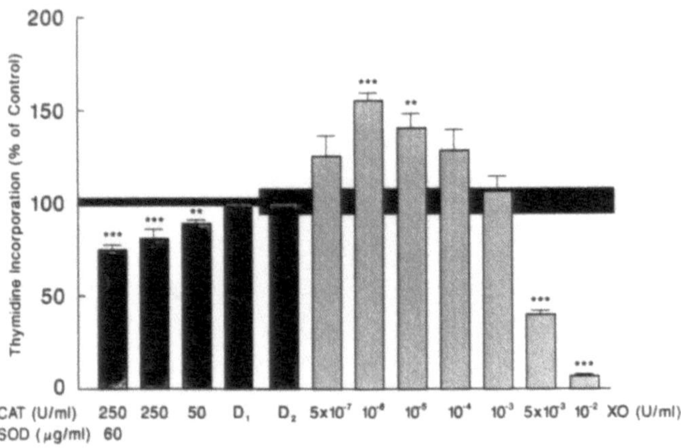

Fig. 3. Modulation of fibroblast proliferation by oxygen free radicals. The results of two separate experiments are drawn on the same axes for comparison. *Right*, exogenous free radicals have been introduced by the addition of increasing concentrations of xanthine oxidase (*XO*) to media containing $10^{-3} M$ hypoxanthine. Control (D_2), 10^{-2} U/ml xanthine oxidase heat denatured at 100°C for 15 min. Mean thymidine incorporated in control group was 13 pmol/10^6 cells. *Left*, no exogenous free radicals have been added and endogenous O_2^- or H_2O_2 has been scavenged by superoxide dismutase (*SOD*) and catalase (*CAT*), respectively. Control (D_1), 250 U/ml heat denatured CAT and 60 µg/ml heat denatured SOD. Mean thymidine incorporated in control group was 53 pmol/10^6 cells. Expressed as mean ± SEM % of control; $n = 6$. *Significantly different from control (*$p < 0.05$; **$p < 0.01$, ***$p < 0.001$ by two-tailed Students's t-test). (From [20])

thymidine incorporation and increased mean cell area, maximum length and cell density (Fig. 3). Both the stimulatory and inhibitory effects of xanthine oxidase were inhibited if xanthine oxidase was heat inactivated for 10 min at 100°C or $10^{-4} M$ allopurinol (a competitive inhibitor of xanthine oxidase) was added, or O_2^- and H_2O_2 scavengers added (60 µg/ml superoxide dismutase and 250 U/ml catalase) [20]. The results were similar for each of the cell lines, and have been confirmed by other authors in other transformed and nontransformed fibroblast cell lines [21].

Superoxide Release by Cultured Fibroblasts

O_2^- release was estimated using the superoxide dismutase inhibitable reduction of cytochrome c [22,23]. For each parameter assessed half of the wells were incubated with 60 µg/ml superoxide dismutase and half without. The final volume of the reaction mixture was 1.0 ml. After incubation at 37°C for 80 min without agitation, reactions were terminated by addition of 1.0 ml of 2 mM N-ethylmaleimide. The amount of O_2^- release was determined by dividing the average difference in absorbance at 550 nm in samples cultured with and without superoxide dismutase by the extinction coefficient for reduction of cytochrome c.

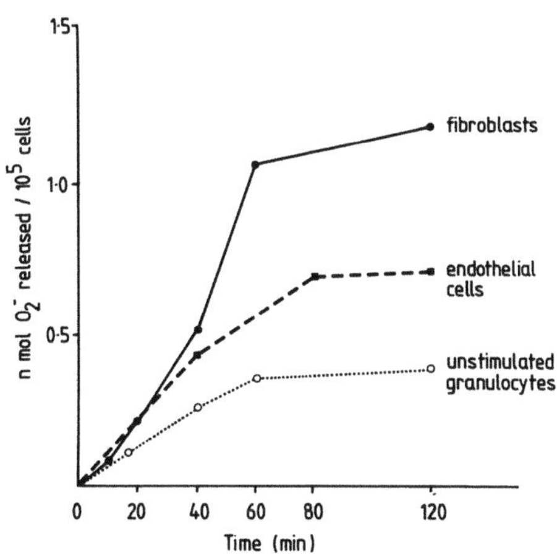

Fig. 4. Time course of O_2^- release by cultured fibroblasts compared with endothelial cells and unstimulated granulocytes. Each point is the mean of a triplicate incubation. (Adapted from [20])

In this system there was a superoxide dismutase inhibitable reduction in cytochrome c that increased with time and cell density. The shape of the O_2^- release vs fibroblast seeding density curve was similar to that previously observed for stimulated granulocytes[23], while the time course of O_2^- release by cultured fibroblasts was similar in form and magnitude to both unstimulated granulocytes and endothelial cells [20,23] (Fig. 4). Superoxide release doubled when cultured fibroblasts were agitated at 2 cycles/s. It is important to note that the stimulatory effect of phorbol myristate acetate (PMA) on O_2^- release by fibroblasts was 10- to 15-fold less than that observed in hagocytic cells. The lower magnitude of O_2^- release compared with phagocytes is in keeping with its role in connective tissues. The source of O_2^- release by cultured fibroblasts is likely to be a plasma membrane bound NADPH oxidase [24]. Xanthine oxidase catalyzed reactions were not a significant source of O_2^-, as addition of $10^{-4} M$ allopurinol in the presence of $10^{-4} M$ hypoxanthine did not alter O_2^- release.

Modulation of Fibroblast Proliferation by Oxygen Free Radicals

The rate of O_2^- release by cultured fibroblasts was equivalent to that which stimulated fibroblast proliferation, while the rate of O_2^- release by phagocytic cells was equivalent to that which damaged and inhibited fibroblast proliferation. Furthermore, fibroblast proliferation could be reduced by inhibiting endogenous free radical release (Fig. 3). These and other observations of inhibition of fibroblast chemotaxis with free radical scavengers [25] suggest that oxygen free radicals may have the ability to modulate fibroblast proliferation and chemotaxis.

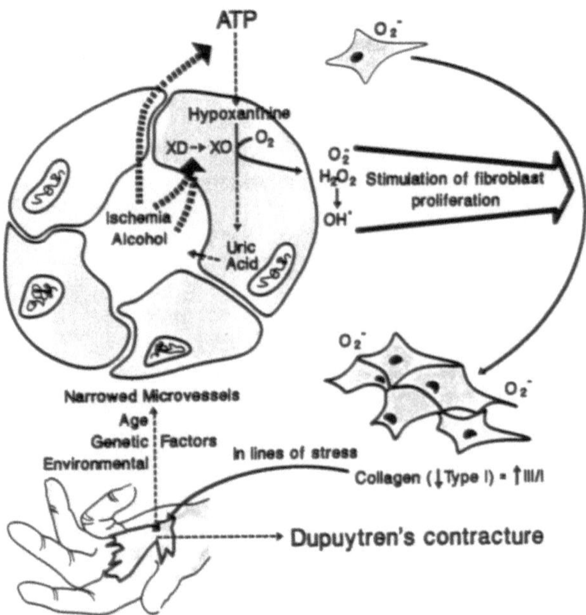

Fig. 5. Hypothesis for Dupuytren's contracture. (Adapted from [10])

Hypothesis

These biochemical and morphological observations have thrown new light on Dupuytren's contracture. They suggest that a number of factors (genetic, age, sex, race) may lead to the characteristic thickening of endothelial cells, lamination of the basal lamina and narrowing of the lumen of microvessels in the palmar fascia. Localized ischemia and alcohol cause adenosine triphosphate (ATP) breakdown to the purine bases, hypoxanthine and xanthine, and the conversion of xanthine dehydrogenase to xanthine oxidase with resultant oxygen free radical (O_2^-, OH˙) and H_2O_2 release.

HIV infection and cigarette smoking are also associated with oxidant stress. Oxygen free radicals may damage pericytes and lead to pericyte regeneration, with consequent further layering of basal laminae, and fibroblast proliferation. Oxygen free radicals released by the fibroblasts themselves may also further stimulate fibroblast proliferation. The collage produced by fibroblasts in areas of high cell density (nodules) is initially highly disorganized and relatively depleted of type I collagen but gradually becomes aligned in lines of stress resulting in the characteristic fibrous "cords" that are palpated beneath the palmar skin and extend into the fingers of patients with Dupuytren's contracture. Progressive fibroblast proliferation and collagen deposition may further compromise microvessels with a positive feedback effect consistent with the progressive nature of the condition (Fig. 5).

Clinical Application

The above scenario suggests that agents which decrease oxygen free radical release may inhibit or prevent Dupuytren's contracture. Allopurinol (a competitive xanthine oxidase inhibitor) has shown early promise in mild contractures, while a group of patients who are likely to consume large amounts of steroidal and nonsteroidal anti-inflammatory agents (patients with rheumatoid arthritis) have a very low prevalence of Dupuytren's contracture [9].

Acknowledgements. We thank the patients and surgeons of the Nuffield Orthopaedic Center for tissue samples and the Rhodes trust for support for GACM.

References

1. Hueston JT (1960) The incidence of Dupuytren's contracture. Med J Aust 2:999
2. Larkin JG, Frier BM (1986) Limited joint mobility and Dupuytren's contracture in diabetic, hypertensive, and normal populations. Br Med J 292:1494
3. Noble J, Heathcote JG, Cohen H (1984) Diabetes mellitus in the aetiology of Dupuytren's disease. J Bone Joint Surg [Br] 66:322–325
4. Attali P, Ink O, Pelletier G, Vernier C, Jean F, Moulton L, Etienne J-P (1987) Dupuytren's contracture, aochohol consumption, and chronic liver disease. Arch Intern Med 147:1065–1067
5. Bower M, Nelson M, Gazzard BG (1990) Dupuytren's contracture in patients infected with HIV. Br Med J 300:164–165
6. An HS, Southworth SR, Jackson WT, Russs B (1988) Cigarette smoking and Dupuytren's contracture of the hand. J Hand Surg [Br] 13:872–874
7. Lund M (1941) Dupuytren's contracture and epilepsy. Acta Psychiatr Scand 16:465
8. Stewart HD, Innes AR, Burke FD (1985) The hand complications of Colles' fracture. J Hand Surg [Br] 10:103–106
9. Arafa M, Steingold RF, Noble J (1984) The incidence of Dupuytren's disease in patients with Rheumatoid Arthritis. J Hand Surg 9:165–66
10. Murrell GAC, Francis MJO, Howlett CR (1989) Dupuytren's contracture: fine structure in relation to etiology. J Bone Joint Surg [Br] 71:367–373
11. Brickley-Parsons D, Glimcher MJ, Smith RJ, Albin R, Adams J (1981) Biochemical changes in the collagen of the palmar fascia in patients with Dupuytren's disease. J Bone Joint Surg [Am] 63:787–797
12. Murrell GAC, Francis MJO, Bromley L (1991) The collagen changes of Dupuytren's contracture. J Hand Surg [Br]
13. Flint MH, Gillard GC, Reilly HC (1982) The glycosaminoglycans of Dupuytren's disease. Connect Tiss Res 9:173–179
14. Rabinowitz JL, Ostermann L, Bora FW, Staeffen J (1983) Lipid composition and de novo lipid biosynthesis of human palmar fat in Dupuytren's disease. Lipids 18:371–373
15. Murrell TGC, Murrell GAC, Pilowsky E (1986) Resolution of Dupuytren's contracture with allopurinol. Proceedings of the 10th Federation of European Connective Tissue Societies, 28 July–1 Aug, Manchester, p 125
16. Murrell GAC, Murrell TGC, Pilowsky E (1987) A hypothesis for the resolution of Dupuytren's contracture with allopurinol. Specul Sci Technol 10:107–112
17. Babio BM, Curnutte JT, Kipnes RS (1975) Biological defense mechanisms. Evidence for the participation of superoxide in bacterial killing by xanthine oxidase. J Lab Clin Med 85:235–244

18. McCord JM, Roy RS, Schaffer SW (1985) Free radicals and myocardial ischemia. Adv Myocardiol 5:183–189
19. Murrell GAC, Francis MJO, Bromley L (1987) Free radicals and Dupuytren's contracture. Br Med J 295:1373–1375
20. Murrell GAC, Francis MJO, Bromley L (1990) Modulation of fibroblast proliferation by oxygen free radicals. Biochem J 265:659–665
21. Burdon RH, Gill V, Rice-Evans C (1990) Intracellular active oxygen species in the promotion and suppression of tumour cell growth. Free Radic Biol Med 9 Suppl 1:167
22. Weening RS, Wever R, Roos D (1975) Quantitative aspects of the production of superoxide radicals by phagocytizing human granulocytes. J Lab Clin Med 85:245–252
23. Murrell GAC, Francis MJO, Bromley L (1989) Fibroblasts release superoxide free radicals. Biochem Soc Trans 17:483–484
24. Meier B, Seis H (1990) Superoxide release in fibroblasts by and NADPH oxidase is related to cell cycle and proliferation. Free Radic Biol Med 9 Suppl 1:31
25. Wach F, Hein R, Adelmann-Grill BC, Krieg T (1987) Inhibition of fibroblast chemotaxis by superoxide dismutase. Eur J Cell Biol 44:124–127

Clinical Findings and Epidemiology of Dupuytren's Disease

Clinical Findings in Dupuytren's Disease

P. Mailänder, P. Brenner, and A. Berger

History

The clinical findings in Dupuytren's disease should not be described without first remarking on the history of the disease and also on the anatomy of the fascia of the palm and the digits.

In 1614 Felix Platter noted the clinical findings of Dupuytren's contracture in his book about diseases of the body and the soul, which was written in Basel. For a long time, the contracture was interpreted as being a consequence of shrinkage of the flexor tendons. Two English surgeons, Henry Cline, in 1808, and Astley Cooper, in 1822, described the correct siting of the pathology. In 1831, Boyer called the contracture "crispatura tendinum." In 1832 Baron Guillaume Dupuytren (1777–1835) stated that the disease is caused by changes in the palmar aponeurosis. Dupuytren wrote: "La plupart des individus que cette maladie affecte, ont ete obliges de faire des efforts avec la paume de main et de manier des corps durs." Most individuals who are affected with this condition have been obliged to use the palms of their hands constantly and to handle hard objects. Immediately after the first publication of Dupuytren's lecture (in 1835 and 1843), Jean Goyrand contested the relation to manual labor and cited not only bilateral disease in his hospital manager, who had never done a day's hard labor, but also bilateral symmetrical disease in a coachman. In 1844 Caesar Hawkins reported similar findings.

Intrinsic and Extrinsic Theory

Dupuytren's contracture is a disease of the fascia of the palm and the digits (McFarlane 1988). The diseased cords and nodules are the result of pathologic changes in the normal fascia. This represents the *intrinsic theory*, which states that the primary lesion in Dupuytren's contracture lies within the internal fibrous architecture of the palmar aponeurosis. In 1963, Hueston presented the *extrinsic theory*, which stated that the primary lesion in Dupuytren's contracture lies in the palmar, subcutaneous, fibrofatty tissue on the anterior aspect of the palmar aponeurosis, which becomes involved secondarily. In 1959, Millesi defined Dupuytren's contracture as a disease of the tight fibers of connective tissue on the palmar side of the hand which finally leads to contracting cords of fibrous tissue.

Anatomy of the Palmar Fascia

It is important for the surgeon to be well aware of the anatomy of the palmar fascia. The pertinent anatomy of the palmar fascia is described in detail in Gosset (1972), Milford (1968), Stack (1971), and Thomine (1972). The palmar fascia is composed of several components which can be diseased either alone or simultaneously.

The palmar aponeurosis is a triangle-shaped tendinous plate in the center of the palm which consists of the terminal fibers of the palmaris longus. Grapow (1887) described connections between the palmar aponeurosis and the skin of the palm. Legueu and Juvara (1893) distinguished between the pretendinous and intertendinous bands within the palmar aponeurosis. Cunningham (1923) defined the palmar aponeurosis as the central part of the palmar fascia. The fascias of the thenar and the hypothenar are the lateral parts of the palmar fascia. Frohse (1906) found connections between the fibers of the palmar aponeurosis and the fibers of the digital fascia. Kaplan (1938) and Stack (1961) confirmed these connections, but Thomine (1965) disagreed. Gosset (1967) found connections between the split pretendinous bands and the fiber system of the lateral digital parts. The function of the fiber system on the palmar side of the hand is to fix the skin to the structures lying beneath it. The subcutaneous tissue is interspersed with tight fibers of connective tissue, Hueston called it a fibrofatty layer.

McGrouther (1982) showed the relations of the pretendinous bands of the palmar aponeurosis to the distal palmar crease. The second part of the palmar fascia is the superficial transverse ligament of the palm, which was exactly described by Skoog (1948). It has relations to the thenar and basal thumb creases and it is deep to the pretendinous bands of the palmar aponeurosis. The natatory ligament comes from the digital web space into the thumb web more distally.

The Palmar Aponeurosis

The palmar aponeurosis is the most common site of Dupuytren's contracture, and a nodule in this fascia is pathognomonic of the disease.

The pretendinous band of the palmar aponeurosis becomes a contracting cord and, in the process, causes the contracture of the medial phalangeal (MP) joint. In fact the only cause of the contracture at this joint is a pretendinous cord. Luck (1959) suggested that normal tissue should be called "bands" and diseased tissue "cords." The pretendinous cord attaches primarily to the skin at the distal palmar crease. It does not disturb the course of the neurovascular bundle.

The fibers of the natatory ligament pass from side to side at the web space, but some fibers pass distally on either side of each finger. This ligament is frequently diseased in Dupuytren's contracture and contributes to contracture of the proximal interphalangeal (PIP) joint. Abduction of the diseased digits is limited. The natatory ligament reaches the web space of the thumb and terminates at the proximal crease of the thumb. If this part of the ligament is diseased, abduction and extension of the thumb will be limited.

The superficial transverse ligament of the palm is deep to the pretendinous bands of the palmar aponeurosis. Skoog (1967) proposed to preserve this structure because it is not involved in the disease process. The part of the superficial transverse ligament which enters the thumb web and attaches the skin at the base of the thumb should only be excised if a thumb web contracture is present.

The diseases of the pretendinous band, the natatory ligament or the superficial transverse ligament are the causes of disease of the thumb or the first web. These three structures are superficial to the neurovascular bundles and do not disturb theses bundles.

The Digital Fascia

Like the fascial structures of the palm the parts of the digital fascia can become diseased too. Contractures of PIP and distal interphalangeal (DIP) joints are caused by disease of the digital fascia. The components of the normal digital fascia are the lateral digital sheet, which is a condensation of the superficial fascia on either side of the finger. It receives fibers from the natatory ligament and from the spiral band. The spiral band consists of fibers around the neurovascular bundle. The fibers of the spiral band reach the lateral digital sheet deep to the neurovascular bundles. Grayson's and Cleland's ligaments hold the skin of the digit in position during flexion and extension. Cleland's ligaments pass from the side of the phalanges to the skin, dorsal to the neurovascular bundle. They are not involved in Dupuytren's disease. Grayson's ligaments pass from the fibrous tendon sheath to the skin, palmar to the bundles. They are frequently diseased. Thomine (1972) descibed a longitudinally oriented fascia dorsal to the neurovascular bundle, the retrovascular cord.

The contracture of the PIP joint is caused by three patterns of cords. The central cord develops from the fibrofatty superficial fascia that lies between the neurovascular bundles. It is in continuity with the pretendinous cord. The central cord attaches distally to the bone and tendon sheath over the middle phalanx.

The lateral cord is adherent to the skin and it attaches the tendon sheath through fibers of Grayson's ligament. It extends distally and can produce contracture of the DIP joint.

The spiral cord can be a continuation of the pretendinous cord through the spiral band or it may arise at the musculotendinous junction of an intrinsic

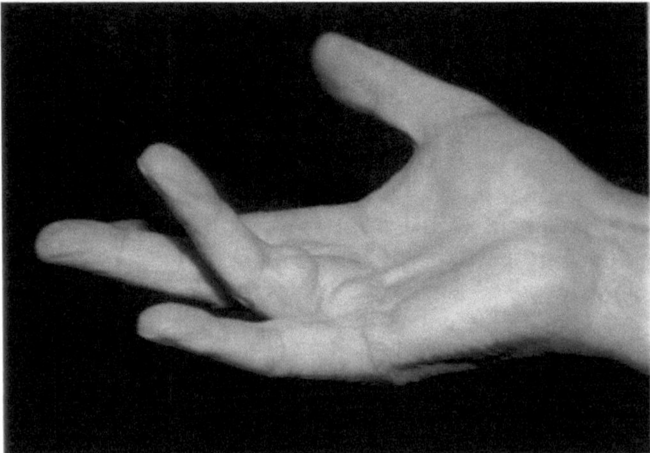

Fig. 1. Contracture of the MP joint

muscle, especially the abductor digiti minimi muscle. The cord attaches distally to the bone and the tendon sheath of the middle phalanx. By increasing contracture of the PIP joint the neurovascular bundle is increasingly displaced.

The retrovascular cord is important for recurrent contracture of the PIP joint. DIP joint contractures can develop by the retrovascular and the lateral cord together.

Clinical Findings

Early stages of Dupuytren's disease show an increased fixation of the skin to the palmar aponeurosis, transverse creases at the hypothenar or punctated fixations of the skin proximal and distal to the palmar crease. With increasing shortening of the connective tissue fibers, a defined part of the skin remains fixed and finally leads to a cord. In the process of the disease a thickened cord causes a flexion contracture of the MP joint by disease of the pretendinous band of the palmar aponeurosis (Fig. 1). In fact, the only cause of contracture at this joint is a pretendinous cord. This attaches primarily to skin at the distal palmar crease. It does not disturb the course of the neurovascular bundle. Nodules which press on nerves can cause the development of pain in the diseased hand.

The PIP joint may develop a contracture by one or all three of the diseased cords. A torsion of the finger can be caused by a cord which is not directed in the midline of the palmar side. If a central cord is present, the diseased fascia can be attached to the fibrous tendon sheath or bone of the middle phalanx. The neurovascular bundle may be attached to the fascia at this level. If Grayson's ligament is diseased, the cord passes to the skin superficial to the

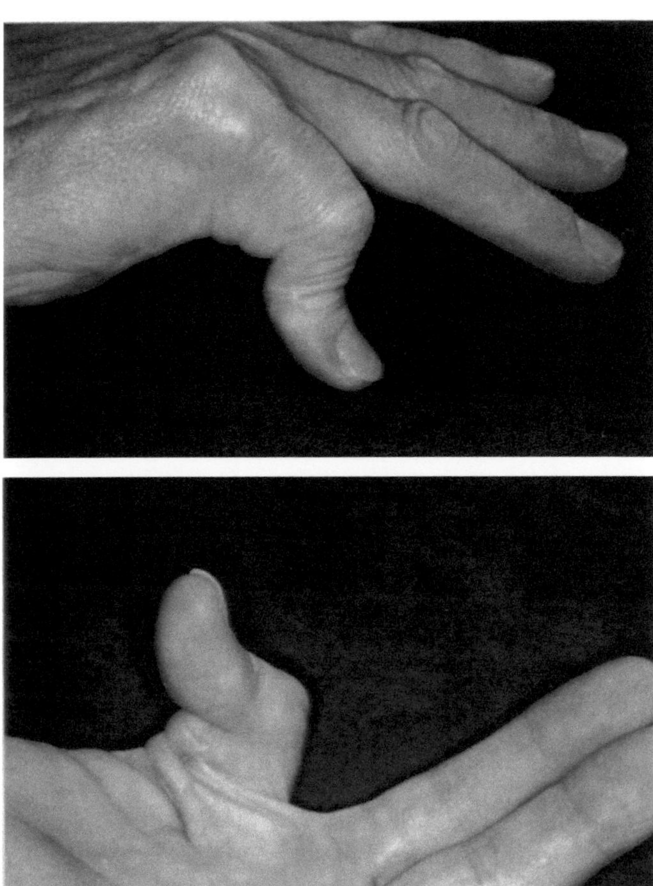

Figs. 2 *(above)*, **3** *(below)*. Hyperextension of the DIP joint combined with flexion of the PIP joint

neurovascular bundle. In PIP joint contracture, a spiral cord contracture may be present and the neurovascular bundle may then be displaced. When the MP and PIP joints are contracted and a spiral cord is present the neurovascular bundle may be displaced in a proximal position between the distal crease of the palm and the proximal crease of the finger.

The ulnar lateral cord in the little finger begins in the hypothenar fascia. In the hypothenar region retraction of the skin and a transverse crease of the skin can develop.

Lateral cord involvement may extend distally to produce contracture at the DIP joint. If the fascia is a continuation of the retrovascular cord rather than the lateral one, it will extend through the branching of the neurovascular bundle.

The hyperextension of the DIP joint is compensatory to PIP joint flexion (Figs. 2, 3). It is usually created by correcting the PIP joint contracture. However, if

Clinical Findings in Dupuytren's Disease   241

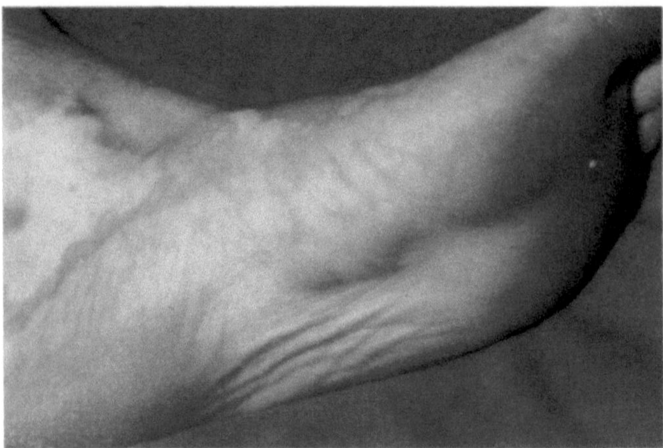

Fig. 4. Nodule on the plantar side of the foot

long-standing, fascial structures such as the oblique reticular ligament and the extensor tendon may be foreshortened and require division.

Due to disease of the natatory ligament, separation of the fingers is limited. Therefore the skin in the web spaces can become macerated and a mycosis can occur.

Garrod (1893) described nodules in the skin at the dorsal side of the PIP joint in patients with Dupuytren's contracture, i.e., knuckle pads. Skoog (1948) found this manifestation in 44% of his patients with Dupuytren's disease. A prognostic value of this manifestation cannot be excluded (Hueston 1963).

Another site of pathologic tissue in the hand is the distal portion of the flexor carpi ulnaris tendon.

If the disease leads to a severe contracture of the PIP joint and this contracture is long-standing, articular structures, e.g., the check rein ligament, the palmar plate, and the accessory collateral ligament, will shorten. In these cases, the joints sometimes show chondral lesions.

What happens to the skin in Dupuytren's disease? In patients with severe long-term contracture, the skin will shorten and a true lack of skin occurs. In some cases ulceration of the skin of the palm is caused by the pressure of a severly contracted digit.

Madelung (1875) and Reeves (1881) described changes in the plantar aspect of the foot that were similar to nodules in the palmar side of the hand (Fig. 4). Ledderhose (1897) reported thickening into the plantar aponeurosis after immobilization of the leg; these changes spontaneously disappeared.

Kirby (1849) described a relation between Dupuytren's disease and induration penis plastica. Hueston (1963) found this ectopic manifestation of Dupuytren's disease in 2.7% and Millesi (1965) in 2.4% of their patients.

References

Boyer C (1831) Traite des maladies chirurgicales. Paris

Cline H (1808) Quoted by J Windsor (1843). Lancet 2:501

Cooper A (1822) A treatise in dislocations and fractures of the joints. London

Cunningham DJ (1923) Textbook of anatomy. Wood, New York

Dupuytren· G (1832) Les lecons orales de clinique chirurgicale faites a L'Hotel Dieu de Paris. Bailliere, Paris

Frohse F (1906) Die Aponeurosis palmaris und digitalis der menschlichen Hand mit besonderer Berücksichtigung ihrer Funktion. Arch Anat Entwickl Gesch 101

Garrod AE (1893) On an unusual form of nodule upon the joints of the fingers. St Barth Hosp Rep 29:157

Gosset J (1967) Maladie de Dupuytren et Anatomie des aponevroses palmo-digitales. Ann Chir 21:554

Gosset J (1972) Maladie de Dupuytren et Anatomie des aponevroses palmo-digitales. Ann Chir 21:554

Goyrand G (1834) Nouvelles recherches sur la retraction permanente des doigts. Mem Acad Roy Med 3:498

Grapow M (1887) Die Anatomie und physische Bedeutung der Palmaraponeurose. Arch Anat 2–3:142

Hueston JT (1963) Dupuytren's contracture. Livingstone, Edinburgh

Kaplan EB (1938) Die Palmarfaszie in Zusammenhang mit der Dupuytren'schen Kontraktur. Surgery 4:414

Kirby J (1849) On an unusual affection of the penis. Dublin Med Press 22:210

Ledderhose G (1897) Zur Pathologie der Aponeurose des Fußes und der Hand. Langenbecks Arch Klin Chir 55:694

Legueu F, Juvara E (1893) Des aponevroses de la paume de la main. Bull Soc Anat Paris 6:383

Luck JV (1959) Dupuytren's contracture. A new concept of pathogenesis correlated with surgical management. J Bone Joint Surg 41A:635–664

Madelung OW (1875) Die Ätiologie und die operative Behandlung der Dupuytren'schen Fingerverkrümmung. Berl Klin Wschr 12:191

McGrouther DA (1982) The microanatomy of Dupuytren's contracture. The Hand 14:215

Milford L (1968) Retaining ligaments of the digits of the hand. Saunders, Philadelphia

Millesi H (1959) Neue Gesichtspunkte in der Pathogenese der Dupuytren'schen Kontraktur. Bruns Beitr Klin Chir 198:1

Millesi H (1965) Zur Pathogenese und Therapie der Dupuytren'schen Kontraktur. Eine Studie an Hand von mehr als 500 Fällen. Ergebnisse der Chirurgie und Orthopädie, vol 47. Springer, Berlin Heidelberg New York, p 51

McFarlane (1988) Green's operative hand surgery. Livingstone, New York, p 553

Platter F (1614) Observationum in hominis affectibus plerisque corpori et animo functionum, laesione, dolore, aliave molestia et vitio in sensi libris tres, 2nd edn. Basel

Reeves HA (1881) Remarks on the contraction of the palmar and plantar fasciae. Br Med J II:1049

Skoog T (1948) Dupuytren's contraction. Acta Chir Scand Suppl 96:139

Stack HG (1961) Anatomy of the fascia of the fingers. The second hand club meeting, Göteborg, 1961

Stack HG (1971) The palmar fascia and the development of deformities and displacements in Dupuytren's contracture. Ann R Coll Surg Engl 48:238

Thomine J (1965) Conjonctive d'envelope des doigts et squelette fibreux des commissures inter-digitales. Ann Chir Plast 10:194

Thomine JM (1972) Le fascia digital – development and anatomie. Tubiana R (ed) La maladie de Dupuytren, 2nd edn. Expansion Scientific Francais, Paris

Skoog T (1967) The tranverse elements of the palmar aponeurosis in Dupuytren's contracture. Scand J Plast Surg 1:51–63

Epidemiology of Dupuytren's Disease

P. Brenner, P. Mailänder, and A. Berger

Introduction

The palmar contracture nowadays associated with Dupuytren's name, had already been described by the Swiss physician Platter (1614) and Sir Astley Cooper (1824) in England before Baron Guillaume Dupuytren made it the subject of his famous lecture on the December 5, 1831 in Paris (Dupuytren 1832, 1834). Despite more than 160 years of investigation, the nature and demography of Dupuytren's contracture are still not entirely clear (Berger et al. 1990).

The prevalence of Dupuytren's malady appears to vary widely in different parts of the word (Early 1962; Strickland et al. 1990). Dupuytren's contracture is virtually confined to Caucasians, mainly of North European extraction, and runs in families (Ling 1963). The digitopalmar fibromatosis is common in Scandinavian countries, frequent in the United Kingdom and Ireland, but less frequent in mediterranean Europe (Egawa 1985; Brouet 1986). Hueston (1987) stated that the disease is almost unknown in Greece and the Middle East.

Egawa et al. (1990) designed a globe with different pale question marks overlying the black-colored continents, pointing to the dearth of information about the epidemiology of Dupuytren's contracture. Consequently, the task of the following presentation is to give a brief survey of the literature concerning geographic and social differences in the prevalence of Dupuytren's disease. Only etiological factors which are of special epidemiological interest will be mentioned.

Dupuytren's Disease Among Caucasians

According to Bunnel (1944) the prevalance of Dupuytren's disease in an unselected American population can be estimated at 1%–2%. In the USA, Dupuytren's contracture is reported to affect mainly whites (Conway 1954). Based on a study among 403 randomly chosen inpatients at a medical and surgical clinc, Rafter et al. (1980) determined an incidence for palmar fibrosis of 17% in an Irish population. In Norway, a skillful examination of hands in a screening programm among 15905 persons was carried out by Mikkelsen

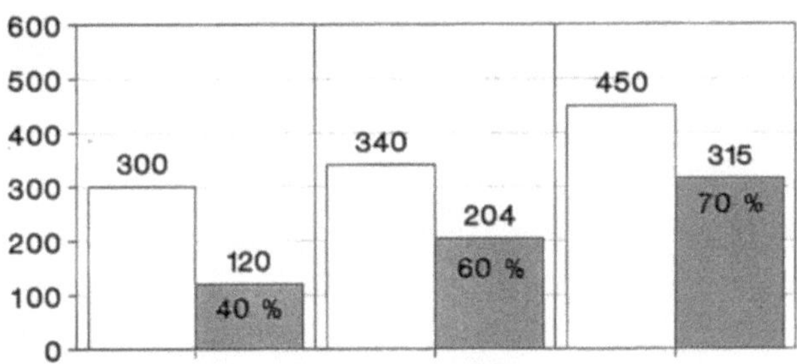

Fig. 1. Survey of blue-eyed Toulonese with Dupuÿtren's disease (DD). *Left*, control group; *middle*, DD patients, not operated; *right*, DD patients, operated. The *hatched columns* represent the blue-eyed proportion of Toulonese. (From Brouet 1986)

(1972). Dupuytren's contracture was found in 901 individuals, 9.4% of the men and 2.8% of the women. Mackenney (1983) examined 919 patients attending orthopedic clinics in England for evidence of Dupuytren's disease. He determined the male prevalence to be 5% and the corresponding value for females 3.5%. In a thorough study including 80 000 patients in Munich, Schnitzler (1935) reported a prevalence of 1.7% with regard to Dupuytren's malady. While the incidence of Dupuytren's disease in a general population of the Federal Republic of Germany can only be estimated, we nowadays may profit from the statistics of former German Democratic Republic. Here we can refer to exact data: Beck (1954) recognized Dupuytren's contracture in 2.39% of the general population of East Germany. If we calculate, based upon the aforementioned figures, the prevalevance of Dupuytren's disease in the reunited Federal Republic of Germany, with 79 670 000 inhabitants (von Baratta 1991), than at least 1 354 390 and as many as 1 904 113 Germans suffer from digitopalmar contracture.

It is interesting that contracture tends to be more prevalent in countries with small homogeneous populations. Dupuytren's fibrosis is seemingly determined by a dominant gene with high penetrance, especially in males; usually men of Celtic or Scandinavian ancestry are affected (Woolridge 1988).

Thus, the prevalence of Dupuytren's disease in mediterranean countries is low; furthermore, the frequency varies from the north to the south. Brouet (1986) pointed at a striking difference concerning the prevalence of Dupuytren's contracture among French Mediterraneans. Due to the Norman invasion of the Mediterranean coast and Sicily in 1066 by the brother of William the Conqueror, there are blue-eyed Toulonese of Nordic stock with a higher incidence of palmar fibrosis and dark-eyed Toulonese with a lower prevalence of Dupuytren's malady. Figure 1 demonstrates a 40% incidence of blue eyes in the control group; the prevalence is impressively increased in patients with Dupuytren's contracture. These ethnic findings are furthermore supported by the geographic distribution of the patients' families. The city of Toulon is situated in the extreme south east of France with a maximal frequency of 17% Comparable but lower percentages are listed for Brittany and Normandy where the invaders also landed (Fig. 2).

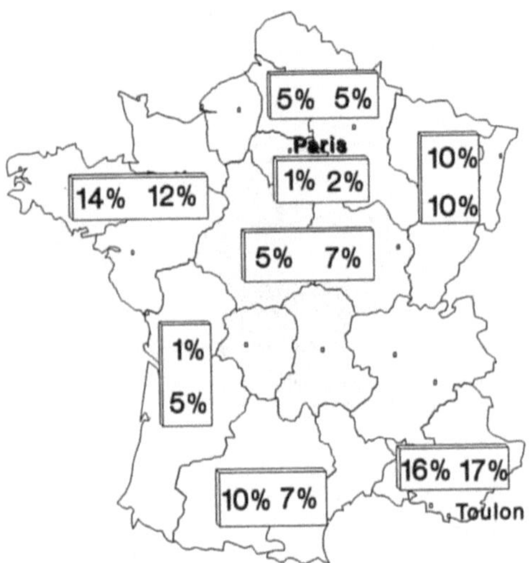

Fig. 2. Distribution of family origin in 650 cases of Dupuytrens disease. Operated patients, *n* = 250, percentages on *left*; nonoperated patients, *n* = 400, percentages on right. (From Brouet 1986)

Dupuytren's Disease in Asia

According to Chow et al. (1984) the incidence of Dupuytren's disease in non-Caucasians is low. Palmar contracture appears only rarely in Asian people of pure stock. Concerning the prevalence of Dupuytren's disease on the Indian subcontinent, Srivastavas et al. (1989), in an overview of the available literature, found only ten male cases, three from Pakistan and the remaining seven from North India. Vathana et al. (1990) ascertained a published prevalence of 19 cases of Dupuytren's disease among the Thai population, very few considering that Thailand has 55 million inhabitans. The Commitee on Dupuytren's Disease of the International Federation of Orthopaedists reported only 13 Chinese affected with Dupuytren's malady, while 132 cases of palmar fibrosis were collected from Japan (Vathana et al. 1990). Among the total of 13 142 cases at the Soft Tissue Tumor Registry at the Second Department of Pathology, Kyushu University, Ushijima et al. (1984) found only 42 cases of palmar fibromatoses during their clincopatholgical study. Tsuge (1990) about 80 Japanese patients with Dupuytren's contracture, which he treated over 25 years in private practice as a hand surgeon. Obviously, Japan, with such a low incidence of Dupuytren's contracture, is an unusual geographic area. Ewaga (1985) analyzed a total of 3852 Japanese, ranging from 20 to 95 years old. The mean average age for his group was 62.7 years. All participants in the study lived in the areas of Osaka and Kobe. In all, some 2.9% of males and 0.9% of females were found to have Dupuytren's disease. The author determined that the sex ratio in Japan is comparable to that in northern European countries. Linguistic studies have vividly demonstrated a possible ethnic relationship between the Japanese population and peoples from the region northwest of the

Ural mountains. Linguistic and genetic features parallel people's migration behavior (Cavalli-Sforza et al. 1981; Cavalli-Sforza 1990) and thus, at least in part, explain the similarities in sex distribution between Japan and northern Europe regarding Dupuytren's disease.

Dupuytren's Disease in Blacks

Dupuytren's disease in Blacks, American Indians, and Gypsies is believed to be rare (Zachariae 1971; Makhlouf et al. 1987). However, Yost (1955) reported a prevalence of 2.4% among Afro-Americans based on an analysis of 5062 patients at a large municipal hospital in Brooklyn, New York. These data were ignored for a long time. Since that time, a number of cases in Black men have been described (Furnas 1979; Plasse 1979; Makhlouf et al. 1987), but none of these reports presented scientific and conclusive evidence that the affected individuals were pure Negro stock. Furnas (1979) suspected a small but definite prevalence of Dupuytren's disease even among pure Blacks. Finally, Mennen (1986) examined approximately 6000 Blacks who were hand patients in Pretoria (South Africa) and found only four otherwise normal patients with Dupuytren's contracture, corresponding to a prevalence of 0.0007%. Since none of the "classical" Caucasoid genes occurred in any of the examined black patients, Mennen (1986) claimed that there is no Caucasoid admixture in their backgrounds.

Affliction with Dupuytren's Disease with Progessive Age

Most publications show a comparatively steady increase of Dupuytren's disease with advancing age (Skoog, 1948; James and Tubiana 1952; Millesi 1965). Affliction in early childhood is extremely rare, as demonstrated among others by Berger and Gurr (1985). Conway (1954), for instance, reported that the prevalence was only five men with Dupuytren's disease among one million soldiers, age 21–30 years, during the First World War, The prevalence of Dupuytren's contracture in central Europe in patients <30 years of age ranges from 0 to 5.8%; between 30 and 39 years of age, 2.1%–11.8%; 40–49 years, 12.9%–31.5%; 50–59 years, 24.4%–44.1%; 60–69 years, 16.8%–37.1% and >70 years, 5.2%–14.9% (Geldmacher 1963; Nigst 1971; Stuhler, 1975; Brouet 1986; Forgon and Farkas 1988).
In the UK, Early (1962) determined an incidence of 18.1% for men and 9% for women over age 75. In North America, analyzing a population of the same age, the prevalence among men was 28.7% and 35% for women (Gordon 1964). Among Australians a frequency of 25.6% in men and 20.4% in women older than 60 years was reported by Hueston (1962). The peak prevalence for male Norwegians occurred between 70 and 75 years, whereas women were affected by Dupuytren's disease at a maximum between 85 and 89 years. With regard to peak prevalence, there was a remarkable index shift, pointing to an

approximately 15 years later manifestation of Dupuytren's disease in women than in men (Mikkelsen 1972).

Sex and Digitopalmar Fibrosis

It is not yet known why women are significantly less often affected by palmar fibrosis than are men. Holzrichter et al. (1982) described this phenomenon as "androtropia." Statistics based on a surgical series of Dupuytren's disease demonstrate a much higher frequency in males than in females (Mikkelsen 1972). The male:female ratio, variously reported as approximately 9:1 or 7:1, changes with progressive age to 3.7:1 (Skoog 1948; Berge and Pohl 1988). Statements concerning the sex ratio must be accepted with considerable reserve. Skoog (1948) and McFarlane (1990), for instance, explained that, due to the earlier affliction of males with Dupuytren's disease, they are also operated on more often at an early stage. Thus, due to surgical statistics, the true male:female ratio has probably been overestimated.

Involvement of the Dominant vs Nondominant Hand

Dupuytren's disease was not coincidental to handedness (Hueston 1987). Figure 3 demonstrates graphically the affliction with digitopalmar fibromatosis and involvement of either the right or left hand, or both hands. According to McFarlane (1990), approximately two thirds showed a bilateral affliction with Dupuytren's disease. Data, including those from patients who have undergone surgery, showing that the right hand is predominantly affected actually indicate only that the majority of patients are right-handed and thus handicapped more by Dupuytren's contracture on the right and thus more commonly operated on. However, equal affliction of dominant and nondominant hands does not support a simple traumatic etiology. The relationship between Dupuytren's disease and heavy manual labor is controversial. One of the initiators of this theme of discussion was Baron Guillaume Dupuytren himself (Strickland et al. 1990).

Family History of Dupuytren's Disease Patients

Goyrand (1834) was the first to clearly point out the link between Dupuytren's disease and its familial appearance. A positive family history of Dupuytren's disease is more common in women than in men (McFarlane 1990). Several studies have investigated the role of inheritance in Dupuytren's disease (Fig. 4.) Twin studies showed an equal affliction in both twins compared to a normal population (Jentsch 1937). Ling (1963; $n = 832$ relatives, $n = 50$ patients) concluded that there must be a single, presumably dominant, gene in Dupuytren's disease. Thieme (1989) searched for the modes of transmission, rejecting

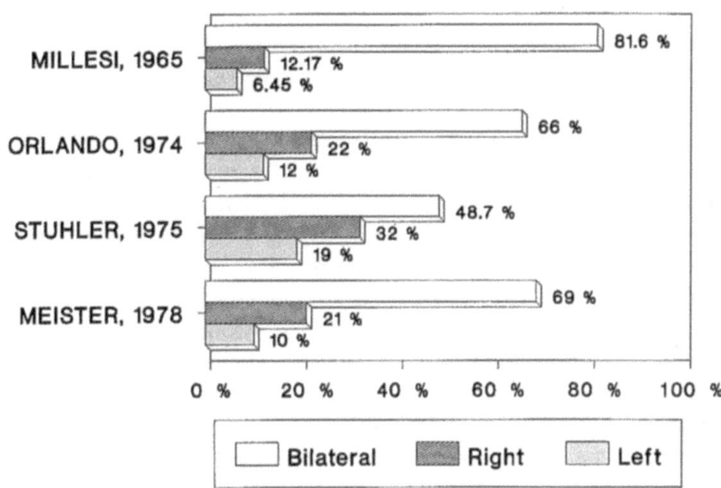

Fig. 3. Affliction with Dupuytren's disease according to handedness according to four studies

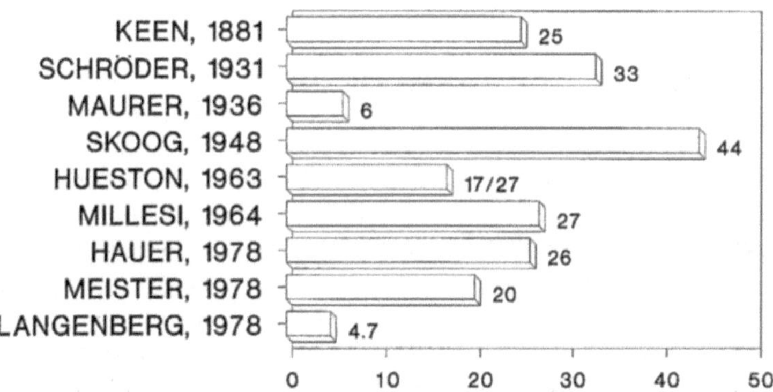

Fig. 4. Percentage of positive family history of Dupuytren's disease in nine studies

sex-linked polygenic and autosomal recessive and concluding that Dupuytren's contracture is an inherited malady with an autosomal dominant form of transmission (McGrouther 1990). A positive familiy history among Japanese with Dupuytren's contracture showed a similiarly low prevalence, indicating either a mild hereditary expression in Asians or that the etiological factors are other than genetic (McFarlane 1990). The possible mode of inheritance is, however, so irregular that some singular or even multiple inductive factors must act on the genetic predisposition (Zachariae 1970). With regard to surgical treatment and relapses, the prognosis of Dupuytren's disease in individuals is poorer if the family history is positive (Hueston 1963; Millesi 1981).

Dupuytren's Manifestation in Alcoholics

Links between alcohol consumption and Dupuytren's disease have long been recognized (Su 1970). Using a cumulative statistic from data of different authers, Mikkelsen (1972) tried to obtain a positive correlation between alcohol abuse and Dupuytren's contracture. Bradlow and Mowat (1986) also reported, that alcoholics with cirrhosis have Dupuytren's contracture significantly more often than noncirrhotic control groups. It would be worthwhile to determine if liver cirrhosis precedes the onset of Dupuytren's contracture or if it is a secondary disease. In a multinational prosective study McFarlane (1990) searched for a fundamental association between Dupuytren's disease and alcoholism. He found that among his series northern Europeans were overrepresented with respect to alcoholism; the alcoholic group more often had disease and a positive family history, greater incidence of other areas involved and more bilateral affliction. Significantly, he could also show that alcoholics had more extensive disease. Hueston denied a positive relationship between Dupuytren's disease and alcohol consumption because the diagnosis of alcoholism by a surgeon is mainly a subjective one.

Dupuytren's Disease in Epileptics

The correlation between epilepsy and palmar fibrosis remains statistically significant. In general, the coincidence between Dupuytren's contracture and other internal diseases should suggest identical etiological pathways (Fig. 5). With regard to a link between epilepsy and palmar contracture, there are two hypotheses: The first suggests that Dupuytren's disease and epilepsy are linked on a hereditary basis, while the second explains increased palmar fibrosis in

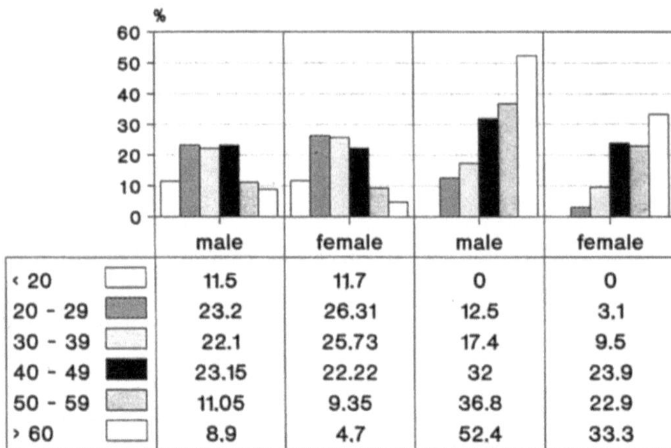

	male	female	male	female
‹ 20	11.5	11.7	0	0
20 - 29	23.2	26.31	12.5	3.1
30 - 39	22.1	25.73	17.4	9.5
40 - 49	23.15	22.22	32	23.9
50 - 59	11.05	9.35	36.8	22.9
› 60	8.9	4.7	52.4	33.3

Fig. 5. Occurrence of Dupuytren's disease in epileptics by sex and age. *Left columns*, data from Lund (1941); *right columns*, data from Stuhler (1977)

epileptics as secondary to drug treatment. The first suggestion is supported by the fact that palmar contracture is more common in idiopathic than in posttraumatic epilepsy, as could be demonstrated for the region of Lower Saxony (Germany) by Stuhler et al. (1977). The prevalence of palmar fibrosis in epileptics increases with the patient's age and duration of epilepsy (Hurst and Badalamente 1990). James (1985) and McFarlane (1990) could prove by means of age-weighted statistics that the incidence of epilepsy in Dupuytren's surgical patients is approximately six times greater than in the general population. The seizures and locations of Dupuytren's disease in the palma manus of epileptics do not differ from the control (nonepileptics or non-Dupuytren's diseased patients). The ring finger is predominantly involved. For the sake of completeness one should mention that Dupuytren's contracture is not related to the ingestion of barbiturates (Lund 1941; Fröscher and Hoffmann 1983). Why the prevalence of Dupuytren's contracture in epileptics is increased remains unclear.

Dupuytren's Disease Among Diabetics

With regard to the prevalence of diabetes mellitus and Dupuytren's disease a striking difference becomes apparent: There are differing rates depending whether one examines patients suffering from Dupuytren's disease and concomitant diabetes or diabetics who eventually show Dupuytren's contracture (Geldmacher 1970). Surgical studies the on association of Dupuytren's contracture and diabetes mellitus were mainly based on a positive history for clinical mellitus only, ignoring the fact that diabetics with palmar fibrosis rarely need surgery (Lamb 1989). Careful investigations for chemical and latent diabetes mellitus are missing. However, studies among diabetics underestimate the prevalence of Dupuytren's disease mainly due to misdiagnosis, for instance, as diabetic chiropathia (Crisp 1991). According to Noble et al. (1984) the true incidence of Dupuytren's contracture in diabetes mellitus probably thus approaches 40%. The prevalence of palmar fibrosis is not greater in insulin-dependent diabetics than in diet-controlled diabetic patients. Instead, obese diabetics have seemingly more manifest Dupuytren's contracture (Stradner et al; 1987, Hurst and Badalamente 1990). The severity and location in diabetic hands are reported to be atypical. In diabetics a milder type of Dupuytren's disease is described. Concerning diabetic women with Dupuytren's ailment, knuckle pads, nodular forms and tethering without finger contracture are more frequent than in controls. Furthermore, palmar fibrosis is predominantly more radial in diabetic hands (Noble et al. 1984). Sex-dependent differences modifying the incidence of Dupuytren's disease are not more striking in diabetics than in the normal population (Mikkelsen 1972; Hurst and Badalamente 1990).
When analyzing correlations between Dupuytren's disease and concomitant morbidity, surgeons must be aware that patients needing hand surgery because of Dupuytren's contracture represent only a limited percentage of the total

Dupuytren's population. Furthermore, it is noteworthy that the majority of individuals with Dupuytren's disease go through life having had any kind of fasciectomy. Finally, we agree with Flint (1990), who said that Dupuytren's disease seems to be the common endpoint of numerous exacerbating factors – physical, biochemical, or metabolic – rather than due to a single pathologic factor. Further epidemiologic data will lead to fruitful hypotheses and thus aid in elucidating the etiology of Dupuytren's disease.

References

Beck W (1954) Untersuchungen über die Häufigkeit der Dupuytrenschen Kontraktur. Monatschr Unfallheilkd 57:69–82

Berge G, Pohl G (1988) Die Dupuytren-Erkrankung im hohen Lebensalter. Behandlungsstrategien und Ergebnisse. Zentralbl Chir 113:313–317

Berger A, Gurr E (1985) Dupuytren'sche Kontraktur im Kindesalter. Hanchirurgie 17:139–142

Berger A, Flory PJ, Brenner P (1990) Klinik und chirurgische Therapie der Dupuytren-Kontraktur. Unfallchirurg 93:181–185

Bradlow A, Mowat AG (1986) Dupuytren's contracture and alcohol. Ann Rheum Dis 45:304–307

Brouet JP (1986) Etude de 1000 dossiers de maladie de Dupuytren. In: Tubiana R, Hueston JT (ed) La maladie de Dupuytren. Expansion Scientifique Française, Paris, pp 98–105

Bunnell S (1944) Surgery of the hand. Lippincott, Philadelphia

Cavalli-Sforza LL (1990) Stammbaum von Vöelern und Sprachen. Spektrum Wiss 1:90–98

Cavalli-Sforza LL, Feldman MW (1981) Cultural transmission and evolution: a quantative approach. Princeton University Press, Princeton

Chow P, Luk KDK, Kung TM (1984) Dupuytren's contracture in Chinese. J R Coll Surg Edinb 29:49–51

Conway H (1954) Dupuytren's contracture. Am J Surg 87:101–119

Cooper AP (1824) Dislocation form contraction of the tendon. In: Cooper AP (ed) A treatise on dislocations and fractures of the joint, 4th edn. Longman, Hurst, Rees, Orme, Brown, and Green, London, pp 486–488

Crisp AJ (1991) Connective tissue and joint disease in diabetes mellitus. In: Pickup JC, Williams G (eds) Textbook of diabetes, vol 2. Blackwell, Oxford, pp 753–761

Dupuytren G (1832) Leçons orales de clinique chirurgicale. Faites à Hôtel-Dieu de Paris. Baillière, Paris, pp 1–24

Dupuytren G (1834) Permanent retraction of the fingers, produced by an affection of the palmar fascia. Lancet 2:222–225

Early PF (1962) Population studies in Dupuytren's contracture. J Bone Joint Surg [Br] 44:602–613

Egawa T (1985) Dupuytren's contracture in Japan. Incidental study on outpatients in private practice of general orthopaedics. J Jpn Soc Surg Hand 2:536–539

Egawa T, Senrui H, Horikii A, Egawa M (1990) Epidemiology of the oriental patients. In: McFarlane RM, McGrouther DA, Flint MH (eds) Dupuytren's disease. Churchill Livingstone, Edinburgh, pp 239–245

Flint MH (1990) The genesis of the palmar lesion. In: McFarlane RM, McGrouther DA, Flint MH (eds) Dupuytren's disease. Churchill Livingstone, Edinburgh, pp 136–154

Forgon M, Farkas G (1988) Ergebnisse nach operativer Behandlung der Dupuytren'schen Kontraktur. Handchir Mikrochir Plast Chir 20:279–284

Froscher W, Hoffmann F (1983) Dupuytrensche Kontraktur und Phenobarbitaleinnahme bei Epilepsie-Patienten. Nervenarzt 54:413–419

Furnas DW (1979) Dupuytren's contracture in a black patient in East Africa. Plast Reconstr Surg 64:250

Geldmacher J (1963) Ergebnisse und Erfahrungen bei der operativen Behandlung der Dupuytrenschen Kontraktur. Chirurg 34:451–457

Geldmacher J (1970) Untersuchungen zur Ätiologie der Dupuytrenschen Kontraktur. Handchirurgic Sonderh 1:10–13

Gordon SD (1964) Dupuytren's contracture; plantar involvement. Br J Plast Surg 17:421–423

Goyrand G (1834) Nouvelle recherches sur la rétraction permanente des doigts. Mém Acad (Paris) 3:489

Hauer G, Wilhelm K (1978) Die Dupuytren'sche Palmarfibromatose. MMW 50:1681–1684

Hill NA (1985) Dupuytren's contracture. J Bone Joint Surg [Am] 67:1439–1443

Holzrichter D, Hrynschyn K, Thama G (1982) Dupuytrensche Kontraktur. In: Baumgartl F, Kremer K, Schreiber HW (eds): Haltungs- und Bewegungsapparat-Erhrankungen. Thieme, Stuttgart, pp 331–338 (Spezielle Chirurgie für die Praxis, vol 313)

Hueston JT (1962) Further studies on the incidence of Dupuytren's contracture. Med J Aust 1:586

Hueston JT (1963) Dupuytren's contracture. Williams and Wilkins, Baltimore

Hueston JT (1987) Dupuytren's contracture and occupation. J Hand Surg [Am] 12:657–658

Hurst LC, Badalamente M (1990) Associated disease. In: McFarlane RM, McGrouther DA, Flint MH (eds) Dupuytren's disease. Churchill Livingstone, Edinburgh, pp 253–260

James J, Tubiana R (1952) La maladie de Dupuytren. Rev Chir Orthop 38:352–406

James JIP (1985) The genetic pattern of Dupuytren's contracture and idiopathic epilepsy. In: Hueston JT, Tubiana R (eds) Dupuytren's disease. Churchill Livingstone, Edinburgh, pp 37–42

Jentsch FR (1937) Zur Erblichkeit der Dupuytren's Kontraktur. Erbarzt 4:85

Keen WW (1881) The etiology and pathology of Dupuytren's contracture of the fingers. Philad Med Times 12:370

Lamb D (1989) Dupuytren's disease. In: Lamb DW, Kuczynski K (eds) The practise of hand surgery. Blackwell, Oxford, pp 635–648

Langenberg R (1978) Dupuytren-Kontraktur – partielle Aponeurektomie noch vertretbar? Zentralbl Chir 112:769–773

Ling RSM (1963) The genetic factors in Dupuytren's disease. J Bone Joint Surg [Br] 45:709–718

Lund M (1941) Dupuytren's contracture and epilepsy. The clinical connection between Dupuytren's contracture, fibroma pantae, periarthritis humeri, helodermia, induration penis plastica and epilepsy, with an attempt at the pathogenetic valuation. Acta Psychiatr Neurol 16:465–491

Mackenney RP (1983) A population study of Dupuytren's contracture. Hand 15:155–161

Makhlouf MV, Cabbabe EB, Shively RE (1987) Dupuytren's disease in blacks. Ann Plast Surg 19:334–336

Maurer G (1936) Zur Lehre der Dupuytrenschen Palmarfascienkontraktur und ihre Behandlung. Dtsch Z Chir 246:685–692

McFarlane RM (1990) Dupuytren's disease. In: McCarthy JG (ed) The hand, part 2. Saunders, Philadelphia, pp 5069–5086 (Plastic surgery, vol 8)

McFarlane RM, Botz JS, Cheung H (1990) Epidemiology of surgical patients. In: McFarlane RM, McGrouther DA, Flint MH (eds) Dupuytren's disease. Churchill Livingstone, Edinburgh, pp 201–239

McGrouther DA (1990) Is Dupuytren's disease an inherited disorder? In: McFarlane RM, McGrouther DA, Flint MH (eds) Dupuytren's disease. Churchill Livingstone, Edinburgh, pp 280–281

Meister P, Wilhelm K, Roeckl C (1978) Palmarfibromatose (Morbus Dupuytren). Vergleichende klinisch-pathologisch-anatomische Reihenuntersuchung. MMW 120:93–98

Mennen U (1986) Dupuytren's contracture in the negro. J Hand Surg [Br] 11:61–64

Mikkelsen OA (1972) Prevalence of Dupuytren's disease in Norway. A study in a representative population sample for the municipality of Haugesund. Act Chir Scand 138:695–700

Mikkelsen OA (1990) Epidemiology of a Norwegian population. In: McFarlane RM, McGrouther DA, Flint MH (eds) Dupuytren's disease. Churchill Livingstone, Edinburgh, pp 191–200

Millesi H (1965) Zur Pathogenese und Therapie der Dupuytrenschen Kontraktur. (Eine Studie an Hand von mehr als 500 Fällen). Ergeb Chir Orthop 47:51–101

Millesi H (1981) Dupuytren-Kontraktur. In: Nigst H, Buck-Gramcko D, Millesi H (eds) Handchirurgie, vol 1. Thieme, Stuttgart, pp 15.1–15.37

Nigst H (1971) Die Dupuytrensche Kontraktur. Ther Umsch 28:818–821

Noble J, Heathcote JG, Cohen H (1984) Diabetes mellitus in the aetiology of Dupuytren's disease. J Bone Joint Surg [Br] 66:322–325

Orlando JC, Smith JW, Goulian D (1974) Dupuytren's contracture: a review of 100 patients. Br J Plast Surg 27:211–217

Plasse JS (1979) Dupuytren's contracture in a black patient. Plast Reconstr Surg 64:250

Platter F (1614) Observationum, in hominis affectibus plerisque, corpori et animo, functionum laesione, dolore, aliave molestia et vitio incommodantibus, libri tres. Liber primus. König, Basel, pp 137–145

Rafter D, Kenny R, Gilmore M, Walsh CH (1980) Dupuytren's contracture – a survery of a hospital population. Ir Med J 73:227–228

Schnitzler O (1935) Die Bedeutung von Berufs- und Sportschäden bei Morbus Dupuytren. MMW 82:248

Skoog T (1948) Dupuytren's contracture with special reference to aetiology and improved surgical treatment, its occurence in epileptics, note on knuckle-pads. Acta Chir Scand Suppl 139:1–190

Srivastavas S, Nancarrow JD, Cort DF (1989) Dupuytren's disease in patients from Indian sub-continent. Report of ten cases. J Hand Surg [Br] 14:32–34

Stradner F, Ulreich A, Pfeiffer KP (1987) Die Dupuytrensche Kontraktur als Begleiterkrankung des Diabetes mellitus. Wien Med Wochenschr 137:89–92

Strickland JW, Idler RS, Creighton JC (1990) Dupuytren's disease. Indiana Med 83:408–409

Stuhler T, Stankovic P, Ritter G, Schmulde E (1977) Epilepsie und Dupuytren'sche Kontraktur – Snytropie zweier Krankheiten. Handchir Mikrochir Plast Chir 9:219–223

Su CK, Patek AJ (1970) Dupuytren's contracture. Its association with alcoholism and cirrhosis. Arch Intern Med 126:278–281

Tsuge K (1990) Die Dupuytrensche Kontraktur. In: Tsuge K (ed) Atlas der Handchirurgie. Hippokrates, Stuttgart, pp 245–249

Ushijima M, Tsuneyoshi M, Enjoji M (1984) Dupuytren type fibromatosis. A clinicopathologic study of 62 cases. Acta Pathol Jpn 34:991–1001

Vathana P, Setpakdi A, Srimongkol T (1990) Dupuytren's contracture in Thailand. Bull Hosp Jt Dis Orthop Inst 50:41–47

Von Baratta M (ed) (1991) Der Fischer Weltalmanach 1992. Fischer, Frankfurt

Woolridge WE (1988) Four related fibrosing diseases. When you find one, look for another. Postgrad Med 84:269–271

Yost J, Winters T, Fett HC (1955) Dupuytren's contracture. A statistical study. Am J Surg 90:568–571

Zachariae L (1970) The electroencephalogram in patients with Dupuytren's contracture. Scand J Plast Reconstr Surg 4:35–40

Zachariae L (1971) Dupuytren's contracture. The aetiological role of trauma. Scand J Plast Reconstr Surg 5:116–119

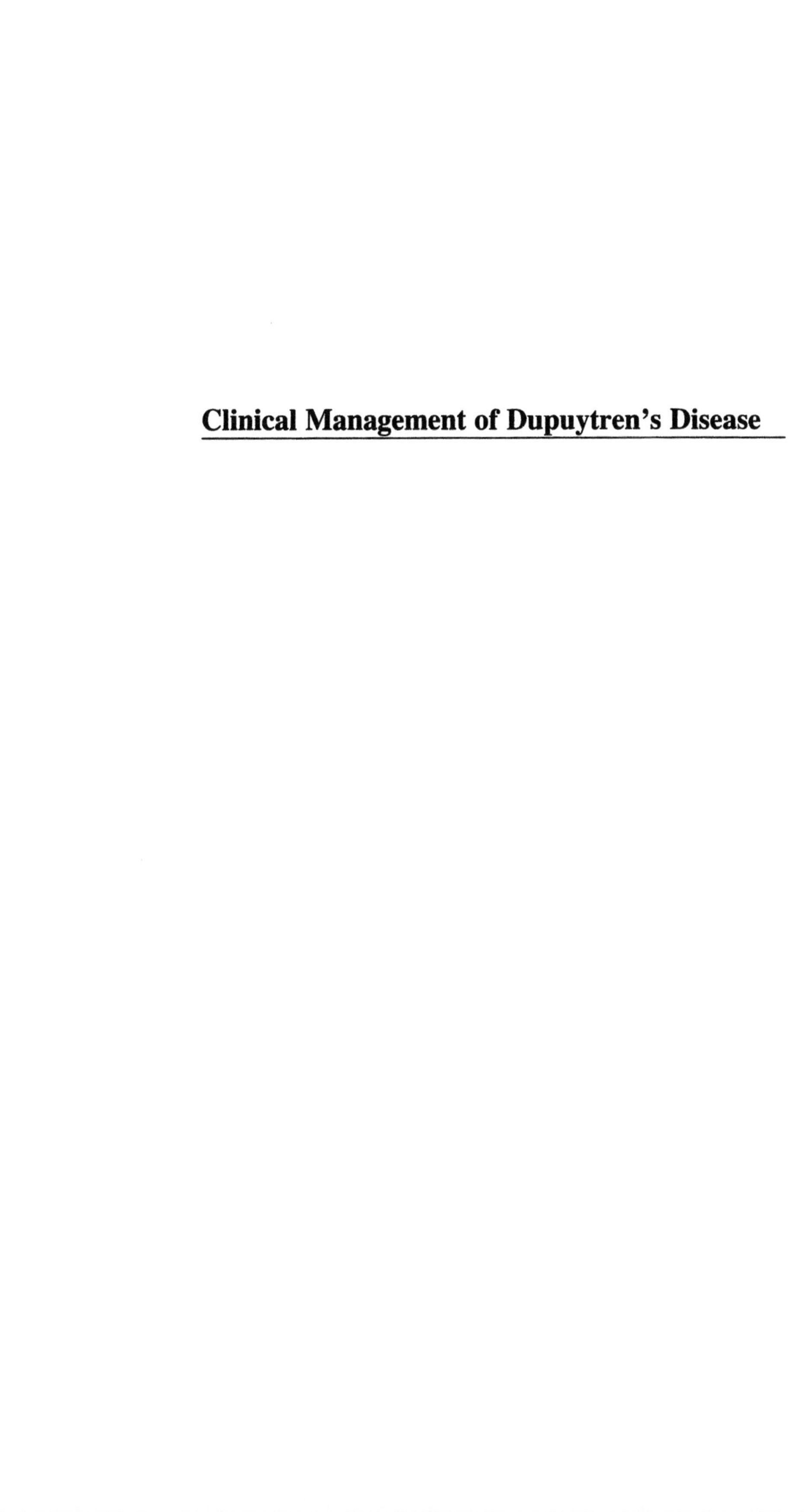

Clinical Management of Dupuytren's Disease

Limited Fasciectomy

J. Geldmacher

Introduction

When we survey the more than 2000 cases of Dupuytren's contracture treated in our clinic since 1956, we find that the severity of disease is reduced compared to 30 years ago. Considering the slow progress of the disease, there is reason to believe that the decreased severity is due to the patients' earlier request for treatment.

Surgery is indicated when we find a widespread alteration of the palmar fascia or when a flexor contracture of the finger joints occurs. We never perform only a fasciotomy and seldom a local excision. In our opinion – in contrast to earlier times – a total fasciectomy (McIndoe et al. 1958; Shaw 1951; Millesi 1981) is indicated if no or at most if a mild contracture of one medial phalongeal (MP) joint exists, because of the higher risk of complications. In 91% of patients, limited fasciectomy, as advocated by Hueston (1961), was done during the last 15–20 years.

In principle we agree with McFarlane (1988) that "no one method to treat Dupuytren's contracture has been established. All methods are equally defensible. One's choice of treatment becomes a decision based on training, technical skill, and one's concept of the disease process." This is also true with respect to the type of incision. Many have been proposed (Geldmacher 1972; McGrouther 1990), but we are guided by the individual findings. The goal is to remove all diseased and potentially diseased tissue; thus the type of incision depends on the extent of the alteration.

The Central Cord

If the lesion is restricted to the palm, it is exposed by a T-shaped incision along the creases of the skin. The root of the palmar fascia is transected at the level of the metacarpal bases and resected along the neurovascular bundles, including the vertical septa in the proximal part. The superficial transversal ligament of the palm beneath the longitudinal cords is never involved and should be preserved if possible, because it supports the deeper structures of the palm (Skoog 1967).

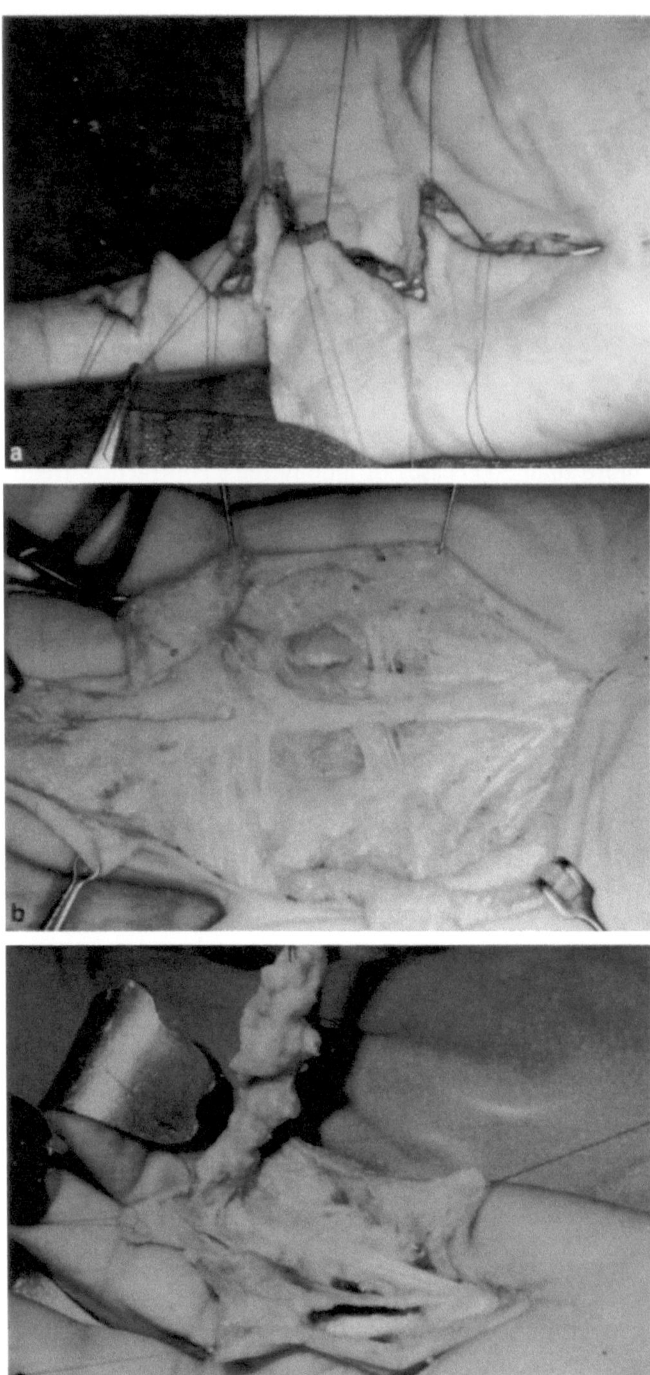

Fig. 1a–c. The central cord: Zig. Zag incision at the base of the finger

If the diseased cord extends into the finger without shortening of the skin, it is exposed by a zig-zag, rectangular, or sinuous continuous incision at the base of the finger (Fig. 1).

If the skin is already shortened and the cords cause a flexion contracture of the MP joint it is preferable to make a longitudinal incision with one or more Z-plasties to obtain a direct exposure of the lesion. This allows precise identification and preparation of the neurovascular bundles.

The base of the finger is the first danger zone of the metacarpodigital ray. Most iatrogenic nerve lesions occur in this area (2.8%). Therefore, we cannot recommend a discontinued incision with sightless preparation deep to a skin bridge in this area (McIndoe et al. 1958). It is well known that in this danger zone there are many alterations of the normal anatomy. Therefore the dissection of the diseased cords and meticulous preparation of the neurovascular bundles is very difficult.

The second danger zone is the area of the proximal interphalangeal (PIP) joint, because of the arrangement of the additional ligamentous structures, as described by Milford (1988), Stack (1962), and Tubiana and Valentin (1964). In normal fingers these are quite difficult to dissect, and in diseased fingers they can usually no longer be identifed and separated (Gosset 1974). The laterodorsal oriented Cleland's ligament is not involved. The other interwoven lateropalmar-placed structures, Grayson's ligament, the transversal part of the retinacular ligament, and the spiral and central cords cause a flexion contracture of the PIP joint and a medial, superficial, and proximal displacement of the neurovascular bundles (McFarlane 1974, 1988; Geldmacher and Köckerling 1985).

Finally, fibers of the oblique retinacular ligament (Landsmeer 1949; Haines 1951), besides the terminal extensor tendon and the distal portion of the lateral fascia of the fingers (Thomine 1974; Gosset 1974; Millesi 1981), can be diseased and produce either an extension or a flexor contracture.

The best way to remove all diseased tissue is by a longitudinal midpalmar incision combined with Z-plasties at the level of the flexion creases of the skin. A remaining flexion contracture of the PIP joint, up to 20°–30° in severe alterations, may be tolerated. Sometimes a palmar capsulectomy (Curtis 1974) is indicated. Although seldom, if the joint itself is damaged an arthrodesis may be required.

The Ulnar Side

The ulnar side of the hand (Fig. 2) is much more often involved by Dupuytren's contracture than the midpalmar region or the radial side. In particular, the fifth finger presents the most severe contractures, the most difficulties in operative treatment, and therefore the worst results.

The fifth finger can be affected alone or in combination with other diseased parts of the hand and often all three joints are contracted, the distal IP joint in flexion or hyperextension. This is caused not only by spiral or pretendinous

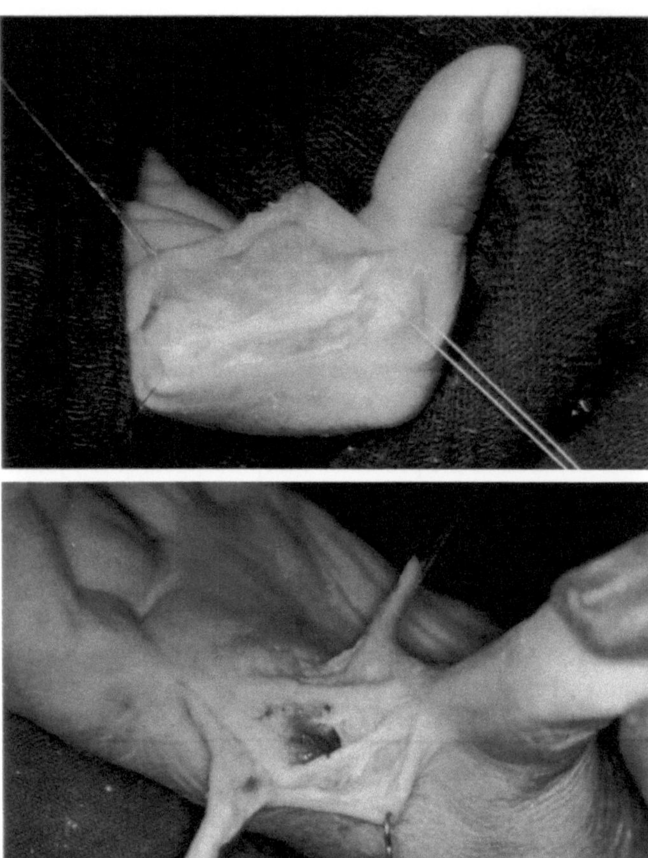

Fig. 2 *(above)*. The ulnar side. A cord extends from the abductor digiti minimi muscle

Fig. 3 *(below)*. The radial side. Pretendinous cord and a cord from the natatory ligament

cords from the palm and the natatory band, but also by the additional cord coming from the abductor digiti minimi. (McFarlane 1988; Barton 1990).
A longitudinal incision runs from the palm to the midline of the finger to free the radial neurovascular bundle step by step. Z-plasties must be localized such that the ulnar cord is removed from the distal end of the abductor muscle belly to the distal end of the cord. Mostly, the cords end at the tendon sheath and bone of the middle phalanx. When they are meticulously resected a hyperextension of the distal phalanx will often also be corrected because the oblique retinacular ligament is not diseased. In long-standing hyperextension contractures this ligament might be shortened and should be divided at the side of the extensor tendon.

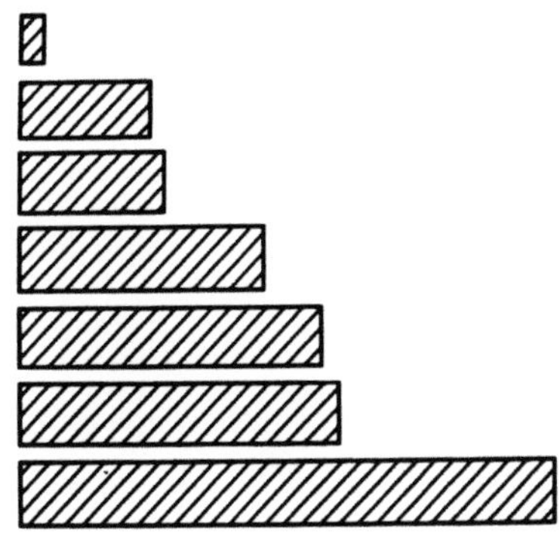

Fig. 4. Intra- and postoperative complications from 2160 operations. *From top to bottom*: injured tendon, $n = 5$, 0.23%; postoperative bleeding, $n = 25$, 1.16%; secondary amputation, $n = 28$, 1.30%; Sudeck's atrophy $n = 47$, 2.18%; infections $n = 58$, 2.68%; nerve injury $n = 61$, 2.82%; skin necrosis $n = 102$, 4.72%, Overall frequency 15.09%

The Radial Side

Dupuytrens disease at the radial side of the hand (Fig. 3) is rare. Cords arise from the transversal ligament of the palmar aponeurosis, the natatory ligament, and the pretendinous band of the palm. There is not much restriction of function except a moderate adduction contracture in long-standing cases. The radial side of the index finger can be involved too. Exposure of the cords in the first web is done by a single Z-plasty of adequate extent.

Radiolateral disease does not restrict function and is easy to remove.

Complication

Most complications are more or less due to extended necroses of the skin owing to disturbed circulation especially in recurrences (4.72%) (Fig. 4). For example, a patient had first been operated on by an inexperienced surgeon, who also had removed the nerves in the diseased region of the palm. We thus performed a secondary nerve transplantation. The result was good but the result of the civil suit expensive.

Another patient was operated on by myself and did not experience postoperative restriction of finger motion. One month after the operation, she began to suffer from continuous burning pain resistant to every therapy. Three months later I operated again because it was not a typical algodystrophia. I found the third palmar A. communis perforating the nerve. After freeing the vessel by longitudinal splitting of the nerve – a kind of "arteriolysis" – the patient was free of pain postoperatively. Perhaps her suffering from pain after the first operation, when the anomaly had been overlooked, was due to constricting scar tissue around the pulsating neurovascular bundle. Finally, postoperative hematoma, although not frequently seen (1.16%), can have serious consequences. To avoid such a complication is the only indication for the "open palm technique" (Fig. 5). We have employed this nearly unsurgical method, which causes a longer period of disablement, only in a few cases. In critical cases we use a thermoinactive protein glue (Tissucol, Immuno GmbH,

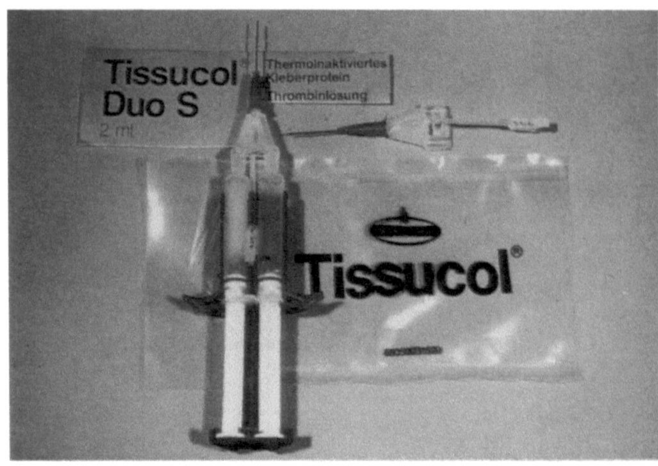

Fig. 5. Fibrin glue for hemostasis

Heidelberg) combined with thrombin solution before suturing the skin (Fig. 5). The two components are mixed by a small electric atomizer while spraying them on the wound area. In 1988, we reported on the initial 40 cases. Meanwhile it has become a routine method. However, the method is no substitute for meticulous coagulation of small vessels during surgery and does not justify removing continuous suction or failure to apply a mild compressing bandage after completing the operation.

There has been immense progress in recognition of cell and tissue alterations caused by Dupuytren's disease; however, the therapeutic consequences of these alterations remain unclear. Nonetheless, there is hope due to the results of research which may allow soon prevention or treatment of this disease before operative intervention is required.

References

Barton NJ (1990) The ulnar side of the hand. In: McFarlane RM, McGrouther DA, Flint MH (eds) Dupuytren's disease. Churchill Livingstone, Edinburgh

Curtis RM (1974) Volar capsulectomy of the proximal interphalangeal joint in Dupuytrens contracture. In: Hueston JT, Tubigna R (eds) Dupuytren's disease. Churchill Livingstone, Edinburgh

Geldmacher J (1972) Die Eingriffe bei der Dupuytren'schen Kontraktur. In: Wachsmuth W, Wilhelm A (eds) Die Operationen an der Hand. Springer, Berlin Heidelberg New York (Allgemeine und spezielle Operationslehre, vol 1013)

Geldmacher J, Köckerling F (1985) Die Flexionskontraktur des Mittelgelenkes beim M. Dupuytren. Handchirurgie 17:4–7

Geldmacher J, Weinzierl G, Flügel M (1988) Komplikationen bei der operativen Behandlung der Dupuytren'schen Kontraktur. Gemeinsame Tagung der handchirurgischen Sektion der Ungarischen Gesellschaft für Traumatologie und der Deutschsprachigen Arbeitsgemeinschaft für Handchirurgie zum 70. Geburtstag von Prof. Dr. J. Manninger, Budapest

Gosset J (1974) Dupuytren's disease and the anatomy of the palmodigital aponeuroses. In: Hueston JT, Tubiana R (eds) Dupuytren's disease. Churchill Livingstone, Edinburgh

Haines RW (1951) The extensor apparatus of the finger. J Anat 85:251–259

Hall-Findlay EJ (1990) The radial side of the hand. In: McFarlane RM, McGrouther DA, Flint MH (eds) Dupuytren's disease. Churchill Livingstone, Edinburgh

Hueston JT (1961) Limited fasciectomy for Dupuytren's contracture. Plast Reconstr Surg 27:569–585

Hueston JT, Tubiana R (eds) (1974) Dupuytren's disease. Churchill Livingstone, Edinburgh (G.E.M. Monograph I)

Landsmeer JMF (1949) The anatomy of the dorsal aponeurosis of the human finger and its functional significance. Anat Rec 104:31–44

McFarlane RM (1974) Patterns of the diseased fascia in the fingers in Dupuytren's contracture: displacement of the neurovascular bundle. Plast Rec Surg 54:31

McFarlane RM (1988) Dupuytren's contracture. In: Green DP (ed) Operative hand surgery, vol 1, 2nd edn. Churchill Livingstone, Edinburgh

McFarlane RM, McGrouther DA, Flint MH (eds) (1990) Dupuytren's disease. Churchill Livingstone, Edinburgh

McGrouther DA (1990) In: McFarlane RM, McGrouther DA, Flint MH (eds) Dupuytren's disease. Churchill Livingstone, Edinburgh

McIndoe AH, Beare RLB (1958) The surgical management of Dupuytren's contracture. Am J Surg 95:197

Milford IW (1988) The hand. Mosby, St. Louis; pp 341–347

Millesi H (1981) Dupuytren-Kontraktur. In: Nigst H, Buck-Gramcko D, Millesi H (eds) Handchirurgie, Thieme, Stuttgart vol 1

Mohr W (1987) Pathologie des Bandapparates. Springer, Berlin Heidelberg New York (Spezielle pathologische Anatomie vol 18)

Shaw MH (1951) The treatment of Dupuytren's contracture. Br J Plast Surg 4:218–233

Skoog T (1967) The superficial transverse fibres of the palmar aponeuroses and their significance in Dupuytren's contracture. Surg Clin North Am 47:443

Stack HG (1962) Muscle function in the fingers. J Bone Joint Surg [Br] 44:889–909

Stack HG (1973) The palmar fascia. Churchill Livingstone, Edinburgh

Thomine JM (1974) The development and anatomy of the digital fascia. In: Hueston JT, Tubiana R (eds) Dupuytren's disease. Churchill Livingstone, Edinburgh

Tubiana R, Valentin P (1964) The anatomy of the extensor apparatus of the fingers. Surg Clin North Am 44:897–906

Fasciotomy and the Open Palm Technique

P. Burge

Fasciotomy

Percutaneous fasciotomy of Dupuytren's disease was employed by Astley Cooper (in 1823), who divided the cord through a small incision. The same procedure was performed though a larger incision by Dupuytren (1832). Many surgeons described the use of fasciotomy during the following 100 years. Luck (1959) advised removal of the nodule in addition to division of the cord. Many authors have commented on the use of fasciotomy in the management of medial phalangeal (MP) joint contracture in elderly patients. During the last 10 years, several studies have helped to clarify its role in the management of Dupuytren's disease.

The indications for fasciotomy, and the surgical technique, were described concisely by Colville (1983), who reported the results of release of 137 fingers in 95 patients. The chief criterion for fasciotomy was a well-defined pretendinous cord with bowstringing across the distal palm. Bowstringing was said to indicate the absence of deep fascial connections. Extensive attachment between the skin and the cord, which prevents the cord from sliding distally after fasciotomy, was a contraindication. Prior to division of the cord, the skin distal to the site of division was separated from the cord with the fasciotomy knife. The combined extension deficit was improved from a mean of 102° preoperatively to 45° immediately postoperatively, 31° at 3 months, 56° at 1 year and (in 107 of 137 fingers) 75° at 3 years. Postoperative night splintage, continued for 3 months, was regarded as essential.

Rowley et al. (1984) followed 107 fingers in 78 hands for 15 months after fasciotomy. In those hands in which MP joint contracture predominated, mean MP joint contracture improved from 46° preoperatively to 8° at 3 months but had increased to 17° at 15 months.

A review of 44 digits in 30 hands at an average of 5.3 years after fasciotomy was conducted by Bryan and Ghorbal (1988). When patients who subsequently required fasciectomy are excluded, the mean MP joint contracture in 26 digits was 36° preoperatively and 31° after an average of 5.3 years. However, the correction was maintained in roughly half of the patients whose contracture was mainly at the MP joint.

These results are less satisfactory in terms of correction of deformity and durability than many surgeons would expect from limited fasciectomy for MP joint contracture. This view is supported by the multicentre survey conducted by McFarlane and Botz (1990). In 739 hands treated by regional fasciectomy of the palm, the average MP joint contracture was 38° preoperatively and 2.6° 1 year postoperatively.

The role of fasciotomy in the management of PIP joint contracture is controversial. Colville (1983) performed fasciotomy at PIP joint level "if necessary" after the cord had been divided in the palm, provided that the cord was well-defined and bowstringing. No permanent digital nerve injuries occurred in his series. Other authors express concern that the digital nerve, which pursues an unpredictable course over the proximal phalanx, may be damaged by fasciotomy. The anatomical studies of McFarlane (1974) and others confirm that extension of disease from the pretendinous cord into the spiral cord can certainly trap the digital nerve between a well-defined cord and the skin over the proximal phalanx, where it is definitely at risk from percutaneous fasciotomy.

The availability of safe anaesthesia in the form of axillary block has diminished the importance of medical unfitness as an indication for fasciotomy. It is evident that those cases which are most suitable for fasciotomy are also quite straightforward to manage by fasciectomy.

Comparison of published series is marred by uncertainty that the patients groups were comparable in terms of age, severity of contracture, skin adherence and the other factors which are known to influence the risk of recurrence. However, the evidence indicates that recurrence of MP joint contracture is more likely after fasciotomy than limited fasciectomy. In elderly or infirm patients, the greater risk of recurrence may be acceptable because of the simple and uncomplicated nature of fasciotomy.

Open Palm Technique

The open palm technique, described by McCash (1964), was similar in respects to the methods employed by Dupuytren and other surgeons in the last century. The open transverse palmar wound was, however, only one aspect of McCash's regimen, which also included closure of transverse incisions in the digits and proximal palm, immobilisation for 7 days and prolonged night splintage. It is the relative safety of the open palm technique which accounts for its widespread popularity over the last 25 years. The open palm method relies on the fact that in a primary case of Dupuytren's disease there is no loss of skin. The apparent shortage of skin that is evident after fasciectomy results from puckering and wrinkling of the palmar skin by virtue of its attachment to the contracted fascia. Contraction of the healing transverse palmar wound draws the skin out to its original length. Lubahn et al. (1984) demonstrated that marks placed on each side of the incision gradually approach each other as the wound heals, confirming that healing occurs by wound contraction and skin relaxation rather than by growth of new epithelium over the open wound.

A description of an operation for Dupuytren's disease must cover the incision, the management of the fascia and the wound closure. The open palm method is simply a technique for dealing with the palmar wound. Although McCash employed additional transverse incisions in the digit and in the proximal palm, other authors have used a variety of digital incisions and types of fascial excision.

Many authors remark on the freedom from pain and on the low incidence of haematoma, skin necrosis and infection which results from free drainage and lack of skin tension in the open palm. Although concern has been expressed that the open wound is liable to infection, this has not been a problem in practice. Serious infection is usually a consequence of haematoma and/or necrosis, which are generally avoided if the wound is open.

Gelberman et al. (1982) compared the open palm method with longitudinal incisions in a controlled study of 75 patients. Complications of infection, haematoma or necrosis occurred in seven of 56 patients with closed zig-zag or Z-plasty incisions but in none of 27 open palm cases. Lubahn et al. (1984) reported a complication rate of 19% in 115 patients with closed palms and 8% in 38 patients treated with the open palm technique. Schneider et al. (1986) found no haematoma, infection or necrosis in 49 patients with open palms but six developed reflex dystrophy. In contrast, the multicentre results reported by McFarlane and Botz (1990) showed a complication rate of 15% in 896 hands managed by palmar closure and 17% in 174 hands in which the palm was left open. The nature of the complications was not stated. It may be relevant that, although contractures of the individual digits were comparable in the two groups, the open palm group contained twice as many hands which received surgery to three rays than the closed group (52% vs 26%).

Correction of contracture was better (17% improvement in total active motion) in open palm cases than in closed cases (10%) in Lubahn's series. The groups were comparable in terms of disease severity but it is unclear whether the open and closed techniques were employed contemporaneously or sequentially. If it was the latter, the effect of other variables cannot be excluded. McFarlane and Botz (1990) found that correction of MP joint contracture was not influenced by palmar wound closure. However, proximal interphalangeal (PIP) joints fared less well in the open palm group even though the preoperative PIP joint contracture was less severe than in closed palm patients.

McCash (1964) recognised that correction of PIP joint contracture by his technique was incomplete. He advised against making an incision distal to the PIP joint, believing that this hampered full use of the hand during convalescence, and preferred to correct PIP joint contracture at a second operation, if necessary.

The transverse palmar incision provides good access for removal of diseased palmar fascia. Access to the digital fascia may be obtained though multiple transverse incisions or through a longitudinal approach (Z-plasty or zig-zag) which may be confined to the digit or connected with the palmar incision. Safe exposure of digital nerves and vessels is more difficult if the approach requires dissection beneath intact skin bridges. Lubahn et al. (1984) and Schneider et al. (1986) indicated that the longitudinal digital incision may be connected with the transverse palmar incision quite safely.

Use of the open palm technique in recurrent Dupuytren's disease is controversial. The open palm method will not overcome a true shortage of skin and it cannot be used as a substitute for skin replacement by full-thickness skin graft or (rarely) by means of a flap. If the palmar incision has a transverse component, however, then this portion may be left open. The author's experience suggests that the advantages of free drainage and lack of tension are valuable in operations for recurrent disease and in primary procedures.

The uncontrolled nature of many reports limits the validity of comparisons between the open palm technique and other methods. It is probable that many reports are biased by a greater proportion of difficult cases in the open palm groups. The evidence for a low incidence of complications in the open palm technique is good. However, many questions are unresolved. Is correction of PIP joint contracture compromised by the open palmar wound? Although pain and swelling of the hand appear to be influenced favourably in the immediate postoperative period, Schneider et al. (1986) noticed loss of flexion in 40% of 49 patients managed by the open palm method. Is delayed palmar healing associated with more prolonged digital swelling and/or fibrosis? Is the risk of recurrence influenced by the open palm technique? What is the role of open palmar wounds in operations for recurrent disease? The resolution of these questions will require large studies in which selection bias is strictly controlled and follow-up is both prolonged and complete.

References

Bryan AS, Ghorbal MS (1988) The long-term results of closed palmar fasciotomy in the management of Dupuytren's contracture. J Hand Surg [Br] 13:254–256

Colville J (1983) Dupuytren's contracture – the role of fasciotomy. Hand 15:162–166

Dupuytren G (1832) Lecons Orales de Clinique chirurgicale, vol 1. Bailliere, Paris

Gelberman RH, Panagis JS, Hergenroeder PT, Zakaib GS (1982) Wound complications in the management of Dupuytren's contracture; a comparison of operative incisions. Hand 14:248–254

Luck JV (1959) Dupuytren's contracture. J Bone Joint Surg [Am] 41:635–644

Lubahn JO, Lister GD, Wolfe T (1984) Fasciectomy of Dupuytren's disease, comparison between the open-palm technique and wound closure. J Hand Surg [Am] 9:53–58

McCash CR (1964) The open-palm technique in Dupuytren's contracture. Br J Plast Surg 17:271–280

McFarlane RM (1974) Pattern of the diseased fascia in the fingers in Dupuytrens's contracture. Plast Reconstr Surg 54:31

McFarlane RM, Botz JS (1990) The results of treatment. In: McFarlane RM, Flint MH, McGrouther DA (eds) Dupuytren's disease. Churchill Livingstone, Edinburgh, pp 387–388

Rowley DI, Couch M, Chesney RB, Norris SH (1984) Assessment of percutaneous fasciotomy in the management of Dupuytren's contracture. J Hand Surg [Br] 9:163–164

Schneider LH, Hankin FM, Eisenberg T (1986) Surgery of Dupuytren's disease: a review of the open-palm method. J Hand Sury [Am] 11:23–27

Skin Grafting in the Management of Dupuytren's Disease

J. Varian

Skin grafts can be split skin or full thickness. Generally speaking, on the palmar surface of the hand it is better to use full thickness skin graft and, therefore, in the management of Dupuytren's disease full thickness grafts are the better choice. They are used in the following situations:

1. To replace skin devitalised during surgery
2. To correct longitudinal skin shortening
3. To replace densely involved skin in recurrent contracture
4. To prevent recurrence in the patient with a strong Dupuytren's diathesis

Split skin graft would be used in the first of these situations, in which there was a delay in diagnosing the skin loss and the graft required to be placed on a granulating area. The other situations require full thickness graft and this article will dwell on the last – the use of skin graft to prevent recurrence. The fact that recurrence does not occur under a skin graft was suggested by Piulachs and Mir-mir (1952). Subsequently, this fact was noted by Hueston (1962, 1969, 1973), Gordon (1964), and Gonzales (1973). It is now widely accepted that excision of the Dupuytren's tissue and the volar skin overlying it with replacement of that skin by full thickness skin graft (dermofasciectomy) does greatly reduce the recurrence rate under the graft, but many surgeons are not convinced that the condition is eliminated by this procedure. In a recent issue of the *Annals of Hand Surgery*, two cases of the appearance of nodules under skin grafts were published, but the nodules in these cases appeared to arise from under the neurovascular bundle. Were they cases of extension or recurrence? Hueston goes further and says that the rarity of recurrence under a graft implicates the dermis in the causation of the disease, and his followers believe that the skin exerts some control over the Dupuytren's process. Others believe that excision of the overlying skin simply removes more effectively the whole of the diseased tissue.

Indications

Before one sets out to remove the skin from the flexor surface of a finger, one must examine very closely one's reasons for carrying out the procedure, so that the operation is not made needlessly extensive and the risks of delayed healing, with its attendant complications of scar contracture and stiffness, are kept to a minimum.

Firstly, upon whom does one operate? This generally depends on the degree of aggression of the Dupuytren's diathesis in that particular patient. A large graft across the palm is occasionally necessary in the salvage case in which recurrence has persisted after several operations. The older the patient the less aggressive the condition usually is and the more one would be inclined to carry out a simple fasciectomy. The younger the patient the more likely recurrence is to occur and, certainly, any patient under the age of 40 who has contracture in their little finger should be treated by primary dermofasciectomy, as recurrence is almost inevitable following simple fasciectomy. Most surgeons who use this procedure reserve it for the treatment of recurrent disease, particularly in those cases in which the skin is intimately involved with the recurrent nodule. However, the procedure is much safer if the flexor sheath remains undamaged (vide infra) and it is sometimes difficult to ensure a complete excision of a recurrent Dupuytren's cord, in which the flexor sheath was damaged at the primary operation, without again injuring the flexor sheath. For this reason, when the likelihood of recurrence is very high, it is better to carry out dermofasciectomy at the first operation.

How much skin must one excise? Most skin grafts are confined to the ring and little fingers beyond the distal palmar crease, and in the majority of these only the little finger will be grafted. There is no need to extend the skin excision proximal to the distal palmar crease, as a recurrent nodule in this area is rare, and furthermore, is unlikely to contract a finger that has been skin grafted, as there will be no fascial band running into the finger through which the nodule can contract it. The skin excision must be taken to the midaxial point at each of the flexor creases in the finger and at the palmar digital crease but the skin excision need not be taken to the midaxial line between these points.

Technique

A standard fasciectomy is carried out through a midline longitudinal approach. The fasciectomy is completed before any skin excision is carried out in case there is major injury to the flexor sheath which would prevent one proceeding with skin grafting. If this occurs, closure by a simple Z-plasty can be carried out. Small nicks in the flexor sheath can be repaired with 8/0 nylon allowing the surgeon to proceed to skin grafting. It is not necessary to preserve subcutaneous tissue as the graft will take well on a bed of flexor tendon sheath and neurovascular bundle. Skin excision is performed as described above. Skin is excised from the distal palm only if there is a nodule underlying the skin in that area.

It is vital that there be complete haemostasis prior to the graft being sutured into place, and the tourniquet is released to ensure that this is the case. Some surgeons then leave the tourniquet down for the rest of the operation but a completely dry bed can be ensured by reinflating the tourniquet for the period of time that the graft is sutured into place.

The skin graft is taken from any of the usual places, but the most convenient is the inner aspect of the upper arm. A pattern is used and the graft is tailored exactly to the defect. Primary closure in this region is easily obtained.

The dressing is held onto the graft using the tie-over technique and the hand is splinted in a plaster of Paris volar slab for a period of 1 week. Splintage is then removed and discarded with removal of the sutures. A light dressing may be applied for the first week while early mobilisation is encouraged, but it is important to ensure that the dressing is not applied in such a way that it abrades the graft. Sutures are left in the donor site for 2 weeks prior to their removal.

Discussion

The above technique has been used by the author since 1975. The cases that were carried out in Derby between 1975 and 1981 were reported by Tonkin et al. in 1984. Since then the author has carried out a further 35 dermofasciectomies in 24 patients, bringing the total number of these operations to 76. The average age of these patients was 49 ranging from 19 to 72. The average follow-up was 4 years (range: 1–9 years). There were 27 primary skin grafts and 49 secondary skin grafts in which there had previously been a fasciectomy and the skin graft had been carried out for a recurrence.

The average flexion contracture pre-op was 67°. This was a measure of the total extension loss, being the sum of the contractures in all three finger joints. The average postoperative contracture was 22°. This represents an average improvement of 67%. The average loss of flexion in the operated finger was a loss of 1 cm between the distal palmar crease and the fingernail compared to the other side which is the same as the range found in the simple fasciectomies that were studied in Derby.

Extension of the disease and recurrence outside the grafted area are both high, as is to be expected in younger patients who have aggressive disease. The recurrence rate outside the grafts was 40%, similar to rates reported by Hakistian (1966) and Honner et al. (1971). Only one patient developed a recurrence under the skin graft and this has recently been published. The recurrence was found to lie under one of the neurovascular bundles and in continuity with a nodule under the skin distal to the graft.

Recovery of sensation in the grafts was, objectively, very poor, but some patients, in whom two-point discrimination was absent, denied any sensory impairment. In no case was sensory loss a cause of complaint or functional loss.

There is no question that the appearance of Dupuytren's nodules under full thickness skin grafts is very rare. The operation is the one of choice in any patient under the age of 40 in whom recurrence is likely, particularly in the little finger. The complications of the operation are few provided that adequate surgical technique and meticulous attention to haemostasis are carried out. In two cases there was failure of part of the graft to take. In each case split skin grafting was carried out 1 week later with no adverse sequelae.

There was secondary skin or scar contraction in five patients. One required surgical correction by Z-plasty.

Many of the patients who require dermofasciectomy as a secondary procedure have some degree of irreversible flexion contracture in the proximal interphalangeal joint, but, provided they can fully extend the metacarpophalangeal joint, this residual contracture is often functionally insignificant. It is important to realise that most young patients who present with an aggressive nodule in their little finger will probably end up, after several operations, with amputation of that finger, unless dermofasciectomy is carried out.

References

Gonzales RI (1973) Open fasciectomy and full thickness skin graft in the correction of digital flexion deformity. In: Hueston JT, Tubiana R (eds) Dupuytren's contracture. Churchill Livingstone, Edinburgh, pp 123–127

Gordon S (1964) Dupuytren's contracture, the use of free skin grafts in treatment. Transactions of the Third International Congress of Plastic Surgeons, Washington, p 963

Hakistian RW (1966) Long term results of extensive fasciectomy. Br J Plast Surg 19:140

Honner R, Lamb DW, James JIP (1971) Dupuytren's contracture. J Bone Joint Surg [Br] 53:240–246

Hueston JT (1962) Further studies on the incidence of Dupuytren's contracture. Med J Aust 1:586

Hueston JT (1969) The control of recurrent Dupuytren's contracture by skin replacement. Br J Plast Surg 22:152–156

Hueston JT (1973) Skin replacement in Dupuytren's contracture. In: Hueston JT, Tubiana R (eds) Dupuytren's contracture. Churchill Livingstone, Edinburgh, pp 119–122

Piulachs P, Mir-mir L (1952) Consideractiones sobre la enfermedad de Dupuytren. Folia Clin Int 2

Tonkin MA, Burke FD, Varian JPW (1984) Dupuytren's contracture: a comparative study of fasciectomy and dermofasciectomy in 100 patients. J Hand Surg [Br] 9:156–162

Varian JPW, Hueston JT (1990) Occurrence of Dupuytrens disease beneath a full thickness skin graft: a semantic reappraisal. Ann Hand Upper Limb Surg 9(5):376–378

Recurrence in Dupuytren's Disease

C. Leclercq and R. Tubiana

Introduction

Recurrence is defined as new Dupuytren's tissue (whether nodules or cords) appearing in a previously operated area. It must be distinguished from extension of the disease to an unoperated area. So far, only very few cases of recurrence have been reported under a skin graft.

In 1984, we conducted a long-term review of patients we had operated on between 1970 and 1976. The medical records of 230 patients were available. We limited this review to 89 private patients operated on by the same surgeon (RT); all the patients were examined by the same physician (CL). Of these patients, 27 had had operations performed on both hands, amounting to a total of 116 hands.

All operations had consisted of regional fasciectomies limited to the tissues involved. Skin coverage had been done by direct closure in 96 cases and by skin graft in 20 cases (17.2%). The skin graft did not necessarily cover the whole area of fascia removal; more often, it only covered a functional area, such as the palmar aspect of the first phalanx, or the often-invaded area surrounding the distal palmar crease. All grafts were full-thickness skin grafts which, in most cases, had been harvested from the lower medial arm. The surgeon had generally opted for skin grafting prior to the operation. In a few cases, this had been necessary because of poor skin condition or lack of skin for direct closure.

In general, the indications for skin grafting were the following:

- Young age or strong diathesis in six cases
- Recurrence in 14 cases
- Severe form (which means a greater than 90° lack of extension in the finger involved) in 13 cases (the total number of cases is higher than 20 because of associations)

All grafts had healed primarily, except for one with a partial necrosis, which had healed secondarily within a few weeks.

Results

Of the 89 patients examined, we were able to review 38, amounting to a total of 50 hands that had been operated upon. The follow-up ranged from 8 to 14 years, with an average follow-up of ten years. Skin grafting had been performed on 11 of the 50 hands reviewed. Recurrence was very high: 33 out of 50 (66%) hands presented either with a recurrent nodule (9) or retraction (24). In all cases, however, the recurrence was significantly less severe than the initial retraction.

Of the 11 patients on whom skin grafting had been performed, nine presented with recurrence upon review. This high figure is easily explained by the initial severity of the disease and/or the strong diathesis. In no case, however, was recurrence observed under the graft. In a few cases, we observed a nodule at the longitudinal border of the graft, but never under it.

Discussion

The rate of recurrence after surgery varies greatly from one series to another (20%–68%). There now seems to be a general consensus that this rate varies with time, i.e., the longer the follow-up on patients who have been operated on, the higher the rate of recurrence will be (Tubiana and Leclercq). In very few instances has the fate of skin grafts been studied specifically. Our findings go along with other published material (Hueston), in which the authors found no instance of recurrence under a skin graft, except in very rare cases (Hueston, 1 case; Varian, 1 case).

This long-term review allowed us to determine precisely which factors seem to influence recurrence and extension of the disease. In this series, the young age of the patients at the time of the first operation and the existence of previous recurrences were the two main factors leading us to predict recurrence (Table 1). The other factors were: family history, ectopic lesions, association with epilepsy, incomplete correction of the retraction, sex (female), and surgical

Table 1. Influence of various factors on recurrences

Factors	Patients (n)	Recurrence (n)	Percent (%)
Age			
<45	16	16	100
45–65	18	12	66
>65	9	4	44
Famiy history			
+	14	11	78
−	24	14	58
Previous recurrence	6	6	100

Table 2. Patients without recurrence or extension

Factors	Patients without recurrence	All patients
Age at operation (mean)	53	48
Family history	11%	36%
Associated diseases	0	5%
Assessment	3.5	4.7
Complete correction of digital retraction	100%	96%
Complications (hematoma, necrosis etc.)	0	0

complications. The study of the cases without recurrence or extension of the disease is interesting to compare with the general enquiry (Table 2).

The almost-total absence of recurrence under a skin graft leads us to favor its use in cases with strong diathesis involving a high risk of recurrence: young patients, severe cases with a major skin involvment, and recurrence of Dupuytren's disease. Although it is time-consuming and demands a perfect surgical technique, it is worth performing in these specific cases.

Refinements of Plastic Surgery in Relapsing Dupuytren's Disease: Incisions, Flaps, Treatment of Perfusion Disorders, Physiotherapy, and Splinting

E. Euler, K. Wilhelm, and T. Kreusser

Staging and Indications for Surgery

Of prime importance for determining the indications for surgery is, in every case, the stage of the contracture as a measurement of the patient's disability [5].

Stage O, noticeable knot formation, precedes stage I, hardening and thickening of the longitudinal fibers. Significant finger contractions or an impairment of hand function are usually not present, so that there is generally no indication for surgery unless a compression syndrome affecting the function of the digital nerves is present or when an ulnar-sided strand of the small finger pulls outwardly and therefore creates impairment.

In stage II, the increasing palmar changes lead to beginning flexion contractures. We do not see a convincing necessity to operate at this stage. The indication to operate often occurs due to complaints and/or functional deficits.

A definite indication for operative intervention exists in the case of increasing induration and cord formation with distinct extension deficit and a resulting handicap for the patient. The patient is most often operated on at this stage.

Patients who have reached stage III without major subjective impairment present at hand surgery with a massive palmar affliction and a severe flexion contracture over 135°, with corresponding functional impairment or complaints. These end-stages of Dupuytren's contractures are the problem cases for hand surgeons.

Patient Population and Indication for Surgery

Data on our patient population dates from the years 1965 to 1982. During these 18 years, we have operated on 1810 hands from 1471 patients in our department of hand surgery [1,4,8,9].

More than half of these 1471 patients were between 50 and 70 years of age (Table 1). Corresponding to what has been reported in the literature, males are affected eight times more often than females. In addition, we also observed that as has been reported, more than half of the patients (63.6%) have a

Table 1. Age of patients with Dupuytren's disease ($n = 1471$)

Age (years)	Percent
21–30	2.4
31–40	11.3
41–50	21.6
51–60	28.7
61–70	26.8
71–80	8.7
81–90	0.5

Table 2. Dupuytren's disease: 1965–1982 ($n = 1471$ patients/ 1870 hands)[a]

Hand	Percent
Right	22.5
Left	13.9
Both	63.6

[a] M:F = 8.1:1.

Table 3. Localization ($n = 1810$ hands/3937 fingers)

Finger	Percent
D1	10.6
D2	8.5
D3	28.1
D4	60.8
D5	54.8

bilateral affliction (Table 2). It is interesting to note that in the majority of these cases, the changes occur first on the dominant hand, whereas in unilateral affliction, the disease usually manifests itself on the right hand, even in left-handers.

When considering the afflicted hands, in more than half of the cases the little finger and in 60% the ring finger were involved (Table 3).

We found, on average, that more than two fingers were afflicted and corresponding to the preference for the ulnar-sided hand segment, the combination of little and ring fingers increased. When one adds the cases in which the middle finger segment is afflicted, one then finds the combination ring little fingers affected in every third hand (Table 4).

In our patient population we have observed stage III or IV in nearly two of every three cases (Table 5). We therefore consider the presence of regular, objective, functional restrictions or neurological symptoms a definite indication for surgery.

Table 4. Combinations of involved fingers (n = 1273 hands/ 2408 fingers)

Fingers	Percent
D4	19.1
D5	16.5
D4 + D5	20.1
D3 + D4 + D5	11.2
D3 + D4	7.0
D1 − 5	3.7
Rest	22.4

Table 5. Stage of disease (n = 1313 hands)

Stage	Percent
I	9.6
II	29.0
III	37.2
IV	24.2

Table 6. Surgery in relapsing Dupuytren's disease

Operation	Range (%)
Second	10.6–11.5
Third	3.5–3.7
Fourth	0.8–1.7

Total: 14.9%–16.9%.

Table 7. Localization of relapse

Relapse	Percent
Inside operated area	52.8
Out of operated area	34.7
Both	12.5

In stage II there are far more aesthetic points of view to be considered other than functional ones as in stage III or IV. This patient group still made up about one third of our patients who were operated on. Given the goal of the operation, namely, a reduction of the contracture to stage 0 [6], we decline an operation in principal at this stage, considering that the disease is progressive and this would yield unfavorable conditions for a second or even third operation in case of a "relapse." We see here an indication only in the case of

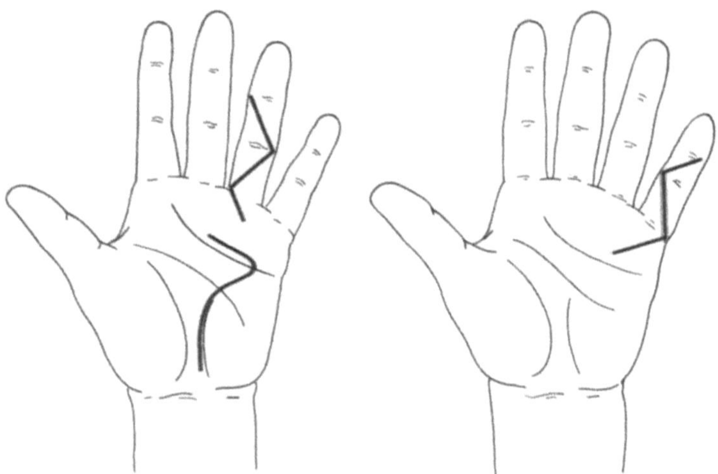

Fig. 1. Skin incisions for surgery in Dupuytren's disease

scarred ulnar deviation of the little finger or conservative pain symptoms due to constricted nerves, a condition which cannot be treated by other means.
About one of six patients underwent one or more reoperations (Table 6 [8,9]). In cases of relapse, we found changes inside the previously operated on area in nearly 50% (Table 7 [1,4,8]).

Incisions

The first difficulties present at the beginning of the operation with the selection of the type of incision. The almost endless number of suggested incision techniques [7] indicate that there is no one valid and ideal skin incision, be it in the palmar region or in the finger region. We can, however, indicate fundamental points, based upon our operative experience.
An analysis of the skin vessels of the palmar side revealed a relatively poorly perfused area in the center of the palm [7]. An undermining of this center should therefore be avoided as far as possible. A longitudinal skin incision in the region of the hypothenar takes this requirement into account and offers the best opportunities for revascularization of the skin margins. The incision bends distally according to the changes in the course of the distal flexion fold after the radial stump angle. This bundle should be kept as small as possible in order to restrict the radially stemming flaps and to limit the separation from the skin vessel coming distally. This incision technique is similar to that described by Bunnell in 1944 [2]. We used this approach in approximately 85% of the operations. Another possibility is that of the zig-zag type of skin incision, which has been described by many, in particular by Tubiana [10,11] (Fig. 1).
Most of the problems arise in the distal palm, and in the region of the finger, due to changes in the composition of the skin in Dupytren's disease. The

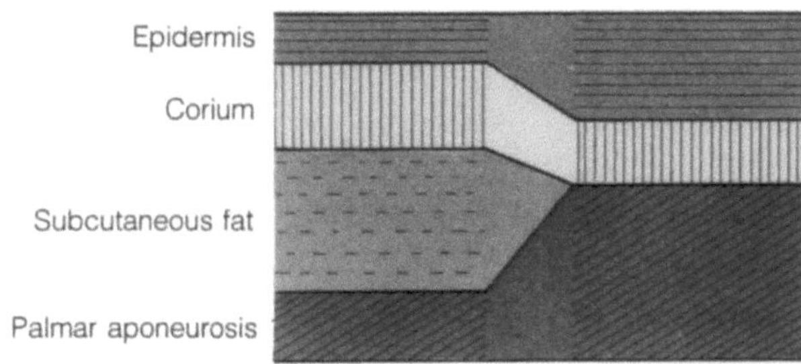

$\triangle$

Fig. 2. Changes of skin in Dupuytren's disease

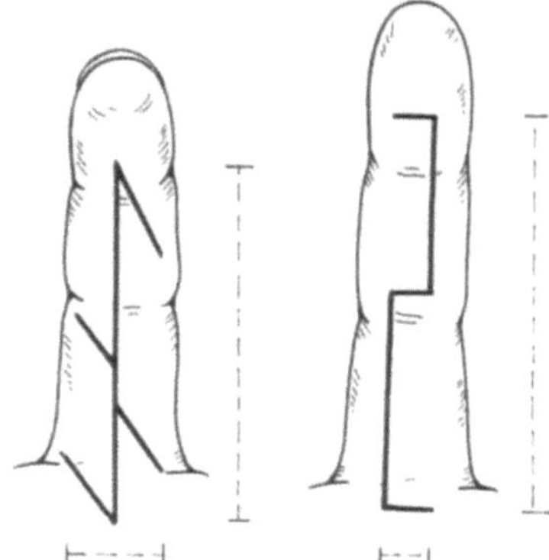

Fig. 3. Z-plasty. (From Iselin and Dickman 1951)

subcutaneous fatty tissue may be completely infiltrated and displaced by fibrotic material,˙whereas the cutis firmly adheres to the changed tissue (Fig. 2) [1]. Furthermore, the skin often shows a shriveled effect longitudinally due to the reduced extension which sometimes has been present for years. Simultaneously, through curved ligamentous projections of the scarred area, a stretching of the skin at the periphery exists. After removal of the knotted tissue, length can be gained at the expense of width. The Z-plasty described by Iselin and Dieckmann [5] incorporates this approach (Fig. 3). The acutely angled skin flap, however, minimizes the risk of a wound margin necrosis.

For this reason we avoid acute angles and use the zig-zag incision, modified after Brunner (Fig. 4). With this technique one gains good visualization of the surgical field and a sufficient mobilization of soft tissue, so that even with considerable contracture in the proximal interphalangeal (PIP) joint, it is possible to achieve skin closure in the case of a distended finger. Furthermore, it allows an extended incision as a VY-plasty, an additional gain in length at the cost of the reserve in width (Fig. 5).

When strong cords which run directly over the long finger in the palm are found, an incision can be selected so that it is brought over the finger. In case of involvement of a second, neighboring finger, for instance D4 and D5, the "Mercedes Star" technique can be used. We, however, use an arched incision, not a straight one. Straight cuts have a tendency to scar contractures and we have found that they should be avoided.

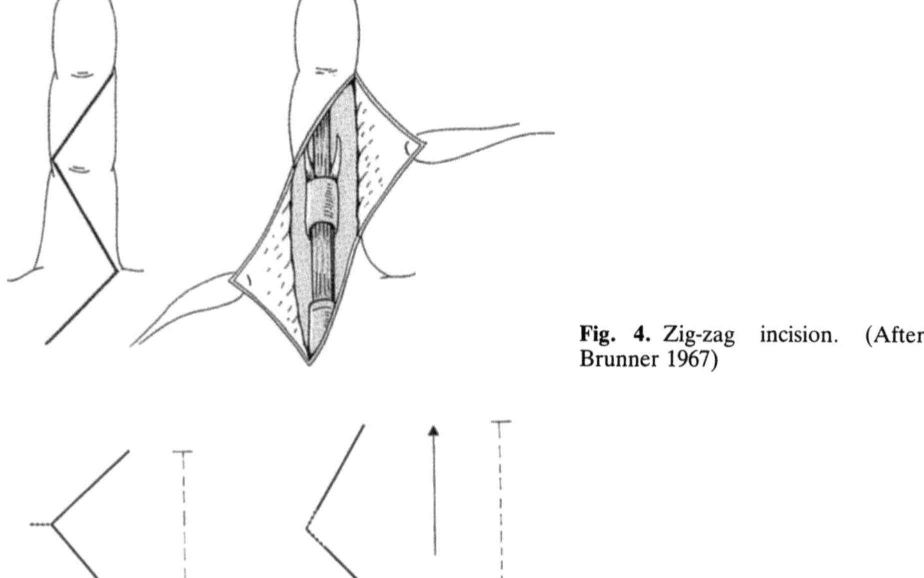

Fig. 4. Zig-zag incision. (After Brunner 1967)

Fig. 5. VY-plasty

Treatment of Joint Stiffness

An additional important point is the treatment of joint stiffness resulting from shrinkage of the flexion side capsular ligament structure, a secondary change in cases of extreme flexion contracture. There are various procedures which can be used in order to avoid a finger amputation. We do not eagerly undertake volar capsulotomy or a partial (or in some cases total) capsulectomy. We want to maintain the fibrocartilage as far as possible in order to avoid an overextension and destabilization of the PIP joint. It is most often sufficient to make an incision of the tractus obliquus which goes towards the palmar side, since these fibers, in particular, are shortened by the flexion contractures (Fig. 6). An overextension or luxation of the PIP joint is, in most cases, thereby avoided. According to our experience, osteotomies in the region of the proximal phalanx head or the middle phalanx base with skeletal shortening, in cases in which straightening of the finger was necessary, present a great traumatization of the tissue. We undertake this only in exceptional cases.

In the case of widespread stiffness of the PIP joint with maximum contracture, a joint resection and skeletal shortening in approximately 30°–40° extension

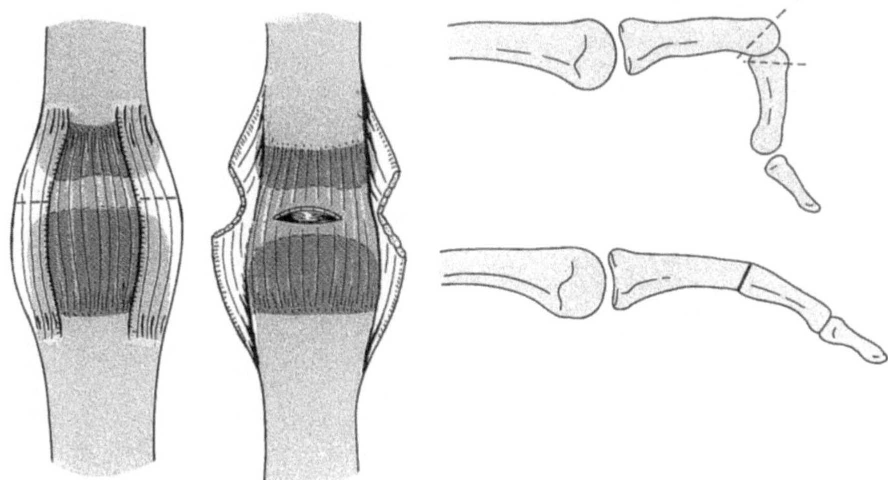

Fig. 6 *(left)*. Incision of the tractus obliquus or partial volar capsulotomy

Fig. 7 *(right)*. Treatment of stiffness of the PIP joint by resection

can achieve correction of finger function. We have found that the traction wire functions as a guide for osteosynthesis (Fig. 7).

Flaps

When one considers the techniques presented up to now, skin transplantations are hardly necessary. When a skin defect is present, it can be closed through full-thickness skin (Wolfe-Krause flap). We use a full-thickness skin transplant taken from the underarm when, due to deep crypt formation or severe adhesion of the damaged tissue with the skin, a secondary loss, due to the operation, leads to thinning of the skin and hole formation. In order to avoid edema under the transplant, we knot a foam patch (Fig. 8). In our patient population this type of skin transplantation is required in about 5% of the cases. Smaller defects of up to 3 mm in diameter are left and close secondarily without problems and without contracting scar formation.

We do not use crossed finger flap plasty, with the removal site from the dorsal surface of the neighboring finger, as described by Eicher and Moberg [3]. We also do not believe that the open palm operation is advantageous, since one must reckon on a prolonged healing process and the development of scar contractures.

Perfusion Disorders

The success of an operation on Dupuytren's contracture is dependent on the later actual use of the finger. A central aspect is therefore finger perfusion. The

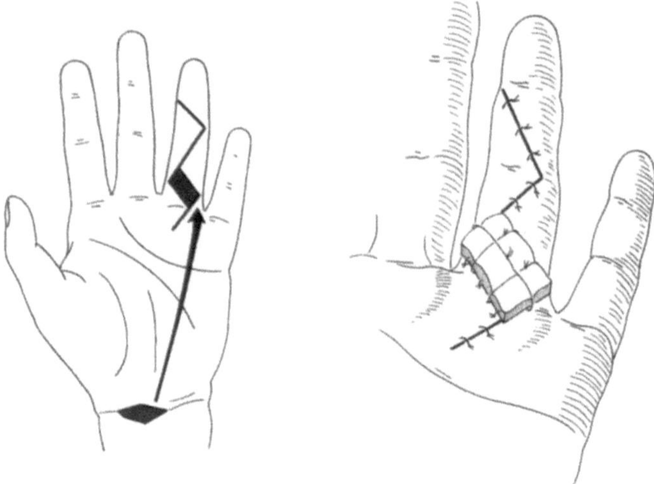

Fig. 8. In case of a skin defect, a full-thickness skin transplant taken from the underarm and knotting of a foam patch to avoid edema under the transplant are required

best way to prevent perfusion disturbance is with a surgical technique which protects, through step-wise freeing and preparation of the vessel, nerve bundles in its course. It is already possible in the preoperative phase to verify a more severe perfusion disturbance stemming from vessel damage or, in the case of vessel breakage, in a finger artery through angiography, which is not infrequently found in relapses after a previous operation. It is in particular in these cases, with intense manifestations of the disease or relapse intervention with a difficult preparation of the vessels, that intraoperative assessment of the perfusion is difficult. Following opening of the tourniquet, we wait for the hyperemia phase, which lasts about 2 min. Thereafter, we stop larger bleeding from soft tissue with electrocoagulation. Following this, if there is insufficient perfusion of the distal part of the extremities with definite capillary pulse, a vessel spasm probably exists when the arteries are intact. Here we can apply the experience from replant surgery of the finger by attempting to resolve the vascular constriction through application of local anaesthetics or nitro spray. We can also positively change the blood flow properties through, for instance, i.v. administration of low molecular weight dextran, thrombocyte aggregation inhibitors (e.g., ASA), or heparin preparations. Furthermore, a strong vessel extension in the longitudinal direction should be avoided through straightening of the finger which can have a major effect upon the blood flow of the fingers, in particular after many years of severe contracture. In these cases the finger must first be kept in a moderate flexion position. Splinting should be first undertaken after 1–2 weeks. In this time the blood flow conditions have improved.

A postoperatively increased palmar pressure can lead to a blood flow disturbance. Prevention of hematoma formation during the operation should therefore be undertaken. We have already mentioned the meticulous hemostasis after opening of the tourniquet. Here we see a considerable advantage over other techniques which the skin closure occurs prior to opening of the tourniquet. In addition, we always insert a Redon drainage, which is removed on the morning of the day after surgery, at the latest 24 h after surgery with removal of the bandages. Furthermore, in the operating room, we insert absorbent gauze in the palm, which, if needed, by slight compression prevents development of a cavity. One should, however, be cautioned not to utilize circular pressure when fixing the absorbent gauze, in order to prevent flow impairment in the form of Sudeck's prophylaxis. We do not recommend the use of steel wool. Furthermore, we apply a dorsal splint for immobilization of the hand immediately in the postoperative phase. We do not have to mention in detail that a clinical control of the blood flow status should be undertaken in the evening after the operation. Postoperative hematoma not only increase the risk of disturbed circulation, but also supports infection, margin necrosis, and delayed healing and encourages development of a Sudeck's dystrophy due to the long immobilization period.

Physiotherapy and Splinting

A longer splint immobilization is necessary, when a hematoma is present, approximately until removal of the stitches. We rarely observe larger hematomas, as they often appear during the operation when the tourniquet is removed after skin closure and bandaging. In these cases we at first wait until the hematoma has liquified on the third to fourth postoperative day, remove a few integumentary stitches, and then attempt to carefully express the hematoma.

Our postoperative regime of exercise encompasses, from the first postoperative day onwards, movement of the finger, in as far as the clinical findings and complaints of the patient allow. After removal of the splints, these exercises increase in the second postoperative week and then carry over to the wrist. Following removal of the stitches 14 days postoperatively, the patient undergoes physiotherapy with trained personnel. Active movement training of the hand and the entire arm and shoulder girdle, and also slight passive extension training of the preoperatively afflicted fingers are undertaken. Lymphatic drainage is used in the case of soft tissue swelling. The use of ultrasound and lasers in the follow-up treatment have been assessed, but we do not have any experience with these.

Finally, we would like to discuss our experience with adjuvant means which are used for extension of the finger. Already during the operation, a splint is applied to the PIP joint in the form of a temporary Kirschner wire ankylosis when, following straightening of the finger, a subluxation of this joint occurs. We prefer a slight flexion of about 20°–30°, as soon as the straightening of the finger leads to a reduced perfusion, due to the stretched vessels. The Kirschner wire is left in place until complete wound healing has occurred.

If the PIP joint which is, after this time, actually passive but in truth actively extended only briefly and returns to its flexion position, we then apply an outer splint placed on the extension side to be used as a night splint for 1–3 weeks. If, due to the severity, a permanent splinting is necessary, exact clinical controls are required since there is a tendency to swelling.

If after the fourth to sixth postoperative weeks, a hardening in the surgical area appears, which from time to time can appear as a relapse but is usually regional edema, we then prescribe a tractor for nightly use. In most cases a subjective and objective treatment success can be achieved. We regularly have the patients demonstrate the mounted splint, so that we are convinced that they fit perfectly.

References

1. Al-Kabbani H (1974) Die Dupuytrensche Fingerkontraktur. Medical dissertation, University of Münich
2. Bunnell S (1944) Surgery of the hand. Lippincott, Philadelphia
3. Eicher E, Moberg E (1970) Möglichkeiten der Vermeidung von Amputation bei schwerer Dupuytrenschen Kontraktur. Handchirurgie 2:56
4. Hübner J (1983) Die Dupuytren'sche Kontraktur-Nachuntersuchungen. Medical dissertation, University of Münich
5. Iselin M, Dieckmann GD (1951) Notre expérience du traitement de la maladie de Dupuytren. Mem Acad Chir 77:251–255
6. Millesi H (1965) Zur Pathogenese und Therapie der Dupuytrenschen Kontraktur. Eine Studie an Hand von mehr als 500 Fällen. Ergeb Chir Orthop 47:51
7. Millesi H (1983) Dupuytren-Kontraktur. In: Nigst H, Buck-Gramcko D, Millesi H (eds) Frische Verletzungen und Rekonstruktionen. Sekundäre Eingriffe. Begutachtung. Thieme, Stuttgart (Handchirurgie, vol 2.)
8. Röckl C (1975) Klinik, Therapie und Histo-Morphologie der Dupuytrenschen Fascienfibrose. Medical dissertation, University of Münich
9. Schönsiegel M (1983) Die Dupuytrensche Kontraktur-Ätiologie, Klinik, Ergebnisse. Medical dissertaiton, University of Münich
10. Tubiana R (1964) Le traitement sélectif de la maladie de Dupuytren. Rev Chir Orthop 50:311–334
11. Wilhelm K, Hauer G (1981) Die Dupuytrensche Kontraktur. In: Heberer G, Schweiberer L (eds) Indikation zur Operation. Springer, Berlin Heidelberg New York, pp 972–975

The Complications and Unsatisfactory Results of Treatment for Dupuytren's Disease

J.T. Hueston

Introduction

A satisfactory result from surgery for Dupuytren's disease makes for a happy patient. Both the surgeon and the patient will be satisfied if there is a painless full correction of deformity with full recovery of flexion allowing resumption of normal hand activities in 1 month and with sustained correction thereafter. An unsatisfactory result, usually due to a complication, makes for an unhappy patient. A complication is something not anticipated by the surgeon. An early complication is due to the surgeon's technique, a late complication is due to the patient's genetic constitution. Examples of these complications are, for the former, lack of communication, incisional scar contracture, skin necrosis, neurovascular injury, wound infection, joint stiffness, and reflex dystrophy; and for the latter, recurrence and extension.

The only way to prevent a surgical complication is not to operate. This truism is so often overlooked that it must be reiterated. The mere presence of Dupuytren's disease (DD) is not an indication for surgery and only a small proportion of all patients with DD require operation. Even then it is often a delicate question of the timing and extent of any surgical intervention. By the same token the only "satisfactory" result is a happy patient not necessarily a happy surgeon.

The object of surgery in DD is to preserve or to restore function to the patient's hand, if possible enough for him to continue with his occupation and hobbies. We must not reduce the function of the hand.

Any operation is an injury, within the control of the surgeon. Like any other injury to the hand, any operation, particularly with a complication, can initiate a series of normal biological changes leading to the gravest loss of hand function.

The future course ('evolution") of DD itself is not yet controllable except in some limited regions. Some patients have an unfavorable prognosis by virtue of a strong diathesis, but this should not be regarded as a surgical complication.

Surgery can change the state of the hand but not as yet the genetic makeup of the patient. Therefore let us consider those unsatisfactory results attributable to the surgeon and those unsatisfactory results attributable to the patient.

The Surgeon's Fallibility

Lack of Communication

A common surgical error is not to explain enough to the patient of what to expect from surgery. Thus, while a palmar nodule alone does not yet require operation, the patient should be told to return when medial phalangeal (MP) deformity appears, because this can usually be fully corrected. However, proximal interphalangeal (PIP) deformity often cannot be fully corrected and a residual 45° deformity may need to be accepted. Thus a hand which pre-operatively cannot be placed flat on a table-top can reasonably be expected to be capable of this after operation even if some PIP flexion deformity persists, because the MP release will usually allow enough MP *hyper*extension to accomodate for the residual PIP flexion.

Full flexion of all digits into the palm is to be expected after operation but cannot be guaranteed.

Such a simple exchange of expectations between surgeon and patient at those very important "hand-holding" consultations before surgery can establish in the patient a trust and confidence that the surgeon will "do his best" and that a mutually satisfactory result can be expected but not guaranteed. The personality type of the patient can be assessed at this stage. Failure to establish trust of mutual expectations *before* surgery is a common cause of a later result that may seem satisfactory to the surgeon but quite unsatisfactory to the patient!

After operation this trust should continue to be fostered by frequent meetings between patient and surgeon–at least twice weekly–rather than an abrupt dismissal to a therapist with no knowledge of the patient's personality or of any peculiarities of the preoperative or intraoperative state of the hand.

Incisional Scar Contracture

Principles govern practice in the choice of incisions. In each patient, indeed in each palm and each digit, this choice depends on the disease distribution and functional requirements of that hand.

Most surgeons develop preferences depending on their training and experience. Respect for the "stationary midlateral line" of each digit will prevent scar contracture producing early secondary flexion which is often mistaken for recurrence.

Longitudinal exposure allows safe proximal indentification of the neurovascular (NV) bundles in the palm–avoiding that dangerous "no man's land", between a transverse palmar incision and a separate digital incision, in which digital nerves can be displaced and endangered. But longitudinal incisions usually need interruption by Z-plasties or by transverse grafts to avoid again postoperative flexion from scar contracture. The V-Y and zig-zag exposures combine longitudinal access with a low risk of scar contracture, but flap tip necrosis over an adherent band is a risk.

Long transverse incisions, first used for total "prophylactic" palmar fasciectomy, and still often used for extensive palmar disease, leave no problem of scar contracture. Marginal skin necrosis in thin flaps occurs rarely, but extensive necrosis can occur if the wound is tightly sutured over a tense haematoma.

Of course if there is no wound closure there can be no haematoma. Hence the seduction of many surgeons by the siren song of the "open palm." Wound contracture is a wonderful thing! However wound approximation by two or three everting sutures allows drainage and healing in 2 weeks rather than the 4–6 weeks deemed "satisfactory" by a surgeon who would, I believe, prefer the shorter convalescence if he were himself the patient!

Skin Necrosis

Elevating skin flaps over extensive invasive DD is fraught with this risk, for the dermis, being directly infiltrated by the DD, may be included in the specimen so that the flap at that point is only keratin and is thus virtually perforated. Magnification will lessen this risk but it may need to be accepted that some DD will be left in the dermal layer to preserve flap vascularity. In an elderly patient or one with a low diathesis this can be safely accepted and the small risk of local recurrence further reduced if the lines of longitudinal stress in the infiltrated dermis are changed or broken by Z-plasty or graft interposition. If the patient is young, with a strong diathesis and with grossly involved dermis in the digit, regional resurfacing by a Wolfe graft after excision of both fascia and skin (dermofasciectomy) may be considered advisable to prevent recurrence. Such locally radical excision is usually reserved for the digits where recurrence can produce early PIP fixation – it is rarely used in the palm.

Z-plasties should not be incised in longitudinal incisions until after fasciectomy is complete, to allow safe placement of the flaps in viable margins. In cases in which flap viability is in doubt, or rarely even in the palm, excision and graft replacement after tourniquet release is to be considered. Primary excision of dead skin is preferable to prolonged slough separation, sepsis and granulation.

Neurovascular Injury

While fasciectomy is well described as a "dissection of the digital nerves", arterial continuity should also be preserved if possible or, as with division of a nerve restored if possible.

In primary disease the connective tissue sheath of the NV bundle is not directly infiltrated and allows modest mobility during dissection. In recurrent disease, because this gliding sheath has often been breached at the primary operation, there may be extreme difficulty in dissecting out the digital nerve and artery intact. It is preferable to leave a little recurrent disease around such an involved NV bundle and to resurface the defect with a Wolfe graft because involution of the DD can follow but leaving the bundle intact. The same compromise works over a fibrous flexor sheath found infiltrated with recurrent disease. It is safer to accept some persistent flexion, to resurface with a Wolfe graft, and to await some slow later resolution beneath the graft rather than to resort to flaps, particularly cross-finger flaps from adjacent digits which may themselves later need dermotasciectomy but have lost the dorsal integument in the earlier cross-finger flap.

Cold sensitivity and even distal gangrene have followed double digital artery damage, where discretion may have left a flexed but more useful and hence "satisfactory" digit. Digital artery damage can often be detected clinically before secondary operation. A digital Allen's test is not difficult. In surgery for recurrence, in which sensory loss has followed the first operation, the patient should not be promised full restoration of sensation but nerve grafts and donor sites should be discussed.

Wound Infection

"Wounds don't get infected and then break down – they break down and then get infected!" This axiom of Gillies applies particularly when nonviable skin flaps have been retained. The risk of operative contamination from intertrigo is greatly reduced by preoperative and intraoperative attention, requiring at

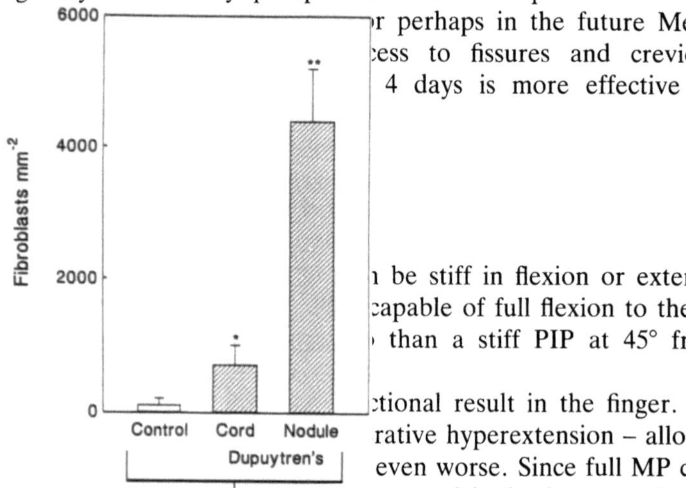

r perhaps in the future Messina's continuous cess to fissures and crevices. Postoperative 4 days is more effective than prophylactic

be stiff in flexion or extension. A PIP joint capable of full flexion to the palm, contributes than a stiff PIP at 45° from arthrodesis or

ctional result in the finger. Full MP release – rative hyperextension – allows accommodation even worse. Since full MP correction is one of ranteed in fasciectomy, the more limited PIP possibilities should be discussed with the patient before the operation.

Uninjured normal joints, after release of the extra-articular DD, can be held extended for up to 2 weeks in a dressing or splint to allow the take of a graft, with little risk of not regaining full flexion within the next month. After volar plate release, the joint is injured and constant personal supervision of splints and movements *by the surgeon who has injured the joint* is needed to retain the patient's confidence to continue with his rehabilitation.

The routine use of regional arm block anaesthesia has allowed even intraoperative discussion with patients when amputation may arise as an option.

Early postoperative PIP joint stiffness associated with a swollen hand is often, on careful examination, found to be related to a *local painful focus*. A tiny, exposed, unhealed neuroma in a suture line is easily excised and sutured under local anaesthetic with complete relief. A scar segment under tension may require release or merely rest. Rarely a carpal tunnel syndrome requires release. Such release of a local painful focus allows early resumption of painless movements and rapid rehabilitation with little risk of reflex dystrophy.

Quite distinct is the fairly sudden onset, commoner by far in women than in men, of pain and fusiform PIP swelling 2 or 3 weeks after a surgically uncomplicated operation and without any painful trigger lesion. Despite a protracted period of personal physical and psychological therapy by the surgeon and his team, and despite recent infusional therapy, at least some permanent loss of power grip can still be expected.

The Diathesis Dictates

Fortunately, but not infallibly, it is frequently possible that the strength of a patient's diathesis can be assessed before operation. Every patient with DD has a diathesis (i.e. an inherited tendency to the disease), but if this is not strong then the rate of natural progress is slow and the risk of postfasciectomy recurrence is low. Thus most patients can be assured, after a proper history taking and an enlightened examination, that there is little risk of further progress in the operated site – and even that the release of longitudinal tension will allow some resolution of residual deposits, particularly proximal ones. This assessment varies enormously with race, from low risk Japanese to high risk young Scots and Irish.

With increasing honesty in the publication of surgical results in the past two decades, it has become clear that some recurrence (i.e. of DD within the area cleared at operation) is seen in about 50% of patients. Probably less than 30% of these "technical" recurrences will require later surgery for recurrent PIP deformity. But these patients "at risk" from a strong diathesis should have this risk explained before operation and the possibility of primary dermofasciectomy offered to avoid the far more difficult and dangerous secondary surgery.

It is the patient – not the surgeon – who determines the recurrence by his diathesis. Recurrence rates differ greatly from one race to another so that national statistics often differ. Each surgeon must learn what to expect in his own area. But that 50% recurrence rates (40%–60%) are reported from expert surgeons in USA, UK, France and Australia, makes a mockery of McFarlane's claim that "recurrent disease is due to incomplete excision at the initial operation".

Extension (i.e. occurrence of DD beyond the operated field) is another manifestation of the same process in these same patients with this same inherited diathesis. As early as 2 weeks after operation the surgeon and/or the patient may notice new nodules elsewhere in the operated hand. These thickenings may be in the first web space, in the palm or in another digit – areas which were perfectly clear before the operation. The operation is an injury to the hand and, just as a fracture or even a superficial burn with swelling may be followed in a month by palmar thickening, so can the surgical injury.

As stated at the outset, the only way to prevent a surgical complication is not to operate. Also, the only way to prevent a recurrence or to postpone an extension is not to operate. Even after an impeccable fasciectomy and early return of function it is the diathesis of each individual – low or high, weak or strong – which will determine the date and rate of recurrence or extension, if any, of the DD.

The Continuous Elongation Technique in Dupuytren's Disease

A. Messina

Introduction

The difficulty of programming surgical treatment in very severe Dupuytren's disease (some surgeons have classified it as "inoperable" because it is impossible for seriously retracted fingers to attain functional recovery) has induced us to search for an indirect surgical solution that avoids necrosis, loss of vascularity, and functional impairment resulting from classical operations (Fig. 1). The continuous elongation technique (TEC) aims to achieve the extension of the retracted fingers, the correction of the deformity, and some functional reconstruction (Fig. 2).

The contracture of the pathological fascia in Dupuytren's disease sometimes progresses without interruption, sometimes rapidly, and sometimes very slowly; the disease can also display a stop-and-go development with alternating periods of inactivity and progress. All this has convinced us that a valid and

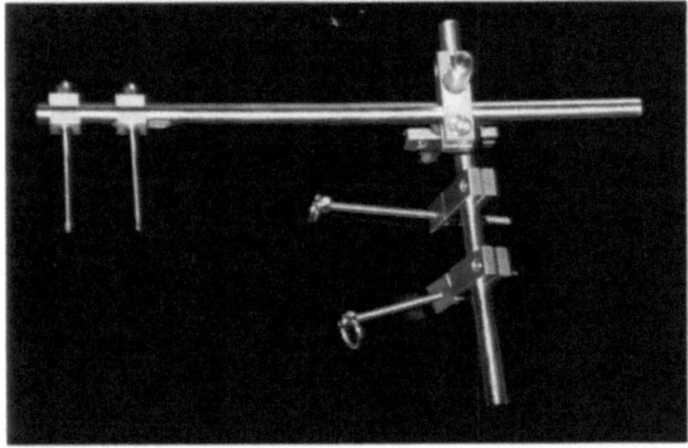

Fig. 1. Last prototype (190 g) for the extension of retracted fingers in severe Dupuytren's contracture treated by TEC. Since 1986 we have temporarily utilized other devices made of available steel materials in 30 patients (Fig. 3); meanwhile, however, the weight and size have been reduced

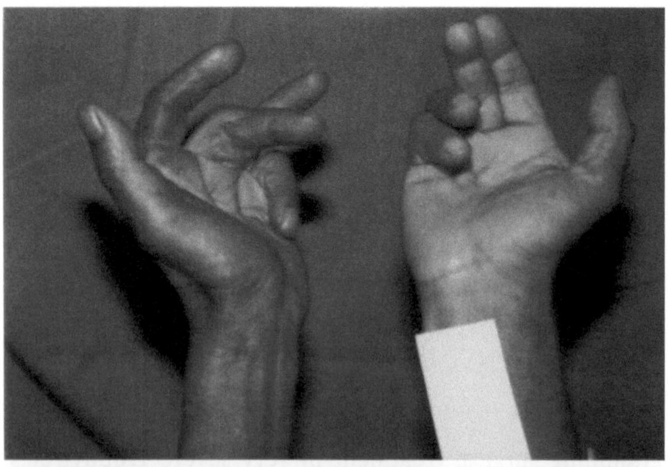

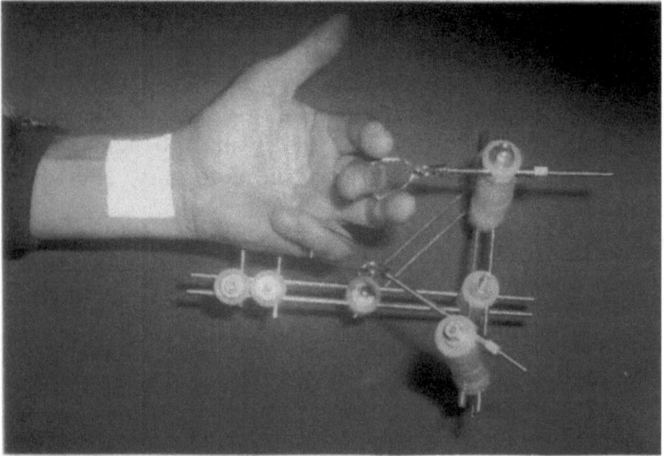

Fig. 2 *(above)*. Patient with severe bilateral Dupuytren's disease asked to have the left little finger, which is flexed and retracted with joint ankylosis and skin loss, amputated

Fig. 3 *(below)*. We suggested applying the TEC device in order to extend the little and middle finger of the left hand

correspondingly exact method of extending these retracted fingers might consist of elongating them "naturally" by applying *continuous* pressure at a *constant intensity*, as can now be carried out by TEC (Messina 1989).

This physiological elongation technique is atraumatic and painless; in a biological way, it induces the retracted tissues to return to the first anatomic stage of the disease (Fig. 3).

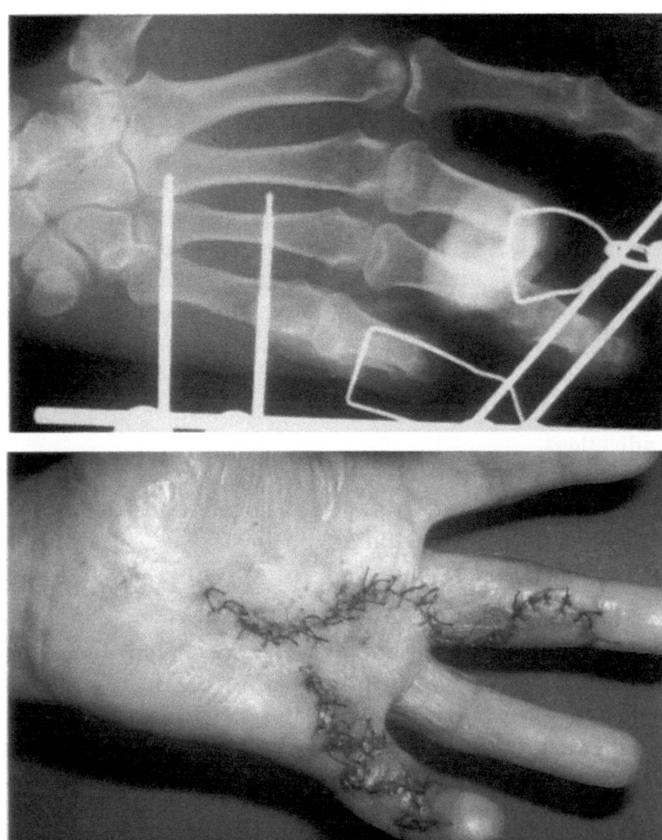

Fig. 4 *(above)*. X-rays of metacarpal pins

Fig. 5 *(below)*. Elongation that was incomplete but sufficient for carrying out a conservative operation to achieve finger functioning. With TEC, the operation is quite simple and short, with a very easy surgical approach

Technique

Two self-drilling pins with continuous threads are inserted on the cubital side of the hand through the skin without an incision (the recommended pin sizes are 2.5, 3.0, and 3.5 mm in diameter). The pins are inserted transversally and orthogonally through the fifth and fourth metacarpal bones at the proximal and distal metaphyses. Clinical and X-ray control of the length and position of the inserted pins confirms that they have completely penetrated both cortices of the fourth and fifth metacarpal bones. In this way, we obtain a very stable and painless assembly which supports the TEC device in order to induce the continuous elongation of the retracted fingers (Messina 1989, 1991).

A Kirschner wire is then inserted transversally either through the distal metaphysis of P2, through the proximal metaphysis of P3 if this is also retracted, or through both metaphyses if IPP and IPD are flexed together in severe contracture. The Kirschner wire is bent to form a traction loop. After skin dressing, the TEC device is assembled on metacarpal pins, and the phalangeal traction loop is connected to a threaded screw, allowing a 2 mm/day lengthening of the retracted finger. The device is regulated with regard to adequate direction and height according to the respective extent of flexion and direction until the complete extension of the retracted finger has been achieved. The pins and Kirschner wire are then removed on an outpatient basis.

Indications

TEC can be indicated in severe Dupuytren's disease (i.e., when maximally retracted fingers are held to be inoperable because of the impossibility of achieving secondary functional recovery) in the following cases:

- Long-term retracted joint stiffness (Fig. 2)
- Advanced stages in patients who have already been operated on
- Loss of volar skin of the fingers or of the hand palmar surface (Fig. 5)
- Severe problems with collateral neurovascular bundles in prolonged contracture of the fingers
- Systemic illnesses (e.g., severe and unstable diabetes, immunodeficiency, or serious cardiopulmonary illnesses)
- Old age
- Indication of amputation of the retracted finger
- Severe recurrence and extension of advanced Dupuytren's contracture (Messina 1991)

TEC can also be indicated in posttraumatic retraction scars accompanying flexion deformity of the fingers (caused by burns, tendon and osteoarticular trauma, skin loss, etc.). In this way, TEC not only circumvents plastic surgery, it also avoids joint interventions such as arthrotomies and capsulotomies as well as sections of retracted collateral ligaments, of check-reins, and of the retracted palmar plate of finger joints.

Advantages

This technique is a *preparatory step* for pathological palmar fascia exeresis in severe and inveterate Dupuytren's contracture. TEC is also an alternative to amputation for severely retracted fingers (Fig. 2). In addition, TEC:

1. Facilitates surgical intervention, greatly reducing trauma and the complexity, length, and difficulties of the operation

2. Simplifies the skin incision and surgical approach; it avoids complementary articular interventions such as capsulotomy and arthrolysis as well as the surgical release of check-reins, of collateral ligaments, and of retracted lateral digital fascia (Fig. 3)
3. Avoids the sudden surgical extension of the retracted finger and the stretching and tearing of collateral neurovascular bundles, which cause devascularisation and trophic problems in fingers that have been retracted for many years in complete flexion (Fig. 2)
4. Is an alternative to plastic surgery for correcting digital or palmar skin loss; this applies particularly to patients requiring a flap or skin graft, to certain cases of severe Dupuytren's contracture, and to some patients with posttraumatic retraction of the finger
5. Surpasses the McCash "open-palm" technique both in theory and in its practical applications (Fig. 5)
6. Provides the option of conserving severely retracted fingers and restoring their functionality; this had previously strained the technical limits of classical operations or been downright impossible
7. Might be a possible solution in some cases of inveterate Dupuytren's contracture; this is confirmed by the disappearance of the pretendinous cord and of the palmar nodule
8. Might benefit posttraumatic retraction scars accompanying flexion, ankylosis, and deformity of the fingers (caused by burns, tendon and osteoarticular trauma, skin loss, etc.)

Summary

The Continuous Elongation Technique (TEC) represents an alternative to finger amputation in severe cases of Dupuytren's disease, as a means of avoiding necrosis, loss of vascularity, and functional impairment resulting from classical operations. This technique is an advanced method and a preparatory step for the excision of pathological palmar fascia in severe and inveterate Dupuytren's contracture. TEC always achieves the extension of fascia of very contracted fingers and, in a very simple way, enables the retracted tissues to revert to the first stage of Dupuytren's disease.

Until now, this type of retraction has been thought to be irreversible. The TEC method, however, has shown that the histomorphologic process can in fact be reversed (Messina 1989). We have named this process the "stop-go back" process, because the retracted collagen tissue returns to the original cellular state of the first stage of the disease.

TEC is a painless technique for treating severe contractures by means of physiological and atraumatic elongation; it is performed with a device fixed on the fourth and fifth metacarpal bones using two self-drilling pins. Finger elongation simplifies the surgical approach and skin incision methods; it avoids plastic surgery to correct skin loss, complementary articular interventions such as arthrolysis (i.e., the surgical release of palmar plate, of check-reins, and of collateral ligaments), as well as the danger of immediate extension of inveterate contracted fingers. This technique may also be used to treat posttraumatic retraction scars in cases of flexion, ankylosis and deformity of the fingers (caused by burns, tendon and osteoarticular trauma, skin loss, etc.).

References

Messina A (1989) La TEC (tecnica di estensione continua) nel morbo di Dupuytren grave. Dall'amputazione alla ricostruzione. Riv Chirurg Mano 26(2–3):253–257
Messina A, Messina J (1991) The TEC treatment (continuous extension technique) for severe Dupuytren's contracture of the fingers. Ann Hand Surg 10(3):247–250

Subject Index